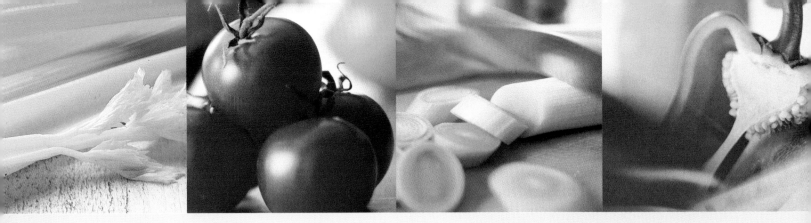

Over 300 scrumptious recipes to help you to enjoy life and stay well

Reader's Digest
DIABETES
Cookbook

Published by the Reader's Digest Association Limited

LONDON • NEW YORK • SYDNEY • MONTREAL

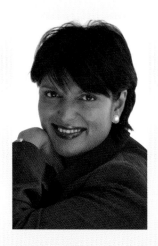

Azmina Govindji BSc RD, consultant for
this book, is a nutritionist, registered
dietitian and author. She was chief
dietitian to Diabetes UK for eight years and
has produced two diabetes education
videos with GMTV's Dr Hilary Jones.
Azmina now works as a freelance
consultant and has written ten books,
including Healthy Eating for Diabetes
with Antony Worrall Thompson, and
The 30-minute Diabetes Cookbook.
Azmina won the Ismaili Community's
National Award for Excellence (2002) for
Outstanding Professional Achievement.

Reader's Digest
DIABETES
Cookbook

was published by
The Reader's Digest Association Limited, London

Consultant
Azmina Govindji

Project editor
Rachel Warren Chadd

Art editors
Jane McKenna
Conorde Clarke

Assistant editors
Caroline Boucher
Marion Moisy

Proofreader
Barry Gage

Indexer
Hilary Bird

READER'S DIGEST GENERAL BOOKS

Editorial director
Cortina Butler

Art director
Nick Clark

Executive editor
Julian Browne

Managing editor
Alastair Holmes

Picture resource manager
Martin Smith

Pre-press account manager
Penelope Grose

Origination Colour Systems Limited, London
Printing and Binding Tien Wah Press Ltd., Singapore

Introduction

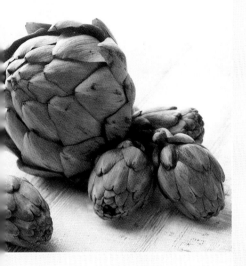

Plenty of cookbooks have great tasting recipes. What makes the *Diabetes Cookbook* different is that it offers creative recipes for delicious dishes, specially designed for people with diabetes. Inside these pages you will find superb combinations of ingredients, wonderful flavours and a diverse range of cooking styles and techniques.

Over the past decade or so, there has been something of a revolution in thinking about diabetes. Gone are the days of limited food choices. In recent years, science has learned that most people with diabetes don't need to be so restricted. Rather, the goal is to eat a diversity of nutrients in proper portion sizes, spread evenly through the day. Sugar is fine, for example, if eaten in small portions and properly balanced with proteins, fats and more beneficial carbohydrates.

The more than 300 recipes inside all represent this new thinking; they are nutritious, diverse and created to help to keep blood sugar levels stable. In addition to the recipes, we've provided a thorough reading section on the art and science of eating for diabetes. You'll discover the newest nutritional information, sample meal plans, ideas for shopping, hints and tips for combining ingredients and much more. This is information that you should read.

You'll also discover another interesting fact: eating well for diabetes is becoming increasingly similar to eating well for almost any health goal or concern. The recipes inside are great for heart health, cancer prevention, hypertension control and everyday well-being. They are rich in nutrients – particularly phytochemicals, the ingredients in fresh produce that have many specific health benefits – and contain the healthy fats that doctors and nutritionists are talking so much about.

So while we have worked hard to deliver the best cookbook possible for people with diabetes, we have also made sure that we are delivering recipes that the entire family can enjoy. To reinforce that, we make a point of detailing many of the health benefits of the recipes that go beyond diabetes management.

Diabetes is a serious disease and is affecting an increasing number of people. Eating healthy, delicious food in proper portions is perhaps the very best way to combat it. We can't imagine a much better treatment than the recipes inside. Give them a try.

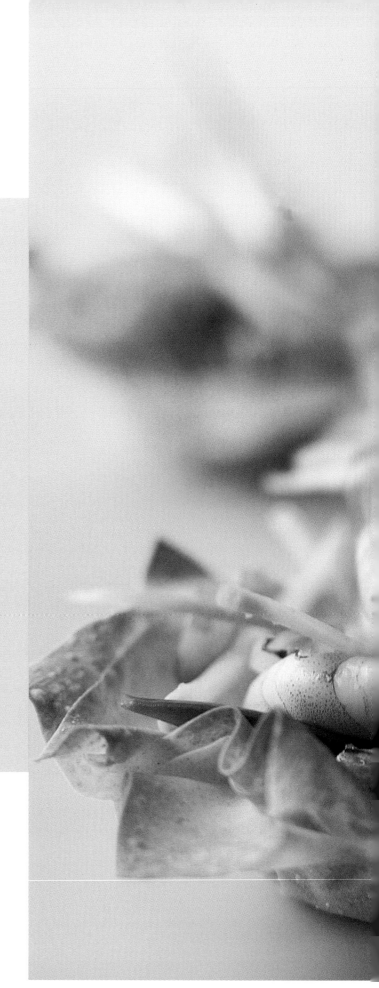

contents

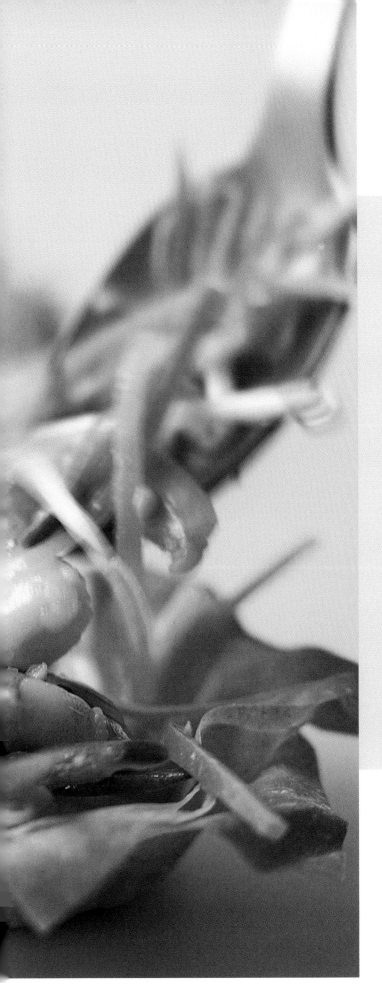

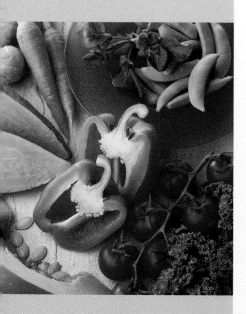

Living well with diabetes

In the past, a diagnosis of diabetes was followed by 'the talk', a particularly frustrating conversation with the doctor about your future. You'll have to watch your diet far more closely now, the doctor would say. Cut out the sugar. Cut back on carbohydrates. Watch the fat. Lots of steamed green vegetables. No indulgent restaurant meals. No more desserts. It was depressing, disheartening, annoying.

What a difference a few years can make. Thanks to ever-improving research, a whole new mind-set has emerged about eating for diabetes. Blandness is out; flavour is in. Rigid restrictions are out; intelligent moderation is in. The new thinking is to eat delicious, healthy, creative food, with a sensible eye towards the right mix of nutrients and the right portion sizes. It's a more open-ended food plan, but with proven results.

This new thinking is part of a bigger, more intuitive approach to treating diabetes. Diabetes is a condition in which your levels of blood glucose (or blood sugar) are abnormally high. Glucose is used by the body for energy, so if you're not using it efficiently, you can begin to feel tired. There are two main causes of diabetes: either the body is no longer creating enough insulin (the hormone secreted by the pancreas that transports glucose from the bloodstream into the cells), or the cells are no longer receptive to the insulin created. In both cases, the result is that there is too much glucose in your bloodstream, and not enough in the cells. Myriad complications can follow.

Today we know that the art of managing diabetes is in good part about controlling blood glucose. There are three key ways to do that:

1. Make sure your body has enough insulin so that your cells can get the fuel they need to function. This may require taking medication such as insulin injections or tablets.

2. Develop lifestyle habits to make your body less susceptible to blood glucose swings and your cells less resistant to insulin. At the top of the list is losing weight and taking more physical activity.

3. Adjust your diet to make sure that you are getting the right nutrients throughout the day, eating regular meals and snacks and reducing fluctuations in your blood glucose levels.

The last item is what this cookbook is all about: developing a way of eating that is healthy, delicious, well balanced, and which helps to keep your blood glucose levels steady. In the pages ahead, you will learn about the science and practice of healthy eating for diabetes. We will explain why the recipes in this book are so appropriate for your condition. And best of all, we'll explain how easy it is to enjoy delicious food with diabetes.

Understanding food

Another aspect of diabetes management that has changed is the demise of a 'one size fits all' nutritional programme. Not only are the scope, impact and cause of the condition different for each person, but each person's lifestyle and priorities differ as well. So it's far more important that if you are newly diagnosed, you ask your GP to refer you to a state-registered dietitian to help craft a unique plan for you. Your eating plan should take into consideration the need for weight loss, the intensity of the condition, personal food tastes and lifestyle issues.

Yet there are core truths about nutrition and diabetes that transcend individual needs and preferences. The key rule is that you must be sensible about your mix of foods, how they are cooked and how often you eat. People with diabetes should eat a balanced healthy diet – low in saturated fat, sugar and salt, with plenty of fruit and vegetables, and the right amounts of starchy foods, such as bread, potatoes, cereals, pasta and rice. Here is an overview of the key nutrients

Diabetes at a glance

All cells use glucose as their main source of energy. Diabetes is a condition in which the process that transfers glucose into your cells breaks down. The result is that glucose builds up in your bloodstream, while your cells are deprived of it. There are two main forms of diabetes:

Type 1 diabetes

This occurs when the body's immune system destroys insulin-producing cells in the pancreas, which can halt insulin production. People with Type 1 diabetes must take insulin injections daily. Without such treatment, glucose levels build up to dangerous levels in the blood, which could lead to heart disease and blindness, and even coma or death. Type 1 diabetes usually occurs in children or young adults and often appears suddenly. It is a lifelong condition and as yet there is no cure. Its symptoms include:

- High levels of glucose in the blood
- High levels of glucose in the urine
- Frequent urination
- Extreme thirst and a dry mouth
- Extreme weight loss
- Weakness and fatigue
- Blurred vision
- Moodiness

Type 2 diabetes

With Type 2 diabetes, the pancreas does produce insulin, but not enough for the body's needs. Often, the body's cells begin to 'resist' insulin's message to let blood glucose inside the cells – a condition called insulin resistance. This form of diabetes is often linked to being overweight, and tends to develop more slowly. It is far more common than Type 1 diabetes. Often there are no obvious symptoms, and diagnosis may be picked up at a routine check-up with the GP. If you believe you could be at risk of developing diabetes, see your doctor. Risk factors include a family history of diabetes, being overweight, being of Afro-Caribbean or South Asian origin, and having gestational diabetes during pregnancy.

that a person with diabetes should consume, to help to give you a better grasp of how to eat healthily for diabetes.

Carbohydrates

The body's main source of energy is carbohydrates. They come in two forms. **Simple carbohydrates** are the kind that are easily digested into glucose, such as table sugar and sugary drinks.

Complex carbohydrates are starches made up of more complex sugars, fibre and a rich assortment of other nutrients. These carbohydrates tend to take longer for the body to digest and contain more beneficial ingredients. They make up the bulk of whole grains and vegetables.

Carbohydrates are easily broken down into sugars, so they have the most impact on your blood glucose levels.

All about the Glycaemic Index

The latest research is based on the theory of the Glycaemic Index (GI), which is a ranking of foods according to their effect on blood glucose levels. The faster a food is broken down during digestion, the quicker the rise in blood glucose levels. Since one of the main aims in the treatment of diabetes is to keep blood glucose levels steady throughout the day, it is best to limit your consumption of foods that cause sharp rises in blood glucose (with the exception of special circumstances, such as when you are ill or taking heavy exercise). Foods that cause a rapid rise in blood glucose will have a high GI, so the key is to consume foods with low GIs on a regular basis.

It was previously thought that if you ate the same amount of carbohydrate, no matter what the food, it would have the same effect on your blood glucose levels. But we now know that different carbohydrates have different effects on blood glucose levels. For instance, 30 g (1 oz) of bread does not have exactly the same effect as the same weight of fruit or of pasta.

USING GI

Each food is given a GI number according to its effect on blood glucose levels. But it's not as simple as just choosing foods with a low number. The GI only tells you how quickly or slowly it raises blood glucose when it's eaten on its own. In practice, we usually eat foods in combination: bread is eaten with butter or margarine; potatoes are eaten with meat and vegetables.

Foods with a high GI are not bad foods. The key to healthy eating is to get the right mix of foods, which will not only ensure a better control of your blood glucose levels, but will also help you to obtain the wide variety of nutrients needed for general good health. Think about the balance of your meals, which should include starchy foods and be low in fat, salt and sugar. The good news is that you can lower the overall GI of a meal by including more low GI foods. Combining foods with different GIs alters the overall GI of a meal, so you should try to incorporate a low GI food into each meal you eat.

Simple carbohydrates – such as sweets and cakes – are so easy to digest that they almost instantly flood your body with blood glucose. It's no wonder, then, that carbohydrates have long been seen as the enemy of people with diabetes. But different carbohydrates affect our blood glucose levels in different ways. It is therefore important to try to understand the glycaemic effect of different foods (see All about the Glycaemic Index, left) so that you can enjoy your favourite foods while still looking after yourself.

Following a strict low-carbohydrate diet may actually do more harm than good because carbohydrates are the best source of fuel for your body. And since carbohydrates, gram for gram, provide only about half the amount of calories of fat, an eating plan that includes complex carbohydrates also gives you much wider food choices with less risk of gaining weight.

The trick is not to avoid reducing 'carbohydrates' to a single category of food. Both bagels and broccoli are mostly carbohydrate but many low-carbohydrate diets do not differentiate adequately between these very different foods. Many plans limit all carbohydrates regardless of the source.

The problem with simple carbohydrates isn't just that they are high in sugar – most people with diabetes can handle such treats every now and then in small portions. Rather, it's that such foods are often high in fat and low in vitamins, minerals and other healthy nutrients.

Use the table below as a rough guide to the GI of popular foods. Note that formulations of processed foods can vary and this will affect the GI.

LOW GI FOODS	MEDIUM GI FOODS	HIGH GI FOODS
Muesli, porridge	Weetabix	Corn flakes, puffed wheat,
Multigrain bread	Shredded wheat	Rice Krispies, sugar-rich
Rye bread	Pitta bread	breakfast cereals
Fruit loaf	Rich tea biscuits	Bagels
Pasta (made from	Digestive biscuits	White/wholemeal bread
durum wheat)	Basmati rice, white	Morning coffee biscuits
Lentils and beans,	Couscous	French fries
including baked beans	New potatoes,	Mashed or baked potato
Sweet potato, sweetcorn	boiled	Rice, white or brown
Oranges, apples, pears,	Ice cream	(except Basmati)
peaches	Honey	Glucose drinks
Yogurt	Jam	Sports drinks

Diabetes UK and the Diabetes Research and Wellness Foundation recommend that starchy carbohydrate foods should be the basis of all your meals. This is because these foods help you to keep your blood glucose levels steady. There are specific starchy foods that are particularly recommended for those with diabetes – these include cereals, potatoes, breads, pasta, rice and oats.

Sugar in context

There is actually no need for people with diabetes to avoid sugar completely. The effect any sugary food or drink has on your blood glucose levels depends not only on how much sugar it contains, but also, for example, on how the food is cooked, what else it contains and what you eat with it. A sugar-rich drink taken between meals is absorbed quickly and causes a sharp rise in blood glucose. However, when you eat sugar as part of a meal, blood glucose levels do not react in the same way because the sugar is absorbed much more slowly.

Sugar substitutes such as aspartame and acesulfame potassium do not affect blood glucose levels. You can use them to sweeten foods after cooking or to sweeten drinks. If you regularly use artificial sweeteners, you should choose a variety of different types.

Complex carbohydrates

By nature, these contain slower-to-digest sugars and tend to have more beneficial nutrients than simple carbohydrates. In particular, they contain lots of fibre.

Fibre, simply put, is the stuff in plants that your body can't digest. It's the husks on the grains, the stringy threads in celery. So what's so good about fibre? Insoluble fibre (found, for example, in whole-grain cereals and in the skin on potatoes) is bulky and absorbs water, so it fills you up faster. It also slows down digestion, prolonging feelings of fullness. This is critical for maintaining healthy weight. Insoluble fibre also binds together waste, keeping you regular. It 'sweeps out' your digestive tract, keeping it clean. Soluble fibre (such as that found in beans and lentils) has been shown to help to reduce cholesterol in your blood, protecting your heart. It also helps to keep blood glucose levels steady. (See page 10 for ways to add fibre to your diet.)

Fibre is not the only beneficial constituent of complex carbohydrates. Compelling new research suggests that eating the right vegetables, whole grains and beans every day may play a role in preventing disease. For instance, the phytochemicals in broccoli may help to prevent certain cancers; onions' allium compounds may help to reduce cholesterol, an important factor for people with diabetes; oats and some soy products may also reduce cholesterol.

Fatty foods

Fats are a class of organic chemicals that scientists refer to as fatty acids or lipids. When digested, they create nearly double the energy of the same amount of carbohydrates or protein. Fat is only a problem when you eat too much of it and especially of the less healthy type. Fat molecules that you eat are stored in your body and this results in weight gain. The build-up of fat-related molecules in your bloodstream is also bad for your heart and circulatory system.

As with carbohydrates, it is wrong to speak poorly of all forms of fat. There are three main categories of fats, and two of those categories offer health benefits so important that you might wish to add them to your diet – in appropriate amounts. The type of fat that is least healthy for you is the type that maintains a solid shape at room temperature. Primarily, this means butter, cheese, and the fat on meat. While this kind of fat (known as saturated) offers incredible amounts of fuel, it has few other health benefits and has the most detrimental effect on your blood cholesterol, which in turn makes you more prone to heart problems.

Fats that are in liquid form at room temperature (primarily plant oils, such as corn, olive or rapeseed oil) are split into two categories: polyunsaturated and monounsaturated. Both have benefits, but the latter are best for you. There is evidence that monounsaturated fat raises your HDL (good) cholesterol, important for people with diabetes because they have an increased risk of heart disease. Monounsaturated fat also has been shown to reduce insulin resistance.

Then there are the fish oils, or omega-3 fatty acids. These are essential to the body and are found in fish such as salmon, herring, mackerel, trout and sardines. Research shows that eating oily fish as part of a healthy lifestyle can help to lower the risks of heart disease. You should consume oily fish once a week.

Trans fatty acids are generally used in the food industry to make unsaturated fatty acids firmer. They are found in manufactured foods such as biscuits and cakes. Studies show that these fats, like saturated fats, can raise your blood cholesterol levels, so watch out for foods which have 'hydrogenated vegetable oils' high up on the ingredients list.

Salt

Eating too much salt is linked with high blood pressure so it is advisable to cut down on salt intake to prevent heart disease. It's estimated that people in the UK eat at least 10 g (two teaspoons) of salt each day. Because most of the salt you eat comes from manufactured foods, it is very likely that you are taking in far more than this amount each day, especially if you consume a lot of processed meals and snacks. For good health, it is recommended that you keep your total daily salt intake to 6 g (just over a teaspoon). Remember that food labels will only give you the sodium content (usually per 100 g), so you need to multiply this figure by 2.4 to get the amount of salt in 100 g of the food.

Some tips for cutting down on salt:
• Measure the amount of salt you add in cooking and gradually reduce the amount. When the recipes in this book suggest adding salt, use an amount that imparts just enough flavour. You will soon get used to eating less salt.

The fibre fill-up

Foods that are fibre-rich tend to be more filling. Because the body does not absorb fibre, high-fibre foods are often also fairly low in calories and so can help you to lose weight. Coupled with the fact that these foods can also help to control blood glucose and cholesterol levels, it makes sense to increase your fibre intake. Here's how:

• Don't skimp on breakfast. A modest meal of whole grains and fruit provides as much as a third of your daily fibre. Compare the fibre content of different breakfast cereals and choose those with more. A product with 3 g of fibre per serving is a good choice, though remember to check the salt and sugar content too. Muesli and porridge are good choices as they contain lots of soluble fibre with a low Glycaemic Index. Eat whole-grain bread instead of white bread and add chopped fruit to your cereal.

• Eat the skins. Scrub and eat the edible skins on fruits and vegetables rather than removing the peel. You lose about a third of the fibre when you remove the skin from a potato. The seeds in berries, kiwis and figs also supply valuable fibre.

• Beans and lentils are a great source of fibre. Try to keep them whole; their skin needs to be broken down in the body before they can be digested, and this means blood glucose rises more slowly. Add beans to a salad, or fill a soft tortilla wrap with heated beans. Baked beans contain sugar, but are a good source of soluble fibre and have about the same Glycaemic Index as a banana, so there's no need to opt for sugar-free varieties.

• Add vegetables. Vegetables such as carrots and celery are good sources of fibre. Add them to casseroles, soups, salads, sandwiches and pasta. Fresh, frozen, or even canned – all are good.

• Switch from white to grainy. Buy whole-grain rather than wholemeal or white when choosing bread. Always check the labels because some so-called brown breads are actually not much higher in fibre than white bread. They get their brown look from colouring or molasses.

• Up the fluid. When you eat more fibre, you need to make sure you are drinking sufficient amounts of fluid (see page 15).

• Avoid adding salt at the table.
• Experiment with herbs and spices, using, for example, freshly ground spices, dried and fresh herbs, paprika and freshly milled black pepper. If you find it hard to get used to a less salty flavour, you can try a salt substitute. Low-salt products (such as unsalted bread and butter) can be used as replacements for salt-rich foods.

• For varied flavours, try lime juice, balsamic vinegar and chilli sauce.
• Read food labels carefully. Salt may appear as sodium, sodium chloride, monosodium glutamate or bicarbonate of soda.
• Cut down on salty foods such as crisps, salted nuts, savoury biscuits and salty pastries. Instead eat fresh fruit, unsalted nuts and unsalted popcorn.

• Salted and smoked foods such as bacon, sausages, smoked fish, some canned fish and other processed convenience foods are often loaded with salt. Whenever possible, eat fresh fish, meats and vegetables. They contain only a small amount of salt naturally.

Be weight wise

The most consistent advice over the years for people with diabetes is the need to keep your weight down. The reason is simple: the more fat you carry, the more insulin-resistant your cells become. Since about 70-80 per cent of diabetics are overweight, this is a key issue. For many people, losing even 4.5 kg (10 lb) is enough to produce beneficial results in blood glucose levels.

The diet industry in the UK is estimated to be worth over £1 billion each year, and most of us are likely to have contributed to this in one way or another. In recent years there has been an explosion in the number of weight-loss plans and theories, yet we don't seem to be getting any slimmer as a population – quite the contrary.

Today high-protein, low-carbohydrate diets are all the rage. The idea is this: when you cut out carbohydrates from your diet, your body no longer has glucose to burn as energy. So instead, it burns body fat, leading to weight loss. The trouble is, protein foods are often rich with saturated fats and many dietitians and nutritionists claim that this type of diet is likely to have long-term

Eating for two

For pregnant women with the temporary condition gestational diabetes, a nutritionally balanced diet is essential to ensure good health and a successful pregnancy. It can help to avoid complications such as high blood pressure.

A mother-to-be actually only needs 200 extra calories a day during the third trimester of pregnancy. You can get this simply by consuming an extra half pint of whole milk. Underweight women, and those who do not reduce their activity levels during pregnancy, may need more. While many women believe they are 'eating for two', excess food leads to weight gain, which makes the diabetes worse. Here are a few tips for healthy eating with gestational diabetes:

* Be diligent about sugar. In pregnant women, sugar is rapidly absorbed into the blood and more insulin is needed to control blood glucose levels. Insulin is temporarily impaired in gestational diabetes, so limit sugary foods.

* Watch the fat. Remember, the weight you gain makes you even more insulin resistant. You only need small amounts of fat in your diet for your own health and foetal growth.

* Eat high-fibre foods. Constipation is often a problem in pregnancy but by increasing your fibre content, you can ward it off (see box on page 10). Make sure you drink enough fluid – at least 1.5 to 2 litres a day.

* Have a bedtime snack. Women with gestational diabetes tend to have low blood glucose levels during the night. This can be prevented by having a bedtime snack that provides both protein and complex carbohydrates.

* Eat steadily. Women with gestational diabetes need at least three daily meals plus a bedtime snack. Another snack may also be added. Try to ensure meal times are evenly spaced. Do not skip meals – this can cause hypoglycaemia, which may harm the foetus and make you feel irritable.

health implications. Recent research has suggested it may lead to kidney problems. Since people with diabetes are more prone to kidney problems, it is not advisable to opt for a high-protein diet.

If you continue to go for the latest quick fix or published diet, you'll continue to fall into the dieting trap. You become lured by the headlines; you're told that the diet is revolutionary and that you'll be slim forever. You'll be promised a huge weight loss in days or weeks, which is far more enticing than the sensible weight loss the

dietitians and medics will encourage. But, you know the facts – it's the steady, sensible weight loss that works and this is far healthier for you.

Then there's the simple theory of weight loss: simply burn more calories in a day than you consume and you'll lose weight. To do that, you exercise a little more, and eat a little less. In this simple approach, you eat a well-balanced, diverse array of food: lots of complex carbohydrates, healthy oils, lean meats and fish. Interestingly, not only does this theory work, it is also almost perfectly in tune the latest thinking about healthy eating for diabetes.

If healthy eating really is about calories, just how many should you eat in a day? Calorie requirements vary from person to person, depending on body size, physical activity and basal metabolic rate. But any diet plan that is set below 1,200 calories a day can make it extra hard to get all the vitamins and minerals you need, and is often not filling enough so you end up stopping the diet. Eating too little can lead to fatigue, which in turn only leads to more overeating.

Essentially, 500 g (1 lb) equals 3,500 calories. So to lose 500 g a week, you should burn an extra 500 calories a day through exercise, or cut 500 calories from your diet, or come up with some combination. To lose 1 kg (2 lb) a week, you will need a 'caloric imbalance' of 1,000 a day, achieved by exercise, diet, or both. It's a pretty simple formula.

It's not all about what's on your plate, however. It's also important to challenge your thinking about weight and health. In June 2002 the Diabetes Research and Wellness Foundation launched Think Well to be Well, a new concept in caring for people with diabetes. Bringing a fresh approach to diet, the concept helps people to take control of their life and to focus on achieving sustainable results.

You can only achieve your ideal weight if you really want to. So, the first step is to make up your mind that this is what you really do want, and then to take action

that is likely to support you in getting the results. It took time to reach the weight that you are, and it will take time to shed it too, so you must be patient.

Think slim, see yourself at that ideal weight, feeling energetic, doing all the things and taking part in the activities that you would love to, with that increased sense of confidence, while enjoying your food as part of a new and healthy lifestyle. Just thinking about 'going on a diet' possibly conjures up food deprivation, preventing pleasurable sensations and more.

Keeping portions under control

The perfect meal is one in which you are served a reasonably sized portion of wonderful, surprising, delicious food. You

Mind that waist

Extensive research has found that if your waist is bigger than your hips (an apple shape), you are more likely to suffer long-term conditions such as heart disease than if your waist is smaller than your hips (pear shaped). This is so significant that the British Dietetic Association Food First Campaign for 2002–2004, called Weight Wise, published the following guidelines:

At risk waist measurement for European men: 94 cm (37 in)
At risk waist measurement for European women: 80 cm (32 in)

shouldn't feel overfull at the end of the meal, but you shouldn't be hungry either. You should feel satisfied and content.

Eating smaller portions of your favourite foods works in many ways. First and foremost, you get to eat the foods you love. It's fine for people with diabetes to eat sugary food, for example; it just needs to be restricted to small portions and eaten after a meal. You'll begin to have a healthier view of food too.

Although the food guidelines today allow people with diabetes to choose from a wide array of foods, portion size still matters. It may seem unlikely that just one extra chicken wing or another teaspoon of oil makes a difference, but they do. Those extra 100 calories make it that much more difficult to lose weight or manage blood glucose.

Some examples of a 'correct' portion:
• 3 tbsp breakfast cereal, or 2 tbsp muesli
• 85 g–100 g (3 oz–3½ oz) roast beef, ham, lamb or chicken
• 115 g–140 g (4 oz–5 oz) cooked fillet of white or oily fish (not fried in batter)
• 2 heaped tbsp boiled rice or pasta
• 1 medium-sized potato or sweet potato
• 25 g (1 oz) Cheddar cheese, or 40 g (1½ oz) low-fat Cheddar cheese
• 1 small pot of yogurt
• Fruit and vegetables: see page 14

Another guideline is to eat more frequently. In other words, instead of having three big meals a day eat smaller meals more frequently, plus lots of healthy snacks. Studies indicate that staggering your food throughout the day not only helps to stabilise blood glucose levels but may also lower cholesterol levels. Of course, your body is unique, and the nature of your diabetes will affect the frequency with which you should eat. Work with a registered dietitian to come up with a good plan for dividing your meals up throughout the day.

The importance of fruit and vegetables

Most of us are poor at eating our full of fruit and vegetables. Fresh produce rarely plays a dominant role in our meal planning. Yet it is an extremely important part of a balanced eating plan. Research studies have also consistently shown that eating regular amounts of fresh fruit and vegetables can bring immense health benefits.

Orange and yellow-coloured fruits are higher in beta-carotene, which is converted into vitamin A in the body. All fruits contain some vitamin C, especially the citrus variety. The antioxidant vitamins found in fruit (A, C and E), are thought to protect against numerous infections and possibly even against some cancers. Fruits also tend to have a low Glycaemic Index, raising blood glucose slowly (see page 8).

Vegetables don't raise blood glucose very much and so add few calories. In fact, they are generally the most nutrient-dense, low-calorie foods you can eat. And if you fill up on vegetables, you will have less room for less healthy, calorie-loaded foods.

How long can I store vegetables and fruit before all the goodness goes?

Heat and light can destroy the vitamins in fresh fruit and vegetables. Store fruit in the fridge or in a cool, dark place and don't keep it too long. It is most nutritious when fresh. Once you start peeling and chopping fruit, nutrients can be lost, so eat it whole if you can.

Will mashing or juicing fruit and vegetables affect the nutrients?

Mashing disrupts the fibre and changes the inherent physical make-up of the fruit or vegetable. This raises the Glycaemic Index, which reduces some of the benefits. But as long as you eat the fruit or vegetable (or drink its juice) quickly, you're still maintaining the nutritional value. Drink fruit juice, even unsweetened varieties, with a meal. This helps to slow down the rise in blood glucose.

Boiled veg and fruit salads can be so boring and uninspiring...

There are hundreds of interesting ways of using fruit and vegetables, as you'll find in the recipes in this book, and you don't need to go abroad or to specialist shops to try out the more unusual kinds. Most are available from your local supermarket, and their exotic flavours can be used to liven up savoury meat dishes, puréed into tropical drinks or even mixed into tempting ice cream and sorbets. Try, for instance, papaya and avocado salad (page 202) or Caribbean butternut squash and sweetcorn stew (page 171).

How much fruit and vegetables do I need to eat to get a benefit?

For good health, you should aim to eat 400 g (just under 1 lb) of vegetables and fruit a day. This equates to about five 80 g (3 oz) portions. Remember that potatoes are classified as starchy carbohydrates, so they don't count.

What's a portion?
- 1 medium fruit, such as apple, banana, orange
- 1 large slice melon, pineapple
- 2 plums, apricots, satsumas
- 2-3 tbsp fresh fruit salad or canned fruit
- 1 tbsp dried fruit
- 1 glass (150 ml/5 fl oz) fresh fruit juice
- 2-3 tbsp raw or cooked vegetables
- 1 dessert bowl of salad

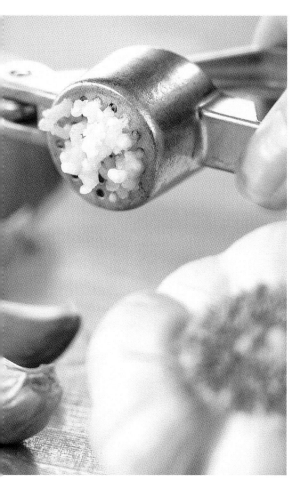

Do juice, dried fruit and vegetables in ready meals 'count' towards my five daily portions?
As you can see from the list of portions, dried fruit and fresh fruit juice do count. However, it is best to choose juice as only one of your five portions, since the valuable fibre has been removed. Pulses, such as beans and lentils, are also counted just once a day. This is because they don't contain the range of nutrients you get from other sources such as green leafy vegetables, carrots and tomatoes.

So, 80 g (3 oz, about half a can) of baked beans counts as a portion, and interestingly, since there might well be 80 g of tomatoes in a serving of canned tomato soup or 80 g of vegetables in a bought stir-fry, then you can, in theory, achieve your five portions a day by eating bought ready-prepared foods. However, it makes good nutritional sense to have a mixture, so that you get a variety from different food sources.

Can I eat as much fruit as I like?
This will depend on individual circumstances. If you test your blood glucose levels, then be aware of how different foods react in your bloodstream. Fresh fruit is brimming with natural sugars, and so can raise blood glucose levels faster and higher than vegetables. The trick is to determine how fruit raises your own glucose levels. One way to do this is to eat a standard portion of fruit, then test your glucose level a couple of hours later. Some fruits may raise your blood glucose more than others. Monitoring is the only way to know.

How nutrients heal

As mentioned earlier, many natural foods are filled with micronutrients – organic chemicals with extraordinary healing powers and important benefits to your body. Since having diabetes may increase the risk of high cholesterol, heart disease, kidney problems and high blood pressure, you'll want to be sure to eat foods that play a role in the prevention of these problems. Examples include:

- **Garlic** This can lower cholesterol levels and blood pressure. The phytochemical it contains is called allicin. In fact, members of the allium family – onions, garlic, leeks, and shallots – can all contribute to lower cholesterol and lower blood pressure.
- **Red wine** It is widely reported that red wine may play a role in preventing heart disease. But drinking alcohol regularly may not be the best idea for a person with diabetes (see A bit of the bubbly, page 15). Scientists now suspect the benefits of red wine are actually from the non-alcoholic flavonoids, particularly in the grape skins. The phytochemical in the skins is called resveratrol. So there seems to be some benefit to eating a small portion of red grapes or a small glass of grape juice, or indeed a glass of red wine with your meal.
- **Oatmeal and soya** The evidence for eating oatmeal and soya to lower cholesterol is strong.

- **Lutein** The phytochemical, found in spinach and other dark green leafy vegetables, may help to fight macular degeneration, a major cause of vision problems.
- **Folic adic** (from fruit, vegetables, pulses and whole grains) acts to lower the levels of a chemical known as homocysteine in the blood. High levels of homocysteine are a risk factor for development of heart disease, strokes and peripheral vein disease.

Fluids

Every system of your body needs fluid – in fact, your lean muscle, blood and brain are each more than 70 per cent water. Water is the most important ingredient your body needs every day. It regulates body temperature, transports nutrients and oxygen, carries away waste, helps to detoxify the kidneys and liver, dissolves vitamins and minerals, and cushions the body from injury. Even mild dehydration can lead to problems such as fatigue and constipation. Drinking adequate water may also help to prevent some diseases such as kidney stones, and may be associated with a lower incidence of colon cancer. And yet, most people do not drink enough.

Water is best, but milk, unsweetened fruit juices, low-calorie squash, tea and coffee all contribute to your fluid intake. Alcohol does not count, as it acts as a diuretic and can increase

A bit of the bubbly

Is there room for alcohol in your diet if you have diabetes? Yes, unless your GP has asked you to avoid it for a specific medical reason. But it does make sense to bear a couple of points in mind. First, alcohol lowers blood glucose levels owing to its effect on the liver. Secondly, it is high in calories – almost as high as fat – but with few nutrients. Here are some useful tips in managing alcohol consumption:

Pair alcohol with food. Food acts like a sponge, helping to absorb some of the alcohol and in turn minimising its effect on blood glucose. Likewise, sip your drink slowly to further slow absorption. Or add a sugar-free mixer to make it go further.

Don't drink when your blood glucose is low. By taking consistent daily blood glucose readings, you will be in a much better position to make an intelligent decision as to whether to drink or not. If your blood glucose is already low, avoid causing more problems and don't drink alcohol.

Observe the safe drinking limit: guidelines for people with diabetes are a maximum of 21 units a week for men (or 3 units a day) and 14 units a week for women (or 2 units a day). Note that these are the maximum recommended amounts, and drinking far less is preferable.

Try to space your drinking throughout the week and to have two or three alcohol-free days each week.

One unit of alcohol is equal to:
- ½ pint beer or lager
- 1 pub measure of sherry, aperitif, liqueur or spirit (vodka, gin)
- 1 standard glass of wine

Alcohol can cause hypoglycaemia (a 'hypo', or low blood glucose, see box on page 303) if you are taking insulin or certain tablets for your diabetes; the higher the alcohol content (such as in spirits, for example) the more likely it is to cause a hypo. The following guidelines may help to prevent this:
- Avoid drinking on an empty stomach. Always have something to eat with a drink and especially afterwards if you have been out drinking – the hypoglycaemic effect of alcohol can last for several hours.
- Choose low-alcohol drinks; avoid special diabetic beers or lagers, as these are higher in alcohol.
- If you enjoy spirits, try to use the sugar-free/slimline mixers.
- If you track the carbohydrate you eat, do not include the carbohydrate from alcoholic drinks.

Drink less alcohol if you are trying to lose weight, and no more than seven units of alcohol a week.

fluid loss. In fact, add an extra glass of water for each glass of alcohol you drink.

Develop a regular routine by keeping water bottles near you as a reminder, or get into the habit of leaving your

desk at work to go for a refill. And don't wait until you are thirsty. You may be already dehydrated. You'll need to drink extra water in dehydrating conditions such as hot, humid or cold weather or high altitudes, and when you are exercising.

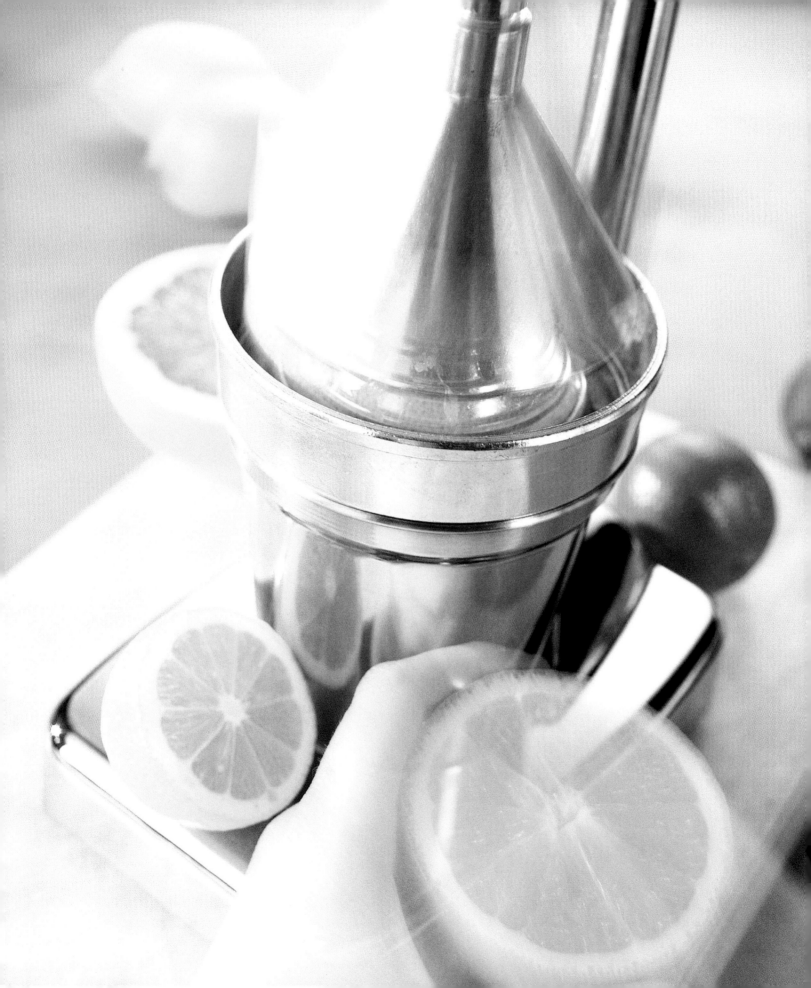

Breakfast

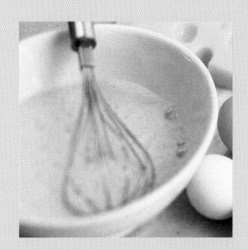

Drop scones

Drop scones, also called Scotch pancakes, are easy and fun to make, and perfect for tea or even as a simple dessert. Served with creamy fromage frais and sweet, succulent berries, they are quite irresistible.

Preparation time **10 minutes**   Cooking time **15–20 minutes**   *Makes about 24 drop scones*

125 g (4½ oz) self-raising flour

2 tsp caster sugar

1 egg, beaten

1 tbsp melted unsalted butter

150 ml (5 fl oz) semi-skimmed milk

4 tsp sunflower oil

To serve

100 g (3½ oz) blueberries

1 tsp clear honey

100 g (3½ oz) raspberries

200 g (7 oz) fromage frais

1 Put the flour in a bowl and stir in the sugar. Make a well in the centre, and add the egg, melted butter and a little of the milk. Gradually stir the flour into the liquids and add the remaining milk a little at a time, to make a fairly thick, smooth batter.

2 Heat a large shallow dish in a low oven, then turn off the heat and line the dish with a tea towel (this is for keeping the cooked drop scones warm). Heat a griddle or large, heavy-based frying pan over a moderate heat and grease it with 1 tsp of oil.

3 Using a dessertspoon, pour the batter from the pointed end (rather than the side of the spoon) to make neat, round drop scones. Depending on the size of the griddle, you should be able to cook 4–6 scones at once, but make sure you leave enough space round them so you can turn them easily. Cook for about 2 minutes or until almost set and bubbles are breaking on the surface; the scones should be golden brown underneath.

4 Using a palette knife, turn the scones over and cook for a further 1–2 minutes or until golden brown on the other side. Transfer to the prepared dish, wrap in the tea towel and keep warm while you cook the remaining scones. Grease the griddle lightly with 1 tsp oil before cooking each batch.

5 Place the blueberries in a bowl and stir in the honey. Add the raspberries and lightly crush the fruit, leaving some berries whole. Serve the scones warm with the honeyed berries and the fromage frais.

Some more ideas

To make **apple drop scones**, stir 1 cored and finely diced dessert apple into the batter with a pinch of ground cloves. Serve the scones dusted with a little sifted icing sugar.

To make savoury **Parmesan and herb drop scones**, instead of caster sugar add 1 tbsp snipped fresh chives, 1 tbsp chopped fresh oregano and 2 tbsp freshly grated Parmesan cheese to the flour. Serve the drop scones topped with a little soft cheese and halved cherry tomatoes.

Plus points

• Home-made drop scones contain less fat and sugar than bought scones, and serving them with fromage frais instead of butter keeps the total fat content low.

• Milk is a good source of calcium, essential for healthy bones and teeth. It also supplies protein, and vitamins B_2 and B_{12}.

Each serving provides   (one drop scone) kcal 55, protein 2 g, fat 2 g (of which saturated fat 1 g), carbohydrate 6 g (of which sugars 2 g), fibre 0.5 g. Useful source of vitamin B_{12}.

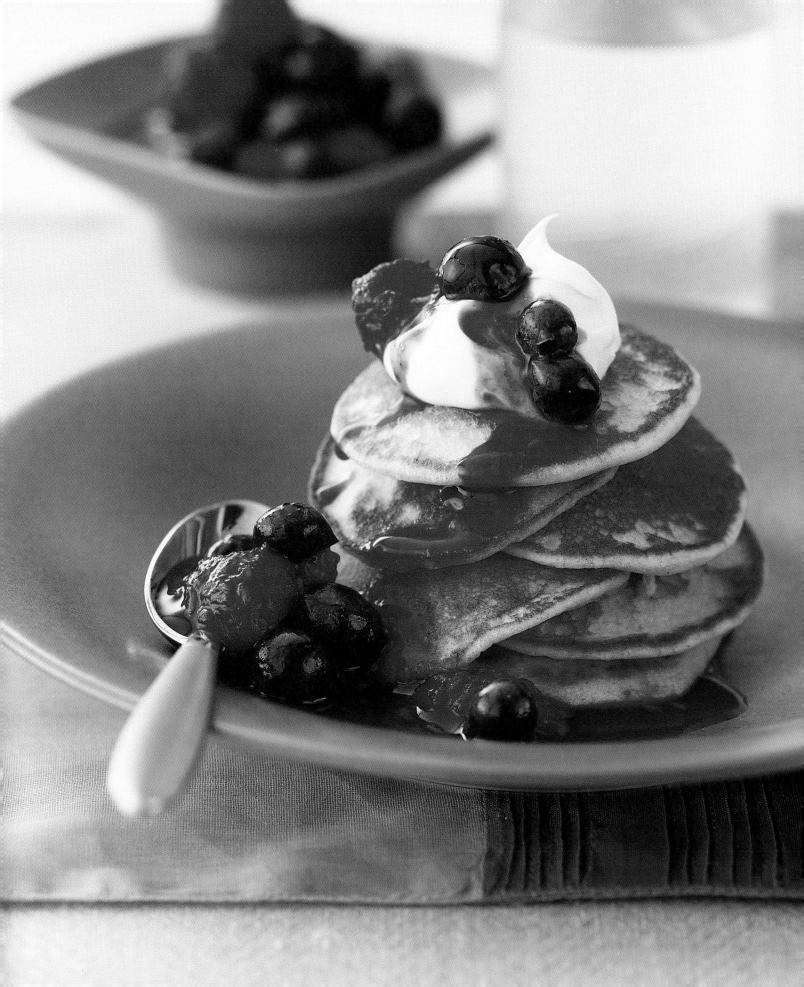

Blueberry popovers

Similar to Yorkshire puddings, popovers are a much-loved American classic, and the sweet version here is perfect for breakfast or brunch. The batter is baked, with fresh blueberries added, in deep muffin or Yorkshire pudding tins, and the popovers are served with sweet, fresh berries to add extra vitamin C.

Preparation time **20 minutes**   Cooking time **25–30 minutes**   *Serves 4 (makes 8 popovers)*

1 tsp butter

125 g (4½ oz) plain flour

pinch of salt

1 tsp caster sugar

2 eggs

250 ml (8½ fl oz) semi-skimmed milk

75 g (2½ oz) blueberries

1 tbsp icing sugar to dust

Mixed berry salad

150 g (5½ oz) raspberries

100 g (3½ oz) blueberries

200 g (7 oz) strawberries, thickly sliced

1 tbsp icing sugar, or to taste

1 Preheat the oven to 220ºC (425ºF, gas mark 7). Using a piece of crumpled kitchen paper and the butter, lightly grease 8 of the cups in a deep, non-stick muffin tray. Each cup should measure 6 cm (2½ in) across the top and be 2.5 cm (1 in) deep.

2 To make the popovers, sift the flour, salt and caster sugar into a mixing bowl and make a well in the centre. Break the eggs into the well, add the milk and beat together with a fork.

3 Using a wire whisk, gradually work the flour into the liquid to make a smooth batter that has the consistency of single cream. Pour into a large jug.

4 Divide the batter evenly among the prepared muffin cups – they should be about two-thirds full. With a spoon, drop a few blueberries into the batter in each cup, dividing them equally.

5 Bake in the middle of the oven for 25–30 minutes or until the popovers are golden brown, well risen and crisp around the edges.

6 Meanwhile, make the berry salad. Purée 100 g (3½ oz) of the raspberries by pressing them through a nylon sieve into a bowl. Add the rest of the raspberries to the bowl, together with the blueberries and strawberries. Sift the icing sugar over the fruit and fold gently to mix in well.

7 Unmould the popovers with the help of a round-bladed knife, and dust with the icing sugar. Serve hot, with the berry salad.

Another idea

For a **baked sweet batter pudding**, make the batter as in the main recipe, then add 4 tbsp fizzy mineral water or cold water. Pour into a 1.4–1.7 litre (2½–3 pint) shallow baking dish that has been lightly greased with butter (omit the blueberries). Bake for 30–35 minutes or until crisp and well risen. Spoon the berry salad into the centre of the hot pudding, scatter over 2 tbsp toasted flaked almonds, dust with the icing sugar and serve immediately.

Plus points

• Blueberries, like cranberries, contain antibacterial compounds called anthocyanins. These are effective against the E. coli bacteria that cause gastrointestinal disorders and urinary tract infections.

• Weight for weight, strawberries contain more vitamin C than oranges do, and more than other berries such as raspberries.

Each serving provides kcal 243, protein 10 g, fat 6 g (of which saturated fat 2 g), carbohydrate 40 g (of which sugars 16 g), fibre 3 g. Excellent source of vitamin C. Good source of vitamin B_{12}. Useful source of calcium, copper, folate, iron, niacin, potassium, vitamin A, vitammin B_1, vitamin B_2, zinc.

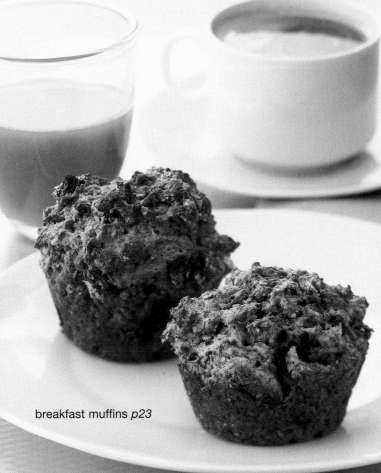
blueberry popovers *p20*

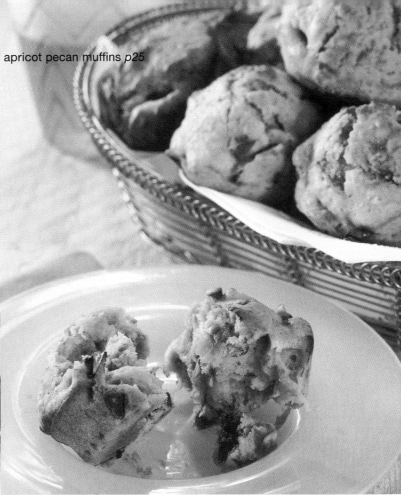
apricot pecan muffins *p25*

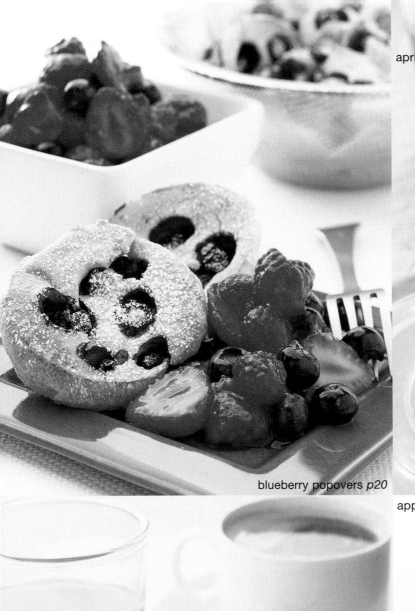
apple and hazelnut drop scones *p22*

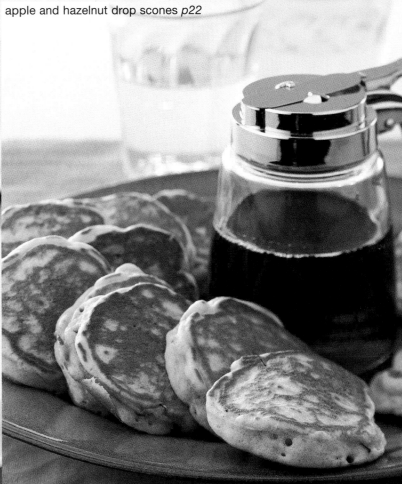
breakfast muffins *p23*

Apple and hazelnut drop scones

Drop scones are an almost instant sweet snack. The thick batter is made by simply stirring together a few basic storecupboard ingredients, and the scones cook in minutes. Here they are flavoured with diced apple and toasted hazelnuts. Top with a little maple syrup and enjoy warm from the pan.

Preparation time **15 minutes**   Cooking time **20 minutes**   *Makes 16 scones*

45 g (1½ oz) skinned hazelnuts, chopped

200 g (7 oz) plain flour

½ tsp bicarbonate of soda

pinch of salt

2 tbsp caster sugar

1 large egg

250 ml (8½ fl oz) buttermilk

1 dessert apple, about 150 g (5½ oz), cored and finely chopped

1 tbsp sunflower oil

4 tbsp maple syrup

1 Heat a small non-stick frying pan, add the hazelnuts and cook until golden brown, stirring and tossing constantly. Take care not to overcook the nuts as they burn easily. Tip them into a small bowl.

2 Sift the flour, bicarbonate of soda, salt and sugar into a large mixing bowl. Make a well in the centre. Lightly beat the egg with the buttermilk and pour into the well. Gradually whisk the flour mixture into the buttermilk mixture to make a smooth, thick batter. Add the apple and toasted hazelnuts, and stir in with a large metal spoon.

3 Lightly brush a griddle or heavy frying pan with a little of the sunflower oil, then heat over a moderate heat. Depending on the size of the griddle or pan, you can cook about 4 scones at the same time. For each one, drop a heaped tablespoon of batter onto the hot surface. Bubbles will rise to the surface and burst. Gently slip a small palette knife under the drop scone to loosen it, then cook for a further minute or until the underside is golden brown. Turn the scone over and cook the other side for 1–2 minutes or until golden.

4 Remove the scones from the griddle or frying pan and keep warm under a clean cloth. Cook the rest of the batter in the same way.

5 When all the drop scones are cooked, quickly heat the maple syrup in a small saucepan just to warm it. Drizzle the syrup over the drop scones and serve immediately.

Another idea

Make fresh berry drop scones by adding 100 g (3½ oz) blackberries or raspberries to the batter in place of the apple, and seasoning with a good pinch of ground mixed spice. Omit the hazelnuts, if you prefer.

Plus points

• Buttermilk is the liquid left over after cream has been turned into butter by churning. Contrary to its name, buttermilk does not contain butterfat, but it does provide protein, minerals and milk sugar or lactose, as well as a delightfully piquant taste.

• Apples are a good source of soluble fibre in the form of pectin. Eating apples with their skins offers the maximum amount of fibre. Research has shown that eating apples can also benefit the teeth, as it appears to help to prevent gum disease.

photo, page 21

Each serving provides (one drop scone) kcal 106, protein 3 g, fat 3 g (of which saturated fat 0.5 g) carbohydrate 18 g (of which sugars 8 g), fibre 1 g. Useful source of vitamin E.

Breakfast muffins

American-style muffins are perfect for breakfast, providing the energy boost the body needs to start the day. This particular recipe is packed full of good ingredients that add fibre, vitamins and minerals too.

Preparation time **15 minutes**   Cooking time **15–20 minutes**   *Makes 12 muffins*

85 g (3 oz) plain wholemeal flour

150 g (5½ oz) plain white flour

2 tsp bicarbonate of soda

pinch of salt

¼ tsp ground cinnamon

55 g (2 oz) dark molasses sugar

30 g (1 oz) wheatgerm

170 g (6 oz) raisins

225 g (8 oz) plain low-fat yogurt

4 tbsp sunflower oil

1 egg

grated zest of ½ orange

3 tbsp orange juice

1 Preheat the oven to 200°C (400°F, gas mark 6). Grease a 12-cup deep muffin tray – each cup should measure 6–7.5 cm (2½–3 in) across the top and be 2.5–4 cm (1–1½ in) deep.

2 Sift the wholemeal and white flours, bicarbonate of soda, salt and cinnamon into a bowl, tipping in any bran left in the sieve. Stir in the sugar, wheatgerm and raisins, and make a well in the centre.

3 Lightly whisk together the yogurt, oil, egg, and orange zest and juice. Pour into the well in the dry ingredients and stir together, mixing only enough to moisten the dry ingredients. Do not beat or overmix.

4 Spoon the mixture into the muffin tray, dividing it equally among the cups. Bake for 15–20 minutes or until the muffins are well risen and just firm to the touch. Leave them to cool in the tray for 2–3 minutes, then turn out onto a wire rack. The muffins are best eaten freshly baked, preferably still slightly warm from the oven, but can be cooled completely and then kept in an airtight tin for up to 2 days.

Some more ideas

Substitute chopped prunes or dried dates for the raisins.

For **carrot and spice muffins**, replace the cinnamon with 1½ tsp mixed spice. Stir 100 g (3½ oz) grated carrot into the flour mixture with the wheatgerm, and reduce the amount of raisins to 115 g (4 oz).

To make **blueberry and walnut** muffins, instead of raisins use 200 g (7 oz) blueberries, and add 100 g (3½ oz) chopped walnuts.

Plus points

● Breakfast is a good opportunity to top up the fibre intake for the day. These muffins are another good choice, as they offer plenty of dietary fibre from the wholemeal flour, wheatgerm and raisins.

● Wheatgerm is the embryo of the wheat grain so contains a high concentration of nutrients, intended to nourish the growing plant. Just 1 tbsp of wheatgerm provides around 25 per cent of the average daily requirement for vitamin B_6. Wheatgerm is also a good source of folate, magnesium, vitamin E and zinc.

photo, page 21

Each serving provides   (one muffin) kcal 180, protein 4 g, fat 5 g (of which saturated fat 1 g), carbohydrate 31 g (of which sugars 17 g), fibre 2 g. Useful source of calcium, iron, selenium, vitamin B_1, vitamin B_6, vitamin E, zinc.

Summer berry muffins

Fresh summer berries not only add delicious flavour and colour to these tempting American-style muffins, they also make them more nutritious. These muffins are lower in fat and calories than standard bought versions. Serve them either warm, fresh from the oven, or cooled – an ideal addition to a lunchbox, or for breakfast on the go.

Preparation time **10 minutes**   Cooking time **20 minutes**   *Makes 9 muffins*

115 g (4 oz) plain wholemeal flour

85 g (3 oz) plain white flour

1 tbsp baking powder

pinch of salt

140 g (5 oz) mixed fresh berries, such as blueberries and raspberries

55 g (2 oz) butter

55 g (2 oz) light soft brown sugar

1 egg, beaten

200 ml (7 fl oz) semi-skimmed milk

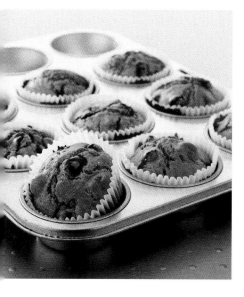

1 Preheat the oven to 200°C (400°F, gas mark 6). Use paper muffin cases to line a 9-cup muffin tray – each cup should measure about 7 cm (scant 3 in) across the top and be about 3 cm (1¼ in) deep.

2 Sift the flours, baking powder and salt into a bowl, tipping in any bran left in the sieve. Gently fold in the mixed berries.

3 Melt the butter gently in a small saucepan, then add the sugar, egg and milk and mix until smooth. Pour this over the flour mixture and gently fold the ingredients together, just enough to combine them. The mixture should remain quite lumpy.

4 Spoon the mixture into the muffin cases, filling each about two-thirds full. Bake for 18–20 minutes or until the muffins are risen and golden brown.

5 Transfer to a wire rack to cool slightly, then serve warm or allow to cool completely before serving. The muffins can be kept in an airtight tin for 1–2 days.

Some more ideas

Instead of a mixture of white and wholemeal flour, use all white or all wholemeal flour.

For a hint of spice, add 1½ tsp ground mixed spice, ginger or cinnamon with the flour.

Replace the berries with other fresh fruit, such as chopped apples, apricots, peaches or strawberries, or dried fruit, such as sultanas, raisins, chopped apricots, dates or figs.

To make **pear and cinnamon oatmeal muffins**, mix 200 g (7 oz) self-raising wholemeal flour, 55 g (2 oz) medium oatmeal, 1 tsp baking powder, 1½ tsp ground cinnamon and a pinch of salt in a bowl. Fold in 2 peeled and chopped dessert pears. In a separate bowl, mix together 55 g (2 oz) melted butter, 55 g (2 oz) caster sugar, 2 eggs and 150 ml (5 fl oz) orange juice. Pour this over the flour mixture and fold the ingredients together. Spoon into 9 muffin cases and bake as in the main recipe.

Plus points

• Combining wholemeal flour with white flour increases the fibre content of these muffins and adds valuable nutrients such as B-group vitamins.

• Fresh berries offer dietary fibre and make a good contribution to vitamin C intake. Raspberries also supply vitamin E. Blueberries, like cranberries, contain a compound that helps to prevent urinary tract infections.

Each serving provides (one muffin) kcal 166, protein 4 g, fat 6 g (of which saturated fat 4 g), carbohydrate 24 g (of which sugars 9 g), fibre 2 g. Useful source of calcium, selenium, vitamin A, vitamin E.

Apricot pecan muffins

Delicious American-style muffins are popular for breakfast and brunch, as well as for sweet snacks at any time. Packed with fresh fruit and nuts, and delicately spiced with cinnamon, the muffins here are lower in fat and sugar than bought muffins, and contain no trans fats or preservatives.

Preparation time **25 minutes**   Cooking time **20–25 minutes**   *Makes 12 large muffins*

250 g (8½ oz) plain flour

85 g (3 oz) strong bread flour

2 tsp baking powder

pinch of salt

115 g (4 oz) light soft brown sugar

1 tsp ground cinnamon

3 tbsp wheat bran

½ tsp grated lemon zest

240 ml (8 fl oz) semi-skimmed milk

2 eggs

55 g (2 oz) unsalted butter, melted and cooled

225 g (8 oz) ripe but firm apricots, stoned and diced

55 g (2 oz) pecan nuts, chopped

1 Preheat the oven to 200°C (400°F, gas mark 6). Using a piece of crumpled kitchen paper and a small knob of butter, lightly grease a deep muffin tray – each cup should measure 6 cm (2½ in) across the top and be 2.5 cm (1 in) deep.

2 Sift the flours, baking powder, salt, sugar and cinnamon into a bowl. Stir in the wheat bran and lemon zest. Combine the milk, eggs and butter in a jug, mixing well. Pour into the dry ingredients and add the diced apricots and pecans. Stir just until the dry ingredients are moistened, leaving some small lumps of the flour mixture in the dough. Do not overmix.

3 Spoon into the prepared muffin tray, filling the cups two-thirds full. Bake for 20–25 minutes or until risen and golden brown and a wooden cocktail stick inserted into the centre of a muffin comes out clean. Leave to cool in the tins for 2–3 minutes, then turn out onto a wire rack to finish cooling. The muffins are best if served within a few hours of baking.

Some more ideas
To increase the fibre content, use 125 g (4½ oz) each plain white flour and plain wholemeal flour with the strong bread flour.

For **blueberry muffins**, use 225 g (8 oz) fresh blueberries instead of the apricots. Substitute 1 tsp grated orange zest for the lemon zest and omit the pecan nuts.

Chopped strawberries, peaches or nectarines can also be used, but the fruit must not be too ripe and mushy or it will make the muffin mixture too wet.

Use 100 g (3½ oz) raisins or sultanas instead of apricots, with walnuts instead of pecans.

Plus points
● Health experts regularly recommend that we should increase the amount of fibre in our diet. These muffins help to do just that, with fresh apricots providing a wide range of fibre components, including both soluble and insoluble fibre – not only good for digestion, but also helpful in controlling fat and sugar levels in the blood.

● Wheat bran contains the indigestible fibrous part of the wheat grain. It helps to provide the bulk that keeps the digestive system healthy.

photo, page 21

Each serving provides (one muffin) kcal 230, protein 6 g, fat 9 g (of which saturated fat 3 g), carbohydrate 34 g (of which sugars 13 g), fibre 2 g. Useful source of calcium, folate, niacin, vitamin A, vitamin B_1, vitamin B_{12}, vitamin E.

Cinnamon raisin bread

This milk-enriched fruity loaf tastes good plain or can be served spread with a little honey or jam. It's also wonderful toasted for breakfast, when the gentle aroma of warm cinnamon makes a soothing start to the day.

Preparation time **20 minutes, plus 1 hour rising**   Cooking time **30 minutes**   *Makes 1 large loaf (cuts into 16 slices)*

450 g (1 lb) strong wholemeal (bread) flour

1½ tsp salt

2 tsp ground cinnamon

1 sachet easy-blend dried yeast, about 7 g

115 g (4 oz) raisins

45 g (1½ oz) caster sugar

55 g (2 oz) unsalted butter

240 ml (8 fl oz) semi-skimmed milk, plus 1 tbsp to glaze

1 egg, lightly beaten

1 Grease and lightly flour a 900 g (2 lb) loaf tin. Sift the flour, salt and cinnamon into a large mixing bowl, tipping in any bran left in the sieve. Stir in the yeast, raisins and sugar, and make a well in the centre.

2 Gently heat the butter and milk in a small saucepan until the butter has melted and the mixture is just tepid. Pour into the well in the dry ingredients and add the beaten egg. Mix together to make a soft dough.

3 Turn the dough out onto a lightly floured surface and knead for 10 minutes or until smooth and elastic. Shape the dough into a loaf and place in the prepared tin. Cover with oiled cling film or a clean tea towel and leave to rise in a warm place for about 1 hour or until doubled in size.

4 Towards the end of the rising time, preheat the oven to 220°C (425°F, gas mark 7). Uncover the loaf and brush with the milk to glaze. Bake for about 30 minutes or until it sounds hollow when removed from the tin and tapped on the base. Cover the loaf with foil towards the end of the cooking time if the top is browning too much.

5 Turn out onto a wire rack and leave to cool. The bread can be kept, wrapped in foil, for 2–3 days.

Another idea

Use the dough to make maple and pecan Chelsea buns. Omit the raisins and, after kneading, roll out the dough to a 23 cm (9 in) square. Beat together 30 g (1 oz) softened butter and 4 tbsp maple syrup, and spread over the dough. Scatter over 115 g (4 oz) finely chopped dried dates and 55 g (2 oz) chopped pecan nuts. Roll up the dough like a Swiss roll and cut into 9 slices. Arrange, cut side down, in 3 rows of 3 in a greased 18 cm (7 in) square cake tin. Cover with oiled cling film and leave to rise in a warm place for about 30 minutes. Brush the top with milk and sprinkle with 2 tsp demerara sugar. Bake in a preheated 200°C (400°F, gas mark 6) oven for 25 minutes or until well risen and lightly browned. Turn out onto a wire rack to cool before separating into buns. These can be kept in an airtight tin for up to 3 days.

Plus points

• Semi-skimmed milk and egg add protein and other nutrients to this loaf.

• Dried fruit, such as raisins, are a concentrated source of energy. Raisins are also a useful source of fibre and potassium.

Each serving provides (one slice) kcal 156, protein 5 g, fat 4 g (of which saturated fat 2 g), carbohydrate 26 g (of which sugars 9 g), fibre 3 g. Good source of selenium. Useful source of copper, folate, iron, niacin, vitamin B$_1$, vitamin B$_6$, zinc.

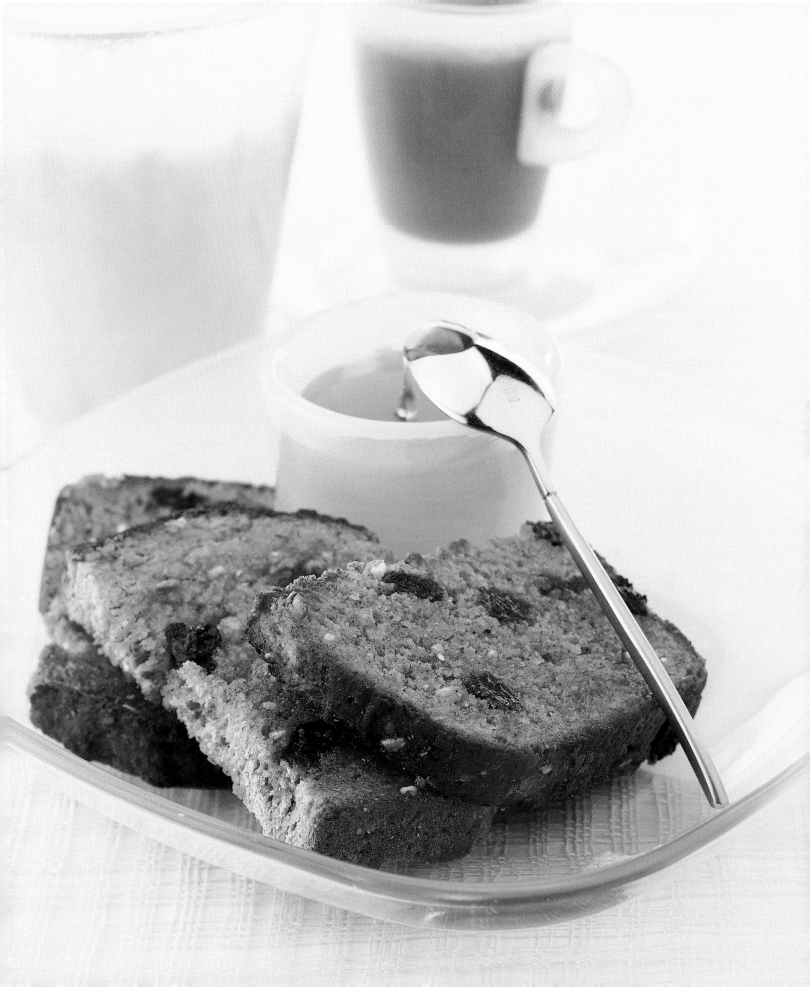

Smoked haddock soufflé

Light, fluffy soufflés rarely fail to impress, yet they are surprisingly easy to make. This recipe uses the fish-poaching milk to make the soufflé base, and fresh herbs and chopped tomatoes are added for a lovely flavour. Serve straight from the oven, with crusty wholemeal bread to accompany.

Preparation time **about 35 minutes**   Cooking time **35 minutes**   *Serves 4*

300 g (10½ oz) smoked haddock fillet

300 ml (10 fl oz) semi-skimmed milk

1 tsp butter

1 tbsp Parmesan cheese

1 tbsp fine dry breadcrumbs

3 tbsp cornflour

3 eggs, separated

250 g (8½ oz) tomatoes, skinned, seeded and diced

1 tsp wholegrain mustard

2 tbsp finely chopped parsley

2 tbsp finely snipped fresh chives

1 egg white

salt and pepper

1 Put the haddock and milk in a saucepan and heat until simmering. Simmer gently for about 8 minutes or until the fish will just flake when tested with a fork. Remove the pan from the heat and leave the fish to cool in the milk. When the fish is cool enough to handle, remove it and flake the flesh, discarding the skin and any bones. Set the poaching milk aside to cool.

2 Preheat the oven, with a metal baking sheet inside, to 190°C (375°F, gas mark 5). Lightly grease a 1.7 litre (3 pint) soufflé dish with the butter. Mix together the Parmesan and breadcrumbs, and sprinkle over the bottom and side of the dish, turning the dish to coat evenly. Shake out any excess crumb mixture and reserve.

3 Mix the cornflour with a little of the reserved, cold poaching milk to make a smooth paste. Heat the remaining milk in a small saucepan until almost boiling, then pour into the cornflour mixture, stirring constantly. Return to the pan and bring to the boil, stirring to make a thick sauce.

4 Pour the sauce into a large mixing bowl. Add the egg yolks, one by one, beating them thoroughly into the sauce. Stir in the flaked haddock, tomatoes, mustard, parsley, chives, and salt and pepper to taste.

5 In a clean, dry mixing bowl, whisk the 4 egg whites until stiff enough to hold soft peaks. Fold a quarter of the whites into the sauce mixture to lighten it, then gently fold in the remaining whites.

6 Spoon the mixture into the prepared soufflé dish and sprinkle the top with the reserved Parmesan and breadcrumb mixture. Set the dish on the hot baking sheet and bake for about 35 minutes or until well risen and golden brown. Serve at once.

Plus points

• Haddock is a useful source of vitamin B$_6$. This vitamin helps the body to make use of protein from food and to form haemoglobin, the pigment in red blood cells.

• Milk is an excellent source of many essential nutrients, the majority of which are concentrated in the non-fat part of milk. Semi-skimmed and skimmed milk therefore contain more of these nutrients than full-fat milks do.

• Thickening the soufflé base with cornflour, instead of the more traditional method using butter, helps to reduce the total fat content of this recipe.

photo, page 31

Each serving provides   kcal 250, protein 25 g, fat 9 g (of which saturated fat 3 g), carbohydrate 19 g (of which sugars 6 g), fibre 1 g. Excellent source of vitamin B$_{12}$. Good source of niacin, selenium, vitamin A. Useful source of calcium, copper, folate, iron, potassium, vitamin B$_1$, vitamin B$_2$, vitamin B$_6$, vitamin C, vitamin E, zinc.

Huevos rancheros

For a fun weekend brunch, serve this Mexican-style dish of poached eggs, warm flour tortillas, a fresh tomato and chilli salsa, and toppings of grated cheese, yogurt, spring onions and fresh coriander.

Preparation and cooking time **35 minutes, plus 30 minutes marinating**   *Serves 4*

4 large or 8 small flour tortillas, about 160 g (5¾ oz) in total

1 tsp vinegar

4 eggs

85 g (3 oz) Edam cheese, coarsely grated

6 tbsp 0% fat Greek-style yogurt

4 spring onions, chopped

chopped fresh coriander to garnish

lime wedges to serve

Tomato and chilli salsa

5 tomatoes, finely chopped

1 plump, mild fresh red chilli, seeded and finely chopped

½ small red onion, finely chopped

1 small garlic clove, finely chopped

2 tbsp finely chopped fresh coriander

1 tbsp extra virgin olive oil

2–3 tsp lime juice, to taste

salt and pepper

1 First make the salsa. Place the chopped tomatoes in a bowl and stir in the chilli, red onion, garlic and coriander. Add the oil and lime juice to taste. Set aside to marinate for about 30 minutes, then season with salt and pepper to taste.

2 Preheat the oven to 180°C (350°F, gas mark 4). Wrap the stacked-up tortillas in foil and put them in the oven to warm for 10 minutes, or according to the packet instructions.

3 Meanwhile, half fill a frying pan with water. Heat until just starting to simmer, then reduce the heat so the water does not boil. Add the vinegar. Break the eggs into the water, one at a time, and poach for 3–4 minutes. Towards the end of cooking, spoon the water over the yolks. When cooked, remove the eggs with a draining spoon and drain on kitchen paper.

4 Place the warmed tortillas on plates (1 large or 2 small ones each). Spoon over a little salsa, then put the eggs on top and season with salt and pepper to taste. Let everyone help themselves to the rest of the salsa, the grated cheese, yogurt and spring onions, plus chopped coriander for sprinkling over the top and lime wedges for squeezing.

Another idea

Add quick home-made **refried beans**, for a very hearty brunch dish. Heat 1 tbsp sunflower oil in a saucepan. Add 1 finely chopped garlic clove and ¼ tsp ground cumin, and cook for a few seconds. Stir in 1 can of pinto or borlotti beans, about 410 g, drained, and 120 ml (4 fl oz) water. Cover and simmer for 5 minutes or until the beans are soft enough to mash. Roughly mash them with a fork, then cook uncovered for a further 3 minutes. If the mixture is too liquid, cook for a few more minutes. Season to taste.

Plus points

- Tortillas, or wraps, are a great alternative to commonly eaten breads, and are another way to boost starchy carbohydrate intake.

- Tomatoes are a rich source of vitamin C, most of which is concentrated in the jellylike substance around the seeds.

photo, page 31

Each serving provides   kcal 451, protein 21 g, fat 17 g (of which saturated fat 6 g), carbohydrate 55 g (of which sugars 6 g), fibre 3 g. Excellent source of vitamin A, vitamin B_{12}. Good source of calcium, niacin, vitamin C, vitamin E, zinc. Useful source of copper, folate, iron, potassium, selenium, viatmin B_1, vitamin B_2, vitamin B_6.

Stuffed eggs en salade

The hollows in hard-boiled egg halves make perfect containers for a tasty filling – here carrot and chive – and the eggs look so pretty served on a bed of ribbon vegetables and lamb's lettuce. All you need is some interesting bread, such as pan gallego with sunflower, pumpkin and millet seeds, to make a satisfying brunch.

Preparation and cooking time **25 minutes**   *Serves 4*

6 large eggs, at room temperature

1½ tbsp low-fat mayonnaise

1½ tbsp plain low-fat yogurt

½ tsp mustard powder

100 g (3½ oz) carrot, finely grated

2 tbsp snipped fresh chives

Tarragon dressing

1 tbsp extra virgin olive oil

1 tsp tarragon vinegar

¼ tsp Dijon mustard

salt and pepper

Orange and green salad

1 carrot

1 small bulb of fennel

2 courgettes

85 g (3 oz) lamb's lettuce

1 First hard-boil the eggs. Place in a large saucepan, cover with tepid water and bring to the boil. Reduce the heat and simmer for 7 minutes. Remove the eggs with a draining spoon and place in a bowl of cold water to cool.

2 Meanwhile, make the dressing. Put the olive oil, vinegar and mustard in a screw-top jar with salt and pepper to taste. Shake well, then set aside.

3 Shell the eggs and cut each in half lengthways. Scoop out the yolks into a bowl using a teaspoon. Set the whites aside.

4 Add the mayonnaise, yogurt, mustard powder, grated carrot and half of the chives to the egg yolks, and mash together. Season with salt and pepper to taste. Using a teaspoon, spoon the egg yolk filling into the hollows in the egg white halves, mounding it up attractively.

5 Using a swivel vegetable peeler or a mandolin, shave ribbons lengthways from the carrot, fennel and courgettes. Put the vegetable ribbons in a mixing bowl with the lamb's lettuce. Shake the dressing again, then pour over the salad and toss together.

6 Divide the salad among 4 plates and top each with 3 stuffed egg halves. Sprinkle the top of the eggs with the remaining chives, and serve.

Some more ideas

For a lightly curried filling, mix the egg yolks with 3 tbsp reduced-fat soft cheese, 1 tsp curry paste, 2 finely chopped spring onions and the grated carrot.

Add 2–3 finely chopped radishes to the stuffing mixture.

Plus points

• Eggs have often been given a 'bad press' because of their cholesterol content. In fact, for most people, eating eggs and other foods rich in cholesterol has little detrimental effect on blood cholesterol levels.

• Preparing vegetables just before use helps to minimise vitamin loss.

• By mixing mayonnaise with yogurt, rather than using mayonnaise alone, the fat and calorie contents of a dish such as this can be reduced.

Each serving provides kcal 210, protein 12 g, fat 15 g (of which saturated fat 3.5 g), carbohydrate 6 g (of which sugars 5.5 g), fibre 3 g. Excellent source of vitamin A, vitamin B_{12}. Good source of folate, vitamin B_2, vitamin E, zinc. Useful source of calcium, copper, iron, niacin, potassium, selenium, vitamin B_1, vitamin B_6, vitamin C.

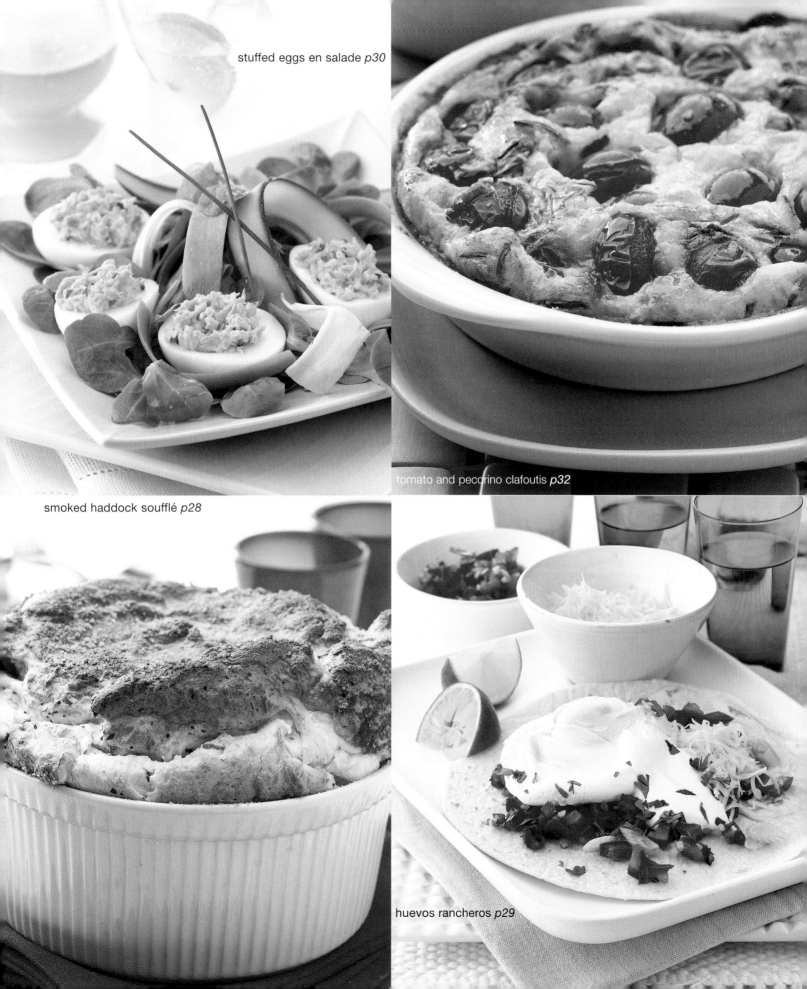

stuffed eggs en salade *p30*

tomato and pecorino clafoutis *p32*

smoked haddock soufflé *p28*

huevos rancheros *p29*

Tomato and pecorino clafoutis

For this savoury version of a classic French batter pudding, sweet cherry tomatoes are baked in a light, fluffy batter flavoured with grated pecorino cheese. Make individual clafoutis, or one large one, and serve for a delicious and sophisticated brunch.

Preparation time **20 minutes**   Cooking time **30–35 minutes**   *Serves 4*

vegetable oil spray

450 g (1 lb) cherry tomatoes

4 tbsp snipped fresh chives

75 g (2½ oz) mature pecorino cheese, coarsely grated

3 large eggs, plus 3 egg whites

45 g (1½ oz) plain flour

3 tbsp half-fat crème fraîche

300 ml (10 fl oz) semi-skimmed milk

1 Preheat the oven to 190°C (375°F, gas mark 5). Spray with oil 4 shallow ovenproof dishes, each 12–15 cm (5–6 in) in diameter. Divide the cherry tomatoes among the dishes, spreading them out, and sprinkle over the chives and the cheese.

2 Break the eggs into a bowl and whisk them together with the whites, then gradually whisk in the flour until smooth. Add the crème fraîche, then gradually whisk in the milk to make a thin, smooth batter. Season with salt and pepper to taste.

3 Pour the batter over the tomatoes, dividing it evenly among the dishes. Sprinkle on an extra grinding of pepper. Bake for 30–35 minutes or until set, puffed and lightly golden.

4 Remove the clafoutis from the oven and leave to cool for a few minutes before serving, as the tomatoes are very hot inside.

Some more ideas

Bake one large clafoutis, using a lightly oiled 23 cm (9 in) round ovenproof dish that is about 5 cm (2 in) deep. Increase the baking time to 35–40 minutes.

For a **Red Leicester and onion clafoutis**, cut 250 g (8½ oz) red onions into thin wedges and fry in 1 tbsp extra virgin olive oil for about 5 minutes or until golden. Stir in 1 tbsp fresh thyme leaves towards the end of the cooking. Scatter the onions over the bottom of a lightly oiled 23 cm (9 in) round ovenproof dish that is about 5 cm (2 in) deep. Coarsely grate 85 g (3 oz) Red Leicester cheese and sprinkle all but a small handful of it over the onions. Make the batter as in the main recipe and pour over the onions. Give the mixture a stir, then sprinkle over the remaining cheese and a few sprigs of fresh thyme. Bake for 35–40 minutes or until puffed and golden.

Plus points

● Pecorino is a hard Italian cheese made from sheep's milk. Like Parmesan, it is quite high in fat, but need only be used in small quantities as it has a rich, strong flavour.

● Using egg whites helps to reduce the number of whole eggs needed, while still maintaining volume.

● Tomatoes contain lycopene, a valuable antioxidant that may help to protect against prostate, bladder and pancreatic cancers if tomatoes are included in the diet regularly.

photo, page 31

Each serving provides kcal 310, protein 20 g, fat 20 g (of which saturated fat 9 g), carbohydrate 17 g (of which sugars 8 g), fibre 1.5 g. Excellent source of calcium, vitamin B_{12}. Good source of niacin, vitamin A, vitamin B_2, vitamin C, vitamin E, zinc. Useful source of copper, folate, iron, potassium, selenium, vitamin B_1, vitamin B_6.

Strawberry yogurt smoothie

This refreshing drink is perfect for summer when strawberries are plentiful and full of flavour and vitamins. It takes only a few minutes to prepare, so is ideal as a nourishing start to the day or as a light snack-in-a-glass at any time. You could also dilute it with more orange juice, to serve in place of sugary fruit squashes.

Preparation time **5 minutes**   *Serves 4*

450 g (1 lb) ripe strawberries, hulled

grated zest and juice of 1 large orange

150 g (5½ oz) plain low-fat yogurt

1 tbsp caster sugar, or to taste (optional)

To decorate (optional)

4 small strawberries

4 small slices of orange

1 Tip the strawberries into a food processor or blender and add the orange zest, juice and the yogurt. Blend to a smooth purée, scraping down the sides of the container once or twice. Taste the mixture and sweeten with the sugar, if necessary.

2 For a really smooth consistency, press through a nylon sieve to remove the pips, although this is not essential.

3 Pour into glasses. If you like, decorate with small strawberries and slices of orange, both split so they sit on the rim of the glass.

Some more ideas

Add a sliced banana to the strawberries. This will thicken the texture of the smoothie and will also add natural sweetness, so be sure to taste before adding sugar – you may not need any.

Swap the strawberries for dried apricots, to make a smoothie with a useful amount of beta-carotene and a good amount of soluble fibre. Gently simmer 200 g (7 oz) ready-to-eat dried apricots in 900 ml (1½ pints) strained Earl Grey tea for 30 minutes or until tender. Cool, then pour the apricots and liquid into a blender. Add the orange zest, juice and yogurt and blend until smooth. Taste and

sweeten with sugar if required. Serve sprinkled with a little crunchy oat and pecan breakfast cereal or blueberry and cranberry granola.

Plus points

• Most of the yogurt sold in the UK is 'live', which means that it contains high levels of beneficial live bacteria. Labelling does not always make it clear if yogurt is 'live', but if it is stored in the chiller cabinet of the supermarket you can be fairly confident that it is 'live' – that is, the yogurt has not been heat-treated after fermentation, a process that destroys the beneficial bacteria. The balance of bacteria in the gut is easily upset by stress, medication such as antibiotics, or a poor diet, but a regular intake of 'good' bacteria, such as that provided by 'live' yogurt, can help to maintain a healthy digestive tract.

• Sugary drinks can make your blood sugar rise quickly. The yogurt in this recipe helps to slow down the rise in blood glucose. Aim to drink sugared drinks during meals rather than in between meals.

photo, page 35

Each serving provides   kcal 55, protein 3 g, fat 0.5 g (of which saturated fat 0.2 g), carbohydrate 11 g (of which sugars 11 g), fibre 1 g. Excellent source of vitamin C. Useful source of calcium, folate.

Pimm's melon cup

This salad is inspired by the classic summer drink, which is often garnished with so much fruit that it is almost a fruit salad in itself. A mixture of sweet melon, berries, pear and cucumber is marinated in Pimm's and then served in melon shells. A decoration of pretty borage flowers is a traditional finish.

Preparation time **20–25 minutes**   Marinating time **20 minutes**   *Serves 4*

1 small Ogen melon

1 small cantaloupe or Charentais melon

200 g (7 oz) strawberries, sliced

1 pear, cut into 2.5 cm (1 in) chunks

¼ cucumber, cut into 1 cm (½ in) dice

1 carambola, cut into 5 mm (¼ in) slices

6 tbsp Pimm's

2 tbsp shredded fresh mint or lemon balm leaves

borage flowers to decorate (optional)

1 Cut the melons in half horizontally and scoop out the seeds from the centre. Using a melon baller or a small spoon, scoop out the flesh into a large bowl. Reserve the melon shells.

2 Add the sliced strawberries, pear chunks and cucumber dice to the melon in the bowl. Reserve some slices of carambola for decoration and chop the rest. Add to the bowl.

3 Sprinkle the Pimm's over the fruit. Add the shredded mint or lemon balm and stir gently to mix together. Cover with cling film and set aside in a cool place or the fridge to marinate for 20 minutes.

4 With a tablespoon scoop any odd pieces of melon flesh from the shells to make them smooth. Pile the fruit mixture into the shells and decorate with the reserved slices of carambola and borage flowers, if using.

Some more ideas

For a non-alcoholic version, omit the Pimm's and flavour with 1–2 tsp of a cordial such as elderflower.

Turn this into a **luncheon fruit and vegetable salad**, using just 1 melon (either Ogen or cantaloupe), the strawberries and cucumber plus an apple instead of the pear and 100 g (3½ oz) seedless green grapes. Omit the Pimm's. Make a bed of salad leaves, including some watercress and chopped spring onion, on each plate and pile the fruit on top. Add a scoop of plain cottage cheese and sprinkle with chopped fresh mint and toasted pine nuts.

Plus points

• This delicious combination of fresh fruit provides plenty of fibre and vitamins, especially vitamin C and beta-carotene (which is found in orange-fleshed melon varieties), both important antioxidants.

• Maximum alcohol recommendations for the general population are 3–4 units a day for men and 2–3 units a day for women. Diabetes UK recommend 3 and 2 units respectively.

Each serving provides kcal 101, protein 1.5 g, fat 0 g, carbohydrate 12 g (of which sugars 12 g), fibre 2 g. Excellent source of vitamin C. Good source of vitamin A. Useful source of folate.

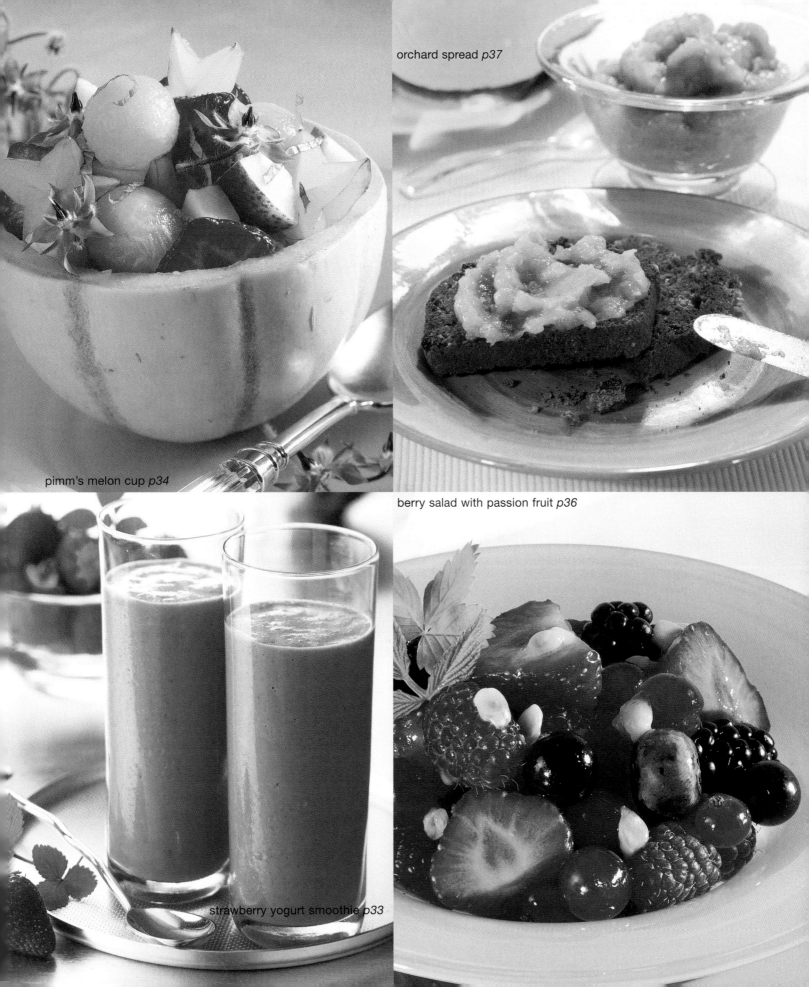

orchard spread *p37*

pimm's melon cup *p34*

berry salad with passion fruit *p36*

strawberry yogurt smoothie *p33*

Berry salad with passion fruit

Berries are the utterly fresh flavour of summer. Tart, sweet and juicy, they come in a wide array of types, ranging from bright and delicate raspberries to fleshy strawberries, plump little blueberries and rich blackberries. The passion fruit is not a distinctive flavour in this dish, but instead it adds a fragrant tart edge.

Preparation time **10–15 minutes**   *Serves 6*

450 g (1 lb) strawberries, cut in half

150 g (5½ oz) raspberries

100 g (3½ oz) blackberries

100 g (3½ oz) blueberries

100 g (3½ oz) mixed redcurrants and blackcurrants, removed from their stalks

2 passion fruit

1 tbsp caster sugar

juice of ½ lemon or lime

1 Mix the strawberries, raspberries, blackberries, blueberries, redcurrants and blackcurrants together in a bowl.

2 Cut the passion fruit in half. Holding a sieve over the bowl of berries, spoon the passion fruit flesh and seeds into the sieve. Rub the flesh and seeds briskly to press all the juice through the sieve onto the berries. Reserve a few of the passion fruit seeds left in the sieve and discard the rest.

3 Add the sugar and lemon or lime juice to the berries. Gently toss together. Sprinkle over the reserved passion fruit seeds. Serve straightaway or cover and chill briefly.

Some more ideas

Instead of passion fruit, add 3 tbsp crème de cassis. Chill until ready to serve.

Omit the passion fruit and instead serve the berry salad with a peach and apricot sauce: peel and purée 2 ripe peaches and flavour with 2–3 tbsp caster sugar, the juice of ½ lemon and a dash of pure almond extract. Finely dice 8 ready-to-eat dried apricots and add to the peach purée. Serve the berries on plates in a pool of the sauce.

Serve the berry salad spooned over vanilla frozen yogurt.

Plus points

• Comparing the same weight of each fruit, blackcurrants come out on top for vitamin C, with 200 mg in each 100 g (3½ oz), as compared with strawberries with 77 mg, raspberries 32 mg and blackberries 15 mg. These days vitamin C is not only recognised as essential to prevent scurvy (a condition where gums bleed, skin becomes fragile and blood vessels leak into the surrounding tissue, causing bruising), but also for maintaining the immune system and as an antioxidant, preventing the damaging processes that can lead to heart disease and cancer.

• To this feast of summer fruit, rich in dietary fibre and vitamin C, passion fruit also adds vitamin A, which is essential for healthy skin and good vision, and blackberries add vitamin E, an important antioxidant. The effects of vitamin E are enhanced by other antioxidants like vitamin C, so this combination of fruits is particularly healthy.

photo, page 35

Each serving provides kcal 55, protein 1 g, fat 0 g, carbohydrate 12 g (of which sugars 12 g), fibre 3 g. Excellent source of vitamin C. Useful source of folate, vitamin E.

Orchard spread

Use this rich, slightly tart, lightly spiced purée of fresh and dried fruit to replace butter on warm morning toast or muffins. The recipe makes far more than 4 people can enjoy at one breakfast, but the spread keeps well in the fridge. Also try it with grated Cheddar cheese in a sandwich, or instead of pickle or chutney in a ploughman's lunch.

Preparation and cooking time **about 45 minutes**   Cooling time **at least 1 hour**   *Makes 1 kg (2¼ lb)*

500 g (1 lb 2 oz) cooking apples, such as Bramley's, peeled, cored and chopped

250 g (8½ oz) ready-to-eat dried pears

250 g (8½ oz) ready-to-eat dried peaches

360 ml (12 fl oz) apple juice

½ tsp ground mixed spice

1½ tsp lemon juice, or to taste (optional)

1 Place the apples, pears, peaches, apple juice, ground mixed spice and 120 ml (4 fl oz) water into a heavy-based saucepan. Set the pan over a high heat and bring the fruit mixture to the boil, stirring occasionally.

2 Reduce the heat to low and simmer, uncovered, for 30 minutes or until the mixture is reduced to a pulp and no liquid is visible on the surface. Stir frequently to prevent the mixture from sticking to the bottom of the pan.

3 Remove the pan from the heat and allow the mixture to cool slightly. Then taste and stir in the lemon juice if the mixture is too sweet.

4 Transfer the fruit mixture to a food processor or blender and process to a thick purée.

5 Leave to cool completely before serving. The spread can be kept, covered, in the fridge for up to 2 weeks.

Some more ideas

Make a **spiced prune spread** by replacing the dried pears and peaches with 500 g (1 lb 2 oz) prunes and using orange juice instead of apple juice. Omit the mixed spice and instead add the seeds from 3 crushed green cardamom pods.

For a **vanilla peach spread**, replace the dried pears with additional dried peaches and use orange juice instead of apple juice. Omit the mixed spice and include a vanilla pod in the mixture while it simmers.

Other combinations to try include apples and dried cranberries flavoured with finely grated orange zest, and apples and prunes flavoured with ground ginger and very finely diced pieces of stem ginger.

Plus points

● Apples are a good source of soluble fibre (pectin), and they provide vitamin C.

● Dried peaches are a good source of potassium. They also provide useful amounts of iron, carotenes and the B vitamin niacin.

● Both dried peaches and dried pears are good sources of fibre.

● The sweetness of fresh fruit is concentrated in their dried forms, so spreads such as this need no additional sugar to make them as sweet as commercial jams and preserves. Ordinary jam can have about 70 per cent sugar, which weight for weight is double the amount of sugar in this spread.

photo, page 35

Each serving provides (30 g/1 oz) kcal 40, protein 0.5 g, fat 0.1 g, carbohydrate 10 g (of which sugars 10 g), fibre 1 g. Useful source of vitamin C.

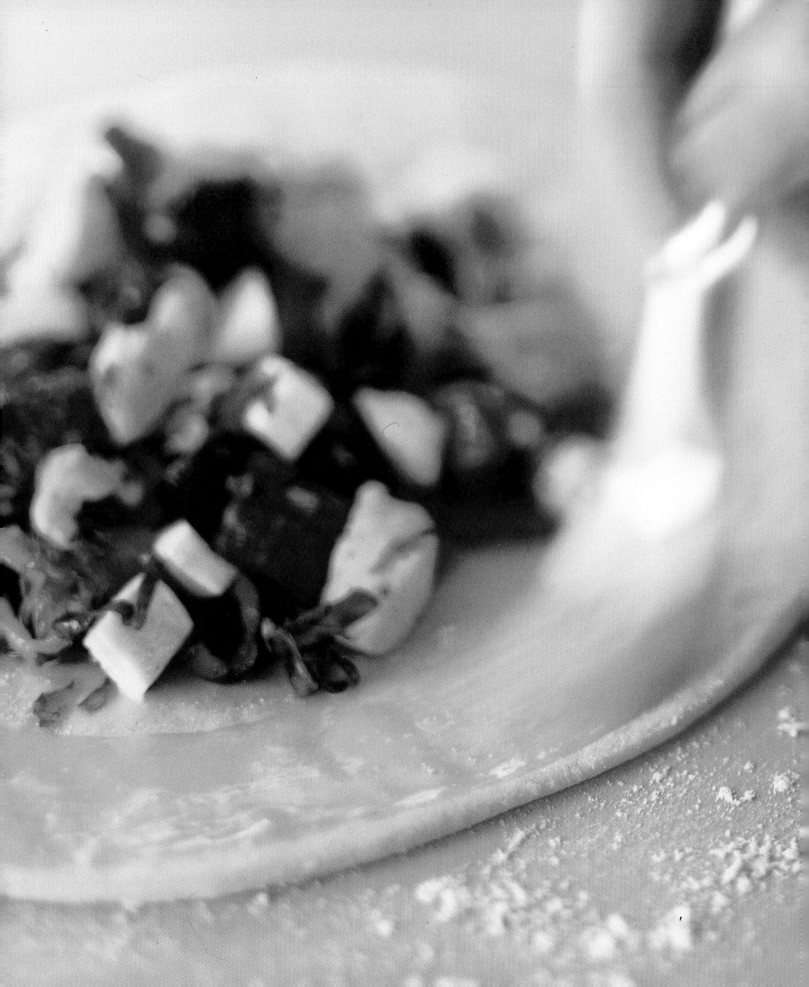

Lunch

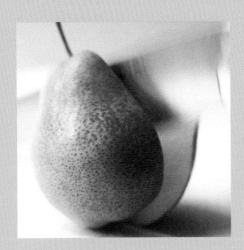

Tarragon chicken salad

Tahini, a paste made from ground sesame seeds, is a favourite ingredient in Middle Eastern cooking. Available from most large supermarkets, it adds a nutty taste and thick creaminess to the dressing for this colourful and nutritious chicken salad. Serve with warmed crusty rolls.

Preparation time **25 minutes**   Cooking time **15 minutes**   *Serves 4*

2 skinless boneless chicken breasts (fillets), about 300 g (10½ oz) in total

360 ml (12 fl oz) chicken or vegetable stock

1 small bunch of fresh tarragon

1 small lemon

3 black peppercorns

2 tbsp tahini

1 head chicory, about 150 g (5½ oz)

140 g (5 oz) baby spinach leaves

2 oranges

30 g (1 oz) flaked almonds, toasted

salt and pepper

Plus points

• Chicken is an excellent source of protein and provides many B vitamins. Removing the skin reduces the fat content a lot, as most of the fat in chicken lies directly beneath the skin.

• Although almonds are rich in fat, most of it is the healthier, monounsaturated type.

1 Put the chicken breasts in a shallow pan, in one layer, and pour over the stock. Remove the tarragon leaves from the stalks and set them aside. Lightly crush the tarragon stalks with a rolling pin to release all their flavoursome oils, then add to the pan. Using a vegetable peeler, remove a strip of zest from the lemon and add this to the pan together with the peppercorns.

2 Set the pan over a moderate heat and bring the stock to the boil. Reduce the heat so the stock just simmers gently and cover the pan. Cook for 15 minutes or until the chicken is white all the way through.

3 Remove the chicken breasts using a draining spoon and leave to cool on a plate. Strain the stock into a jug and discard the tarragon stalks, lemon zest and peppercorns. Set the stock aside. When the chicken has cooled, cut it into thick strips.

4 Put the tahini into a mixing bowl and gradually whisk in 4 tbsp of the reserved stock to make a smooth, creamy dressing. If the dressing is a bit thick, whisk in another 1–2 tbsp of the stock. Squeeze the juice from the lemon and stir it into the dressing. Chop enough of the tarragon leaves to make 1 tbsp, and add to the dressing with salt and pepper to taste.

5 Cut the chicory across on the diagonal into slices about 1 cm (½ in) thick. Arrange the chicory and spinach in a large salad bowl.

6 Peel the oranges, then cut between the membrane into segments. Scatter the segments over the salad leaves, followed by the toasted almonds. Place the chicken strips on top, and spoon over the tahini tarragon dressing. Serve immediately.

Another idea

For an **Oriental chicken salad**, poach the chicken in stock flavoured with 3 thin slices fresh root ginger and 3 black peppercorns. Combine 150 g (5½ oz) shredded Chinese leaves, 100 g (3½ oz) cos lettuce, torn into pieces, and 50 g (1¾ oz) watercress in a large salad bowl, and set the sliced chicken on top. Scatter over 3 peeled and diced kiwi fruit. For the dressing, whisk together 2 tbsp tahini, 1 crushed garlic clove, 1 tsp finely chopped fresh root ginger, the grated zest and juice of 1 lemon, 1 tbsp light soy sauce, a good pinch of five-spice powder and 3–4 tbsp of the reserved poaching stock until smooth and with a light coating consistency. Spoon the dressing over the salad, sprinkle with sesame seeds and serve with warm pitta breads.

Each serving provides   kcal 330, protein 26.5 g, fat 21.5 g (of which saturated fat 2.5 g), carbohydrate 10 g (of which sugars 8 g), fibre 5 g. Excellent source of copper, niacin, potassium, vitamin C, vitamin E. Good source of calcium, folate, iron, zinc. Useful source of selenium, vitamin B_2.

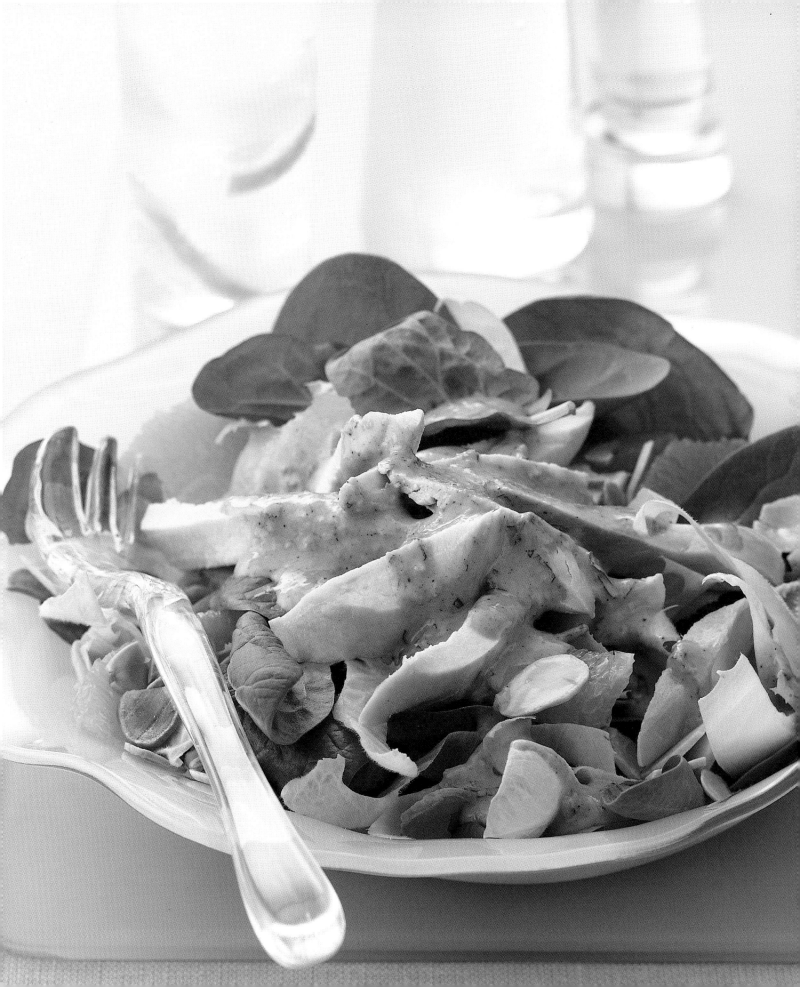

Watermelon and feta salad

A summery cheese salad, this has been devised with a nod towards the Mediterranean. The salty tang of creamy feta cheese is contrasted with bright pink and orange fruit, luscious and full of sweet flavour. A mix of salad leaves adds a slightly peppery taste, and toasted seeds give crunch. With bread, this is good for lunch.

Preparation time **15 minutes**   *Serves 6*

400 g (14 oz) watermelon flesh

2 nectarines or peaches

170 g (6 oz) mixed salad leaves, including rocket and frisée

200 g (7 oz) feta cheese

2 tbsp extra virgin olive oil

juice of ½ lemon

pepper

2 tbsp toasted pumpkin or sunflower seeds

1 Cut the watermelon into bite-sized chunks, removing all the seeds as you come across them. Halve the nectarines or peaches and remove the stone, then slice the flesh. Tear the salad leaves into bite-sized pieces, if necessary. Combine the fruit and leaves in a large salad bowl.

2 Crumble the feta cheese over the salad. Add the oil and lemon juice and toss gently until well mixed. Season with plenty of black pepper, but add salt cautiously as the cheese can be very salty. Sprinkle over the seeds and serve.

Some more ideas

Replace the watermelon and peaches or nectarines with 600 g (1 lb 5 oz) of pears, cored and cut into chunks, and use creamy Stilton instead of the feta cheese. Include radicchio and chicory in the salad leaves.

Wensleydale or white Cheshire cheese can be used in the watermelon version instead of feta.

Toasted walnuts can be added to either version in place of the toasted seeds.

Plus points

• Colourful fruits provide a number of vitamins, including vitamin A from beta-carotene, which gives the yellow colour to peaches and nectarines.

• As well as protein, the cheese provides calcium. Note, though, that feta is high in sodium (salt), with more than twice as much as is found in the same quantity of Cheddar. To reduce the salt content, you can soak the feta in milk for 30 minutes beforehand. Use less or no added salt in cooking.

• Toasted pumpkin and sunflower seeds contain a variety of useful minerals, including phosphorus, magnesium and copper, as well as fibre and protein. Both types of seeds are rich sources of fat, but this is mostly the healthy, unsaturated type.

• Sunflower seeds are a particularly good source of vitamin E.

photo, page 45

Each serving provides   kcal 185, protein 7 g, fat 13 g (of which saturated fat 6 g), carbohydrate 9 g (of which sugars 8 g), fibre 1 g. Good source of vitamin C. Useful source of calcium, copper, folate, niacin, vitamin A, vitamin B$_{12}$, vitamin E.

Middle Eastern salad

Based on 'fattoush', the colourful, crunchy salad served throughout the Middle East, this version adds tuna fish for extra flavour and protein. Make sure you grill the pitta bread until really crisp to prevent it from going soggy when mixed with the other ingredients, and serve the salad as soon as possible after making.

Preparation time **about 15 minutes**   *Serves 4*

4 pitta breads, about 55 g (2 oz) each

1½ tbsp extra virgin olive oil

juice of 1 lemon

6 spring onions, sliced

340 g (12 oz) ripe tomatoes, chopped

½ cucumber, diced

1 can tuna in spring water, about 200 g, drained and flaked

2 tbsp coarsely chopped fresh flat-leaf parsley

1 tbsp coarsely chopped fresh coriander

1 tbsp coarsely chopped fresh mint

salt and pepper

1 Preheat the grill to high. Warm the pitta breads under the grill for a few seconds or until puffy, then carefully split them open through the middle and open out each one like a book. Return to the grill and toast for 2–3 minutes on each side or until lightly browned and crisp. Roughly tear the pitta into bite-sized pieces and set aside.

2 Whisk together the olive oil and lemon juice in a large serving bowl, and season with salt and pepper to taste. Add the spring onions, tomatoes, cucumber and tuna, and toss gently to coat with the oil and lemon juice.

3 Add the parsley, coriander, mint and torn pitta pieces to the serving bowl and toss quickly to mix. Serve immediately.

Some more ideas

Make a more substantial salad by adding 1 can black-eyed or aduki beans, about 400 g, drained and rinsed.

For a **Mediterranean-style vegetable salad**, whisk together 1 tsp Dijon mustard, 1 tsp grated lemon zest, 1 crushed garlic clove, 2 tsp red wine vinegar, 1 tbsp extra virgin olive oil, 1 tbsp chopped fresh oregano, and salt and pepper in a large serving bowl.

Quarter 250 g (8½ oz) baby plum tomatoes and add to the bowl. Add 2 medium-sized courgettes, 1 small bulb of fennel and 1 red onion, all coarsely chopped. Toss to coat the vegetables with the dressing. Serve this salad with sardine toasts for extra protein and carbohydrate. Drain 1 can sardines in olive oil, about 120 g, and roughly mash with 2 tsp drained capers. Cut 12 slices of ciabatta or French bread, each about 1 cm (½ in) thick, and toast on both sides. Spread the mashed sardines on one side of each slice. Sprinkle with 1 tbsp freshly grated Parmesan cheese and grill until golden brown, about 1 minute.

Plus points

• Tomatoes, like so many other fruits and vegetables, are a good source of the antioxidants beta-carotene and vitamin C. They also contain lycopene, a carotenoid compound that acts as an antioxidant and which is thought to be important in helping to prevent the development of cancer.

• Using both the white bulb and leaves of spring onions increases the beta-carotene provided, as this all-important antioxidant is found in the green part of the vegetable.

photo, page 45

Each serving provides kcal 274, protein 18 g, fat 7 g (of which saturated fat 1.5 g), carbohydrate 36 g (of which sugars 5 g), fibre 3 g. Excellent source of selenium, vitamin B$_{12}$, vitamin C, vitamin E. Good source of niacin. Useful source of calcium, copper, folate, iron, potassium, vitamin A, vitamin B$_1$, vitamin B$_6$, zinc.

LUNCH

Citrus and spinach salad

In this colourful salad, the subtle flavour of spinach is enhanced by sweet melon and citrus, and Parma ham adds a savoury touch. You can prepare the dressing in advance, but only assemble the salad at the last moment to preserve as much vitamin C as possible. Serve with French or Italian bread as a light main dish.

Preparation time **15 minutes**   *Serves 4*

1 ruby grapefruit

1 large orange

225 g (8 oz) young spinach leaves

250 g (8½ oz) cantaloupe melon flesh, cut into bite-sized chunks

2 spring onions, white parts only, very thinly sliced

55 g (2 oz) thinly sliced Parma ham, excess fat removed, cut into shreds

Creamy dressing

1 tbsp best-quality balsamic vinegar

1 tbsp extra virgin olive oil

1 tbsp single cream

½ tsp honey

salt and pepper

1 To make the dressing, put the vinegar, oil, cream and honey in a small screw-top jar. Cover and shake until well blended. Set aside.

2 Working over a bowl to catch the juice, peel the grapefruit, removing all the bitter white pith, then cut it into segments between the membranes. If large, cut the segments into bite-sized pieces. Set the grapefruit segments aside on a plate.

3 Using a citrus zester, take fine shreds of zest from the orange and set aside. Working over the bowl containing the grapefruit juice, peel the orange, removing all the pith, then cut it into segments between the membranes and cut the segments into bite-sized pieces, if liked. Add to the grapefruit segments and set aside.

4 Add 1 tbsp of the combined grapefruit and orange juices to the dressing and shake again to blend. Taste and add more citrus juice, if liked. Add salt and pepper to taste.

5 Place the spinach in a large serving bowl. Add the orange and grapefruit segments, the melon and spring onions and toss together. Shake the dressing once more, then pour it over the salad and toss. Scatter the Parma ham and orange zest over the top and serve at once.

Some more ideas

To add a peppery flavour, replace 55 g (2 oz) of the spinach with watercress leaves removed from their stalks. Watercress is an excellent source of vitamin C, as well as beta-carotene.

Replace the balsamic vinegar with a fruit-flavoured vinegar, such as raspberry or lemon.

Make this into a vegetarian salad by omitting the Parma ham. If you want to retain the flavour contrast of the fruit with a savoury, salty ingredient, sprinkle the salad with 55 g (2 oz) of drained and crumbled feta cheese.

Plus points

• This salad is a first-class source of vitamin C. The fruit are loaded with this essential vitamin, as is the spinach. Vitamin C is destroyed when food is cooked or cut, which is why it is better to leave the spinach leaves whole.

• Ruby and pink grapefruit contain the antioxidant beta-carotene, which is converted into vitamin A by the body.

Each serving provides kcal 115, protein 5 g, fat 5 g (of which saturated fat 1 g), carbohydrate 13 g (of which sugars 12 g), fibre 3 g. Excellent source of folate, vitamin A, vitamin C. Useful source of calcium, iron, niacin, vitamin B$_1$, vitamin B$_6$.

44

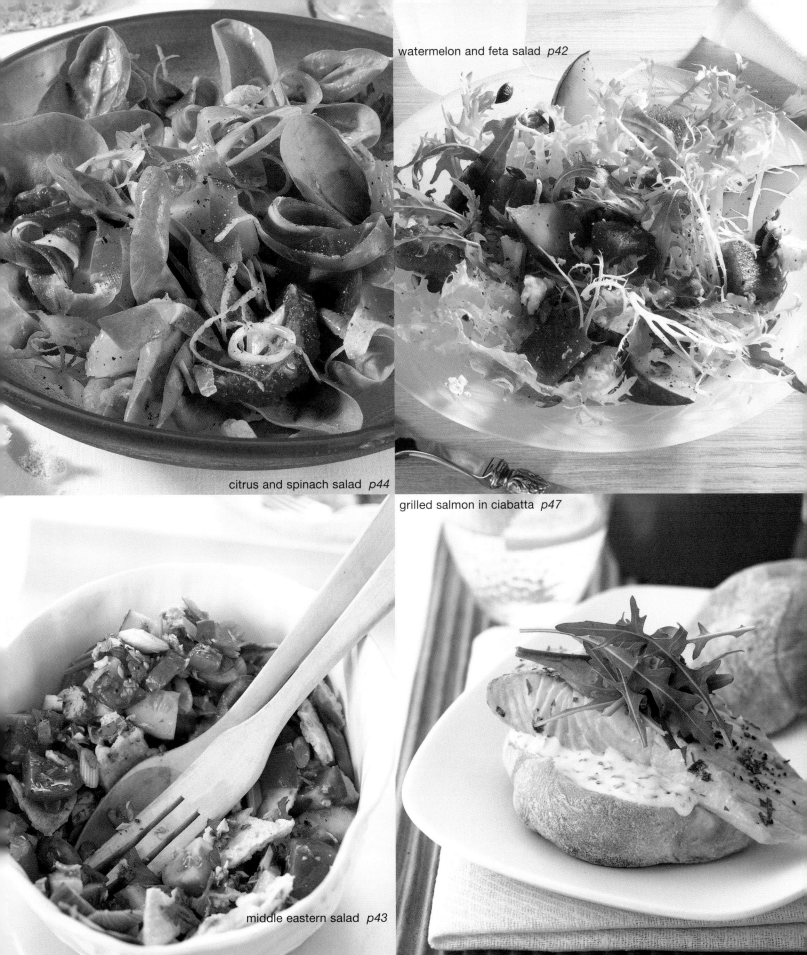

watermelon and feta salad *p42*

citrus and spinach salad *p44*

grilled salmon in ciabatta *p47*

middle eastern salad *p43*

Summer salmon and asparagus

Fresh young vegetables and succulent salmon make this an excellent speedy casserole to prepare for special occasions, especially when home-grown asparagus is in season. Tiny leeks, tender asparagus and sugarsnap peas all cook quickly and look superb. Serve with boiled new potatoes for a memorable meal.

Preparation time **10 minutes**   Cooking time **about 20 minutes**   *Serves 4*

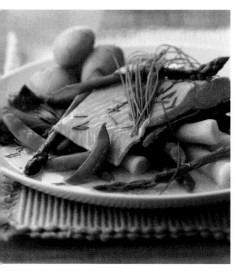

4 pieces skinless salmon fillet, about 140 g (5 oz) each

200 g (7 oz) baby leeks

250 g (8½ oz) tender asparagus spears

150 g (5½ oz) sugarsnap peas

4 tbsp dry white wine

200 ml (7 fl oz) fish or vegetable stock

30 g (1 oz) butter, cut into small pieces

salt and pepper

1 tbsp snipped fresh chives to garnish

1 Run your fingertips over each salmon fillet to check for any stray bones, pulling out any that remain between the flakes of fish. Arrange the leeks in a single layer in the bottom of a large shallow flameproof casserole. Lay the pieces of salmon on top. Surround the fish with the asparagus and sugarsnap peas. Pour in the wine and stock, and dot the butter over the fish. Season with salt and pepper.

2 Bring to the boil, then cover the casserole with a tight-fitting lid and reduce the heat so the liquid simmers gently. Cook the fish and vegetables for 12–14 minutes or until the salmon is pale pink all the way through and the vegetables are tender. Sprinkle the chives over the salmon and serve.

Some more ideas

Mackerel fillets can be casseroled in the same way. Season the mackerel fillets and fold them loosely in half, with the skin outside. Use baby carrots, or large carrots cut into short, thick sticks, instead of the asparagus, and medium-dry cider instead of the wine. Add 2 sprigs of fresh rosemary to the vegetables before arranging the mackerel on top and pouring in the cider and stock.

For a quick **Oriental fish casserole**, use cod or halibut fillet instead of salmon, 4 spring onions instead of the leeks, and 300 g (10½ oz) button mushrooms instead of the asparagus. Arrange the vegetables and fish as in the main recipe, adding 4 tbsp Chinese rice wine or dry sherry with the stock instead of the white wine. Omit the butter; sprinkle 1 tbsp soy sauce, 1 tbsp grated fresh root ginger and 1 tbsp toasted sesame oil over the fish. Garnish with chopped fresh coriander and serve with plain boiled rice.

Plus points

- Asparagus contains asparagine, a phytochemical that acts as a diuretic. The ancient Greeks used asparagus to treat kidney problems. Today naturopaths recommend eating asparagus to help to relieve bloating associated with premenstrual syndrome (PMS).

- Salmon is a rich source of omega-3 fatty acids, a type of polyunsaturated fat thought to help to protect against coronary heart disease and strokes by making blood less 'sticky' and therefore less likely to clot. A diet rich in omega-3 fatty acids may also be helpful in preventing and treating arthritis.

Each serving provides kcal 360, protein 33 g, fat 22 g (of which saturated fat 7 g), carbohydrate 4 g (of which sugars 4 g), fibre 3 g. Excellent source of vitamin B_{12}. Good source of folate, vitamin B_6, vitamin C. Useful source of iron, niacin, selenium, vitamin B_1.

Grilled salmon in ciabatta

Here fresh salmon fillets are marinated, then lightly grilled and served in warm ciabatta rolls with mixed salad leaves and a basil mayonnaise, to create a very tempting and special lunch dish. Lightening the mayonnaise with yogurt reduces the fat without losing out on any of the creaminess.

Preparation time **15 minutes**   Marinating time **30 minutes**   Cooking time **10 minutes**   *Serves 4*

juice of 1 lime

3 tbsp chopped fresh basil

4 pieces skinless salmon fillets, about 85 g (3 oz) each

2½ tbsp plain low-fat yogurt

2½ tbsp reduced-fat mayonnaise

½ tsp finely grated lime zest

4 part-baked ciabatta rolls or wholemeal rolls, about 75 g (2½ oz) each

salt and pepper

mixed salad leaves, such as rocket, Oak Leaf lettuce, baby spinach, red chard and lamb's lettuce, to serve

1 Mix together the lime juice, 2 tbsp of the basil, and salt and pepper to taste in a shallow, non-metallic dish. Add the salmon fillets and turn them in the mixture to coat well all over. Cover and leave to marinate in a cool place for 30 minutes.

2 Meanwhile, mix together the yogurt, mayonnaise, lime zest and remaining 1 tbsp basil in a small bowl. Season with salt and pepper to taste. Cover and chill until required.

3 Preheat the grill to moderate, and preheat the oven to 220°C (425°F, gas mark 7). Lift the salmon fillets out of the marinade and place in the foil-lined grill pan. Brush with a little of the marinade, then grill for 4–5 minutes on each side or until the fish is just cooked and the flesh is beginning to flake, brushing again with the marinade after you have turned the fillets. While the fish is cooking, place the bread rolls in the oven to bake for about 5 minutes, or according to the packet instructions, until crisp.

4 Split the bread rolls in half and spread the cut sides with the basil mayonnaise. Put a cooked salmon fillet on the bottom half of each roll and scatter over a few mixed salad leaves. Place the top half of each roll in place and serve immediately.

Another idea

For **grilled tuna baps** with tomato and ginger relish, use 4 fresh tuna steaks, about 85 g (3 oz) each, and marinate them in a mixture of 2 tsp finely chopped fresh rosemary, the juice of 1 orange, and salt and pepper to taste. Meanwhile, to make the relish, sauté 1 finely chopped small red onion, 1 crushed garlic clove and 1 tbsp finely chopped fresh root ginger in 1 tbsp extra virgin olive oil for 8–10 minutes or until softened. Remove from the heat and add 4 chopped plum tomatoes, 1–2 tbsp chopped fresh basil and salt and pepper to taste. Mix well. Grill the tuna for 3 minutes on each side or until cooked to your taste, then serve in wholemeal or Granary baps with salad leaves and the relish.

Plus points

• Combining mayonnaise with low-fat yogurt not only reduces total fat, it also increases the nutritional value of the dish, in particular adding calcium, phosphorus, and vitamins B_2 and B_{12}.

• Salad leaves such as rocket are useful sources of the B vitamin folate and of beta-carotene.

photo, page 45

Each serving provides   kcal 362, protein 26 g, fat 13 g (of which saturated fat 2.5 g), carbohydrate 36 g (of which sugars 4 g), fibre 3 g. Excellent source of vitamin B_{12}, vitamin E. Good source of niacin, selenium, vitamin B_6. Useful source of calcium, folate, potassium, vitamin A, vitamin B_1, zinc.

Smoked haddock and potato pie

Fish pie is usually popular with children, who may not otherwise be keen on fish. In this version, leek and watercress are added to boost the vitamin value, and sliced potato and cheese make an appealing topping. Try it with roasted tomatoes on the vine, cooked for about 15 minutes alongside the pie, and steamed broccoli.

Preparation time **40 minutes**   Cooking time **25–30 minutes**   *Serves 6*

750 ml (1¼ pints) plus 3 tbsp semi-skimmed milk

500 g (1 lb 2 oz) smoked haddock fillets

1 bay leaf

1 large leek, halved lengthways and sliced

550 g (1¼ lb) potatoes, peeled and cut into 5 mm (¼ in) thick slices

3 tbsp cornflour

85 g (3 oz) watercress, thick stalks removed

50 g (1¾ oz) mature Cheddar cheese, coarsely grated

salt and pepper

chopped parsley to garnish

1 Pour the 750 ml (1¼ pints) milk into a wide frying pan. Add the haddock and bay leaf. Bring to a gentle simmer, then cover and cook for about 5 minutes or until the haddock is just cooked.

2 Lift out the fish with a draining spoon and leave to cool slightly, then peel off the skin and break the flesh into large flakes. Set aside. Strain the milk and reserve 600 ml (1 pint), as well as the bay leaf.

3 Put the leek in the frying pan and add the reserved milk and bay leaf. Cover and simmer for 10 minutes or until the leek is tender.

4 Meanwhile, cook the potatoes in a saucepan of boiling water for about 8 minutes or until they are just tender but not breaking up. Drain. Preheat the oven to 190°C (375°F, gas mark 5).

5 Remove the bay leaf from the leeks and discard. Mix the cornflour with the remaining 3 tbsp cold milk to make a smooth paste. Add to the leek mixture and cook gently, stirring, until slightly thickened.

6 Take the pan from the heat and stir in the watercress, which will wilt. Season with salt and pepper to taste. Add the flaked haddock, folding it in gently. Transfer the mixture to a 2 litre (3½ pint) pie dish.

7 Arrange the potato slices on top of the fish mixture, overlapping them slightly. Sprinkle with the cheese, and season to taste. Bake for 25–30 minutes or until the fish filling is bubbling and the potatoes are turning golden.

8 Sprinkle the top of the pie with parsley and allow to stand for about 5 minutes before serving.

Some more ideas

Use 2 sliced leeks. Omit the watercress and instead, in step 4, add 125 g (4½ oz) baby spinach leaves to the potato slices for the last 1–2 minutes of their cooking time. Drain well. Make a layer of the potatoes and spinach on the bottom of the pie dish. Spoon the hot fish and leek sauce over the top, sprinkle with the cheese and grill under a moderate heat for 5–10 minutes or until bubbling and golden.

For a smoked haddock, pepper and fennel pie, cook 1 seeded and chopped red pepper, 1 small chopped onion and 2 chopped garlic cloves in 1 tbsp extra virgin olive oil in a large frying pan until the onion is soft. Add 250 g (8½ oz) thinly sliced bulb fennel and cook for a further 5 minutes, stirring occasionally. Stir in 1 can chopped tomatoes, about 400 g, with the juice, and season to taste. Cover and

Each serving provides   kcal 271, protein 25 g, fat 6 g (of which saturated fat 3 g), carbohydrate 32 g (of which sugars 7 g), fibre 2 g. Excellent source of iodine, vitamin B$_{12}$. Good source of calcium, niacin, potassium, selenium, vitamin B$_1$, vitamin B$_2$.

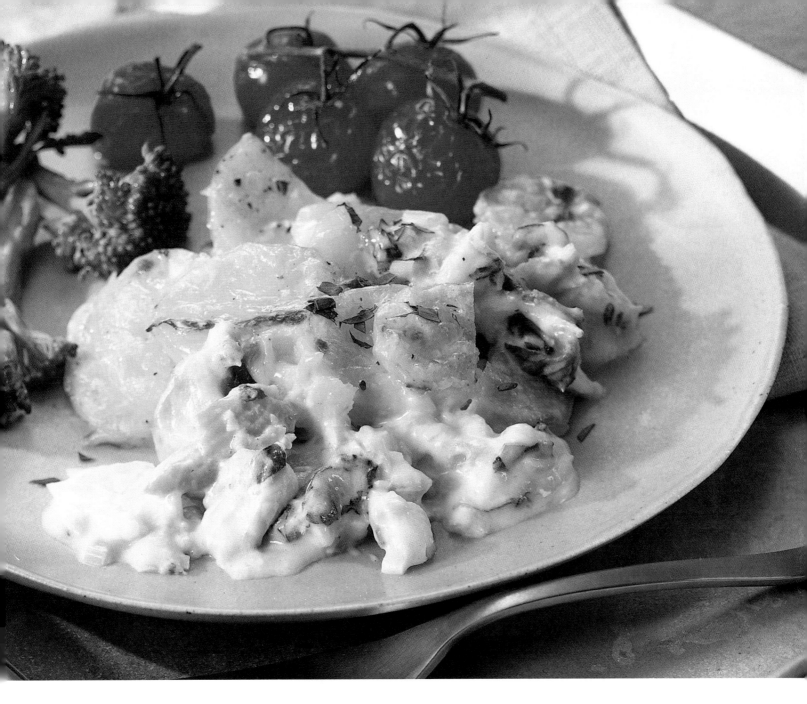

simmer for 25 minutes or until the fennel is tender. Meanwhile, cut the potatoes into chunks and cook for 10 minutes or until tender. Pour the pepper and fennel sauce into the pie dish. Lay the skinned haddock fillets on the top (cut to fit if necessary) and scatter over the drained potatoes. Sprinkle with ¼ tsp crushed dried chillies and 30 g (1 oz) freshly grated Parmesan cheese. Bake for about 20 minutes until golden.

Plus points

• Potatoes do not contain as much vitamin C as many other vegetables, but they are a valuable source of this vitamin because they are eaten so frequently and in such large amounts.

• Smoked haddock is an excellent source of iodine and provides useful amounts of vitamin B_6 and potassium. Undyed smoked haddock is now widely available as an alternative to the vibrant yellow-dyed version, which may cause a reaction in susceptible people. Beware of the sodium content and reduce added salt.

• Watercress, like other dark green leafy vegetables, is an excellent source of many of the antioxidant nutrients, including beta-carotene, vitamin C and vitamin E.

Monkfish and mussel kebabs

To create these succulent mini kebabs, marinated cubes of monkfish fillet and fresh mussels are threaded onto skewers with a selection of colourful vegetables, then lightly grilled. They make an extra special hot nibble to hand round at a celebration party or present on a buffet table.

Preparation time **20 minutes**   Marinating time **1 hour**   Cooking time **8–10 minutes**   *Makes 16 kebabs*

finely grated zest and juice of 1 lemon

juice of 1 lime

1 tbsp extra virgin olive oil

2 tsp clear honey

1 garlic clove, crushed

1 tbsp chopped fresh oregano or marjoram

1 tbsp chopped parsley

200 g (7 oz) monkfish fillet, cut into 16 small cubes

16 shelled fresh mussels, about 125 g (4¼ oz) in total

1 small yellow pepper, seeded and cut into 16 small chunks

1 courgette, cut into 16 thin slices

16 cherry tomatoes

salt and pepper

lime or lemon wedges to garnish

1 Put the lemon zest and juice, lime juice, oil, honey, garlic, chopped oregano or marjoram, parsley, and salt and pepper to taste in a shallow non-metallic dish. Whisk together, then add the monkfish cubes and mussels. Turn the seafood to coat all over with the marinade. Cover and marinate in the fridge for 1 hour.

2 Meanwhile, put 16 wooden skewers in warm water and leave to soak for 10 minutes. Drain. Preheat the grill to moderately high.

3 Onto each skewer, thread 1 cube of monkfish, 1 mussel, 1 piece of yellow pepper, 1 slice of courgette and a cherry tomato. (Reserve the marinade.) Leave the ends of the skewers empty so they will be easy to hold.

4 Place the kebabs on a rack in the grill pan and grill for 8–10 minutes or until the monkfish is cooked and the vegetables are just tender, turning occasionally and brushing frequently with the marinade. Serve hot, garnished with lime or lemon wedges.

Some more ideas

For **prawn and scallop kebabs**, use 16 raw peeled prawns and 16 shelled fresh queen scallops in place of the monkfish and mussels.

To make **tuna or swordfish kebabs**, cut 300 g (10½ oz) fresh tuna or swordfish fillet into 16 small cubes and marinate in a mixture of the finely grated zest and juice of 1 lime, 1 small crushed garlic clove, 1 tbsp extra virgin olive oil, 1 tsp Cajun seasoning, and salt and pepper to taste. Seed 1 red pepper and cut into 16 small chunks, and quarter 4 shallots or baby onions. Thread the marinated fish onto skewers with the prepared vegetables and 16 very small button mushrooms. Grill as in the main recipe.

Plus points

● Monkfish has a huge, ugly head, and only the tail is eaten. The firm flesh tastes rather like lobster. Monkfish is an excellent source of phosphorus and a useful source of potassium, which is vital to help regulate blood pressure.

● Mussels provide several minerals, in particular copper, iodine, iron and zinc. Mussels are also an extremely good source of vitamin B_{12}, needed for the maintenance of a healthy nervous system.

photo, page 53

Each serving provides (two kebabs) kcal 60, protein 6 g, fat 2 g (of which saturated fat 0.2 g), carbohydrate 4 g (of which sugars 4 g), fibre 1 g. Good source of vitamin B_{12}. Useful source of vitamin C, vitamin E.

Chicken and cashew pancakes

Chicken stir-fried with carrots, celery and cabbage, then lightly flavoured with orange and sesame, makes a delicious filling for pancakes. This dish is sure to meet with your family's approval.

Preparation time **15–20 minutes**   Cooking time **about 30 minutes**   *Serves 4*

115 g (4 oz) plain flour

1 egg, beaten

300 ml (10 fl oz) semi-skimmed milk

1 tsp sunflower oil

salt and pepper

Chicken and cashew nut filling

55 g (2 oz) cashew nuts

1 tbsp sunflower oil

300 g (10½ oz) skinless boneless chicken breasts (fillets), cut into strips

1 garlic clove, crushed

1 tsp finely chopped fresh root ginger

1 fresh red chilli, seeded and finely chopped (optional)

2 carrots, cut into thin sticks

2 celery sticks, cut into thin sticks

grated zest of ½ orange

200 g (7 oz) Savoy cabbage, shredded

1 tbsp light soy sauce, plus extra for serving

1 tsp toasted sesame oil

1 To make the pancakes, sift the flour into a bowl and add a little salt and pepper to taste. Make a well in the centre. Mix the egg with the milk, then pour into the well. Gradually whisk the flour into the egg and milk to form a smooth batter.

2 Use a little of the oil to lightly grease a 20 cm (8 in) non-stick pancake pan, and place it on a moderate heat. Pour in a little of the batter and swirl it evenly across the surface, then cook for 2 minutes to form a pancake. Toss the pancake or flip it over with a palette knife and cook on the other side for about 30 seconds. Slide out onto a warm heatproof plate and cover with a sheet of greaseproof paper.

3 Cook the remaining batter in the same way, making 8 pancakes in all and stacking them up, interleaved with greaseproof paper. Grease the pan with more oil between pancakes as necessary. When all the pancakes have been made, cover the pancake stack with foil, sealing it well. Place the plate over a pan of gently simmering water to keep the pancakes warm while you prepare the filling.

4 Heat a wok or large frying pan. Add the cashew nuts and stir-fry them over a moderate heat for a few minutes or until golden. Remove to a plate and set aside.

5 Add the oil to the wok or frying pan and swirl it around, then add the chicken, garlic, ginger and chilli, if using. Stir-fry for 3 minutes.

6 Add the carrot and celery sticks, and stir-fry for a further 2 minutes. Add the orange zest and cabbage, and stir-fry for 1 minute. Sprinkle over the soy sauce and sesame oil, and stir-fry for another minute. Return the cashews to the pan and toss to mix with the other ingredients.

7 Divide the stir-fry filling among the warm pancakes and fold them over or roll up. Serve immediately, with a little extra soy sauce to sprinkle.

Plus points

• Cashew nuts are a rich source of protein, fibre, and minerals such as iron, magnesium and selenium. Cashews are high in fat, but the majority of it is the 'healthy' mono-unsaturated type.

• Stir-frying is a healthy way to cook, because only a little oil is needed, and cooking is done quickly over quite a high heat so that the maximum amount of nutrients in the vegetables is retained.

photo, page 53

Each serving provides kcal 384, protein 29 g, fat 15 g (of which saturated fat 3 g), carbohydrate 35 g (of which sugars 10 g), fibre 4 g. Excellent source of niacin, vitamin A, vitamin E. Good source of calcium, copper, folate, potassium, selenium, vitamin B$_1$, vitamin B$_6$, vitamin C, zinc.

Chicken jamboree

This healthy chicken and vegetable casserole makes an easy mid-week meal. To make it even quicker, you could use supermarket washed-and-cut carrots and broccoli, ready to go from packet to pan. Mixed wild and long-grain rice goes well with the casserole, and adds sustaining and nourishing carbohydrate.

Preparation time **10 minutes**   Cooking time **about 20 minutes**   *Serves 4*

2 tbsp extra virgin olive oil

350 g (12½ oz) skinless boneless chicken breasts (fillets), cut into small cubes

1 small onion, chopped

225 g (8 oz) button mushrooms

1 bay leaf

2 large sprigs of fresh thyme or ½ tsp dried thyme

3 large sprigs of fresh tarragon or ½ tsp dried tarragon (optional)

grated zest of 1 small lemon or ½ large lemon

150 ml (5 fl oz) dry sherry

300 ml (10 fl oz) boiling water

225 g (8 oz) baby carrots

225 g (8 oz) broccoli florets

1 tbsp cornflour

3 tbsp chopped parsley

salt and pepper

1 Heat the oil in a large sauté pan with a lid or fairly deep frying pan. Add the chicken and brown the pieces over a high heat for 3 minutes, stirring constantly. Reduce the heat to moderate. Stir in the onion, mushrooms, bay leaf, thyme, tarragon if used and lemon zest. Cook for 4 minutes or until the onion and mushrooms are beginning to soften.

2 Pour in the sherry and water. Add the carrots and seasoning to taste, and stir to mix all the ingredients. Bring to the boil, then reduce the heat and cover the pan. Simmer for 5 minutes.

3 Stir in the broccoli florets. Increase the heat to bring the liquid back to a steady simmer. Cover the pan and cook for 5 minutes or until the pieces of chicken are tender and the vegetables are just cooked. Remove and discard the bay leaf, and the sprigs of thyme and tarragon, if used.

4 Blend the cornflour to a smooth paste with 2 tbsp cold water. Stir the cornflour paste into the casserole and simmer for 2 minutes, stirring constantly, until thickened and smooth. Check the seasoning, then stir in the parsley and serve.

Some more ideas

Instead of cornflour, use 1 tbsp of semolina or fine oatmeal. Use the oatmeal as for the cornflour; sprinkle the semolina into the casserole, stirring, and continue stirring until the sauce boils and thickens.

Small patty pan squash are good in this casserole. Trim off and discard the stalk ends from 225 g (8 oz) squash and slice them horizontally in half. Add them to the pan with the broccoli. When cooked, the patty pan should be tender but still slightly crunchy.

Plus points

• Broccoli and related cruciferous vegetables (such as cabbage and cauliflower) contain several potent phytochemicals that help to protect against cancer. Broccoli is also an excellent source of the antioxidants vitamins C and E and beta-carotene. It provides good amounts of the B vitamins B_6 and niacin, and useful amounts of folate.

• This recipe uses vegetables to extend a modest amount of chicken. Served with a starchy (complex) carbohydrate, such as rice, it makes a well-balanced meal, especially if followed by fresh fruit for a vitamin boost.

Each serving provides   kcal 260, protein 23 g, fat 10 g (of which saturated fat 2 g), carbohydrate 11 g (of which sugars 6 g), fibre 4 g. Good source of vitamin B_6, vitamin C. Useful source of folate, niacin, selenium.

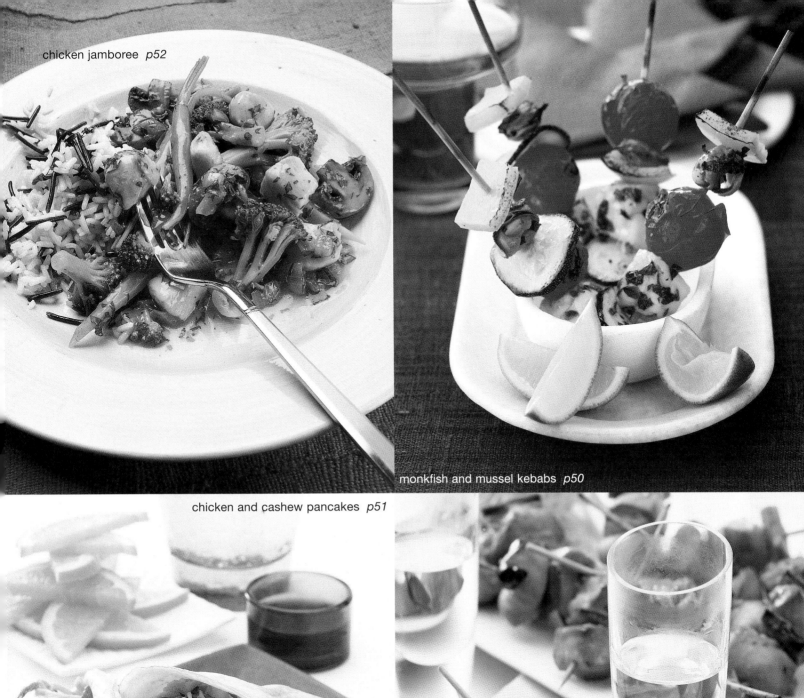

chicken jamboree *p52*

monkfish and mussel kebabs *p50*

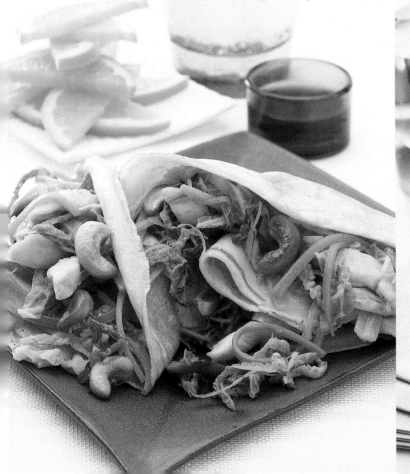

chicken and cashew pancakes *p51*

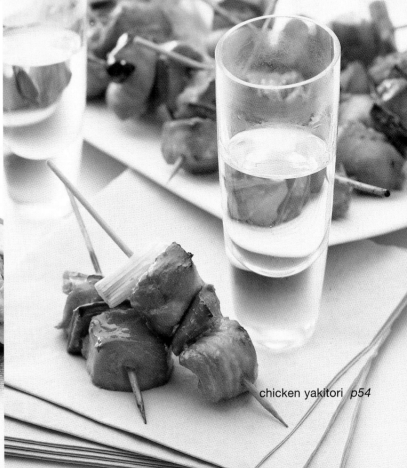

chicken yakitori *p54*

Chicken yakitori

These delicious Japanese-style bites of chicken speared with green pepper and spring onions can be assembled in advance and then grilled just before serving. For the best flavour, leave the chicken to marinate for several hours or overnight, and remember to soak the skewers first so they do not burn under the grill.

Preparation time **20 minutes, plus at least 1 hour marinating**   Cooking time **10–15 minutes**   *Makes 30 kebabs*

3 tbsp shoyu (Japanese soy sauce)

3 tbsp sake or dry sherry

1 tbsp toasted sesame oil

1 garlic clove, crushed

1 tbsp finely chopped fresh root ginger

2 tsp clear honey

500 g (1 lb 2 oz) skinless boneless chicken breasts (fillets), cut into 2 cm (¾ in) cubes

1 large green pepper, seeded and cut into 30 small cubes

4 large spring onions, cut across into 30 pieces

1 Place the shoyu, sake or sherry, sesame oil, garlic, ginger and honey in a shallow dish and stir together to mix. Add the chicken pieces and spoon the marinade over them. Cover and marinate in the fridge for at least 1 hour or overnight.

2 Just before cooking, put 30 short wooden skewers in warm water and leave to soak for 10 minutes. Preheat the grill to moderate.

3 Thread about 2 pieces of chicken onto each skewer, alternating with a piece of pepper and one of spring onion, threaded widthways. Place the kebabs on the grill pan and cook under the grill for 10–15 minutes or until tender, turning from time to time and brushing with the marinade. Serve hot.

Some more ideas

Sprinkle the kebabs with a few sesame seeds towards the end of the grilling time.

An alternative marinade is 3 tbsp hoisin sauce mixed with 2 tbsp Chinese rice wine or dry sherry and 1 tbsp groundnut oil. If liked, add ½ tsp five-spice powder or ½ finely chopped and seeded fresh red chilli.

Instead of green pepper, use pieces of baby leeks, red or orange peppers, courgette or tiny mushroom caps.

For salmon yakitori, use 500 g (1 lb 2 oz) skinless salmon fillet and marinate in a mixture of 3 tbsp shoyu or other soy sauce, 2 tbsp dry sherry, 1 tbsp groundnut oil, 1 crushed garlic clove, 1 tsp clear honey and the grated zest of 1 small orange for about 30 minutes. Thread onto soaked wooden skewers, alternating the cubes of salmon with whole firm cherry tomatoes and pieces of spring onion. Grill for 10–15 minutes, turning and basting frequently with the marinade.

Plus points

• Many party food nibbles are made with pastry and are high in fat and calories. These little kebabs, made with lean chicken and vegetables, offer a lower-fat choice and look really appealing.

• Honey has been used since ancient times as a sweetener and preservative. It has a higher fructose content than sugar, which makes it sweeter, and it is also lower in calories on a weight for weight basis because of its higher water content.

photo, page 53

Each serving provides   (one skewer) kcal 25, protein 4 g, fat 0.5 g (of which saturated fat 0.1 g), carbohydrate 1 g (of which sugars 0.5 g), fibre 0.1 g. Useful source of niacin, vitamin C.

Chinese-style lemon chicken

A savoury lemon sauce seasoned with a hint of sesame tastes fabulous with tender chicken and crunchy Oriental vegetables. Serve plain egg noodles or rice to add some satisfying starchy carbohydrate.

Preparation time **25 minutes**   Cooking time **about 25 minutes**   *Serves 4*

1 tbsp sunflower oil

425 g (15 oz) skinless, boneless chicken breasts (fillets), sliced

1 onion, halved and thinly sliced

1 large green pepper, seeded and cut into thin strips

1 garlic clove, chopped

1 tbsp finely chopped fresh root ginger

2 large carrots, thinly sliced at a slant

1 can water chestnuts, about 220 g, drained and sliced

300 ml (10 fl oz) chicken stock, preferably home-made (see page 212)

3 tbsp dry sherry

2 tbsp cornflour

2 tsp caster sugar

3 tbsp light soy sauce

1 tbsp toasted sesame oil

grated zest of 2 large lemons

juice of 1 lemon

150 g (5½ oz) fine green beans, cut into 5 cm (2 in) lengths

225 g (8 oz) bean sprouts

1 Heat the sunflower oil in a flameproof casserole. Add the chicken and cook for about 1 minute or until the meat is just turning white. Add the onion, pepper, garlic and ginger, and cook over a moderate heat, stirring often, for 5–6 minutes or until the onion is softened but not browned.

2 Add the carrots and water chestnuts. Pour in the stock and sherry, then heat until simmering, but not boiling rapidly. Cover and simmer for 10 minutes, stirring occasionally.

3 Meanwhile, mix the cornflour and sugar to a smooth paste with the soy sauce, sesame oil and lemon zest and juice. Stir the cornflour mixture into the casserole and bring to the boil, still stirring. Add the green beans, cover the casserole and simmer gently for 2 minutes. Stir in the bean sprouts and simmer for a final 2 minutes. Serve the casserole at once, before the bean sprouts soften.

Some more ideas

Fresh shiitake mushrooms are good in this casserole – add 100 g (3½ oz) sliced shiitake with the green beans so that they will be just lightly cooked.

Try 200 g (7 oz) baby corn instead of the water chestnuts and 200 g (7 oz) baby pak choy instead of the bean sprouts. A little chilli spice is good with this vegetable mix, so add 1 seeded and chopped fresh green chilli with the vegetables in step 1.

This is a good recipe for firm meaty fish, such as swordfish. Cut the fish into chunks and add to the casserole in step 2, with the carrots and water chestnuts.

Plus points

● Bean sprouts and other sprouted beans and seeds are rich in vitamins B and C.

● Canned water chestnuts are light and crunchy. Mixed with other vegetables, they can help to extend a modest amount of chicken or meat to make a satisfying meal. They also contribute small amounts of phosphorous and potassium.

photo, page 57

Each serving provides   kcal 320, protein 27 g, fat 12 g (of which saturated fat 2.5 g), carbohydrate 24 g (of which sugars 15 g), fibre 4 g. Excellent source of vitamin C. Good source of iron, vitamin A, vitamin B_6. Useful source of folate, niacin, selenium, zinc.

Chorizo, grilled pepper and tomato bruschetta

This open sandwich of toasted ciabatta bread with a mixed pepper topping is typical of the style of food enjoyed in Mediterranean countries, where bread, along with plenty of fruit and vegetables, is a mainstay of the diet. A little chorizo sausage adds a spicy note to the sweet pepper mix.

Preparation and cooking time **about 30 minutes**   *Serves 6*

1 part-baked ciabatta loaf, about 250 g (8½ oz)

1 red pepper, halved and seeded

1 yellow pepper, halved and seeded

55 g (2 oz) chorizo sausage, thinly sliced

170 g (6 oz) cherry tomatoes, quartered

2 tbsp tomato relish or chutney

15 g (½ oz) fresh basil leaves, roughly torn

1 tbsp extra virgin olive oil

1 garlic clove, crushed

black pepper

1 Preheat the oven to 200°C (400°F, gas mark 6). Bake the ciabatta for 8–10 minutes or according to the instructions on the packet. Remove from the oven and place on a wire rack to cool. Preheat the grill to high.

2 When the grill is hot, place the peppers skin side up on a baking tray and grill for 8–10 minutes or until the flesh softens and the skin begins to blister and char. Transfer the peppers to a polythene bag, seal with a tie and set aside until cool enough to handle.

3 While the peppers are cooling, cook the chorizo sausage in a frying pan for 3–4 minutes or until the oil runs out and the sausage slices start to crisp. Drain on kitchen paper.

4 Place the chorizo in a bowl and add the tomatoes, relish or chutney and basil. Remove the cooled peppers from the bag and peel away their skins. Roughly chop the flesh and add to the bowl. Season with pepper to taste and mix well. Set aside while you prepare the toasts.

5 Preheat the grill to high again. Cut the baked ciabatta across into 3 pieces, then cut each piece in half horizontally. Mix the olive oil with the garlic and brush this mixture onto the cut sides of the ciabatta

pieces. Place them cut side up under the hot grill and toast for 2–3 minutes or until golden and crisp.

6 Top the toasted ciabatta with the pepper and chorizo mixture and serve immediately.

Some more ideas

Use French bread instead of ciabatta.

For a vegetarian topping, omit the chorizo and sprinkle the pepper and tomato mixture with 30 g (1 oz) toasted pine nuts. Or, replace the chorizo with 115 g (4 oz) crumbled feta or goat's cheese.

Plus points

● Like all breads, ciabatta is a good source of starchy carbohydrates and B vitamins. It is sometimes called 'slipper bread' because of its shape.

● Chorizo is a popular Spanish sausage made with pork and pimiento, a Spanish pepper. Chorizo has a high fat content, but this can be substantially reduced by frying the sausage in a dry pan and draining it well.

Each serving provides kcal 188, protein 7 g, fat 6 g (of which saturated fat 1.5 g), carbohydrate 28 g (of which sugars 8 g), fibre 2 g. Excellent source of vitamin C. Good source of vitamin A, vitamin E.

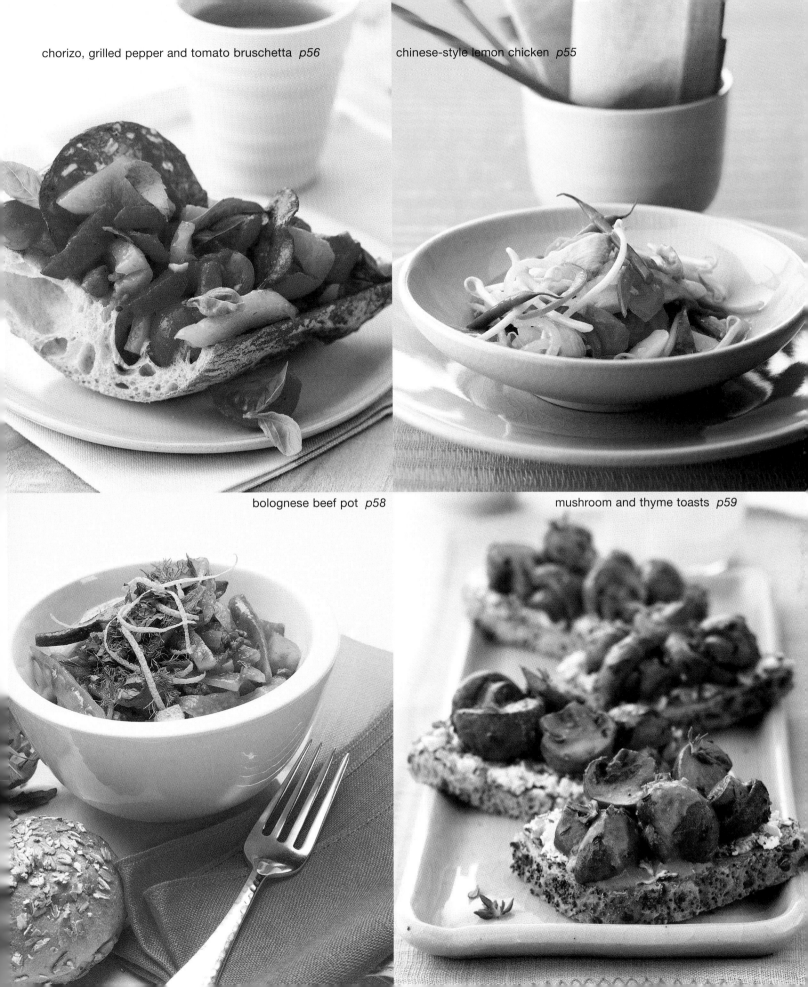

chorizo, grilled pepper and tomato bruschetta *p56*

chinese-style lemon chicken *p55*

bolognese beef pot *p58*

mushroom and thyme toasts *p59*

Bolognese beef pot

Lemon and fennel bring wonderfully fresh flavours to familiar braised minced beef in this Italian-inspired dish, making this as good for al fresco summer dining as for a light supper on a winter evening. Serve plenty of bread or rolls to mop up the deliciously tangy tomato sauce, plus a crisp leafy salad.

Preparation time **10 minutes**   Cooking time **20 minutes**   *Serves 4*

340 g (12 oz) extra lean minced beef

1 onion, chopped

2 garlic cloves, crushed

600 g (1 lb 5 oz) potatoes, scrubbed and finely diced

2 cans chopped tomatoes, about 400 g each

150 ml (5 fl oz) chicken stock, bought chilled or made from a cube

finely shredded zest and juice of 1 lemon

1 tbsp soft light brown sugar

1 bulb of fennel, thinly sliced

100 g (3½ oz) frozen green beans

salt and pepper

To garnish

chopped leaves reserved from the fennel bulb

chopped fresh flat-leaf parsley

1 Place the minced beef, onion and garlic in a large saucepan and cook over a moderate heat for 5 minutes, stirring frequently, until the mince is broken up and evenly browned.

2 Stir in the potatoes, tomatoes with their juice, stock, half the lemon zest, the sugar and a little seasoning. Bring to the boil, then reduce the heat and cover the pan. Simmer for 10 minutes, stirring once or twice to ensure that the potatoes cook evenly.

3 Stir in the fennel, frozen beans and lemon juice. Cover the pan again and simmer for a further 5 minutes or until the potatoes are tender and the fennel and beans are lightly cooked, but still crisp.

4 Taste and adjust the seasoning, if necessary, then spoon the mixture into serving bowls. Garnish with the remaining lemon zest, the chopped fennel leaves and flat-leaf parsley.

Some more ideas

Carrots and canned beans can be used instead of potatoes. Add 1 can cannellini or black-eyed beans, about 400 g, drained and rinsed, and 250 g (8½ oz) finely diced carrots.

Use minced turkey, chicken, pork or lamb instead of beef.

If serving this dish to young children, do not add the lemon juice. Instead, serve with lemon wedges so the juice can be added to suit their taste.

Plus points

● Extra lean minced beef contains 9.6 g fat per 100 g (3½ oz). Provided you use a heavy-based or good-quality non-stick pan, there is no need to add any fat when browning minced meat.

● Tomatoes are a rich source of vitamin C – fresh raw tomatoes contain 17 mg per 100 g (3½ oz) and canned tomatoes about 12 mg.

● Scrubbing potatoes rather than peeling them retains vitamins and minerals found just beneath the skin. The skin also provides valuable fibre.

● Frozen green beans are convenient and versatile for everyday dishes. They are a useful source of fibre and a good source of folate, which is essential for a healthy pregnancy. Folate may also contribute to protection against heart disease.

photo, page 57

Each serving provides   kcal 300, protein 26 g, fat 5 g (of which saturated fat 2 g), carbohydrate 40 g (of which sugars 14 g), fibre 5 g. Excellent source of vitamin B_6, vitamin B_{12}, vitamin C. Good source of folate, iron. Useful source of niacin, potassium, selenium, vitamin B_1.

Mushroom and thyme toasts

Make this whenever you are short of time and want to prepare a satisfying snack quickly. The rich flavour of chestnut mushrooms is enhanced by cooking them with garlic, herbs and a dollop of tangy crème fraîche, and they taste wonderful piled on top of toast spread with low-fat soft cheese.

Preparation and cooking time **25 minutes**   *Serves 4*

125 g (4½ oz) low-fat soft cheese

2 celery sticks, finely chopped

3 tbsp finely chopped parsley

good pinch of cayenne pepper

500 g (1 lb 2 oz) chestnut mushrooms

1 garlic clove, crushed

2 tbsp chopped fresh thyme

2 tbsp half-fat crème fraîche

1 tsp lemon juice

8 thick slices cut from a small loaf of mixed seed bread, about 400 g (14 oz) in total

salt and pepper

1 Put the ricotta, celery, parsley and cayenne pepper in a bowl and mix well together. Set aside in a cool place until needed. Preheat the grill to high.

2 Leave any small mushrooms whole and halve larger ones. Place them in a large, heavy frying pan, preferably non-stick, and add the garlic, thyme, crème fraîche and 1 tsp water. Cover and cook gently for 3–4 minutes or until the mushrooms are just tender and have given up their juices. Add the lemon juice and salt and pepper to taste.

3 While the mushrooms are cooking, toast the bread slices on both sides under the grill. While still warm, spread one side of each piece of toast with some of the soft cheese mixture, then cut it in half.

4 Arrange the toasts on individual serving plates. Spoon the hot mushroom mixture over the toasts and serve immediately.

Another idea

To make devilled mushroom toasts, heat 1 tbsp extra virgin olive oil in a non-stick frying pan, add 1 thinly sliced onion and cook over a moderate heat until softened. Stir in 1 crushed garlic clove, 500 g (1 lb 2 oz) halved chestnut mushrooms and 1 seeded and diced red pepper. Cook, stirring frequently, for 2 minutes, then stir in 1 tbsp Worcestershire sauce, 1 tsp Dijon mustard and 1 tsp dark muscovado sugar. Reduce the heat and cook gently for 5 minutes, stirring occasionally. Add 2 tbsp chopped parsley and season with salt and pepper to taste. Toast the bread and spread with 75 g (3 oz) soft goat's cheese. Spoon the hot devilled mushroom mixture over the toasts and serve immediately.

Plus points

• Though there are more than 2,500 varieties of mushrooms grown throughout the world, not all are edible – indeed some are positively poisonous. Chestnut mushrooms tend to be larger, firmer, browner and stronger in flavour than most cultivated mushrooms. All edible mushrooms are a useful source of several B vitamins.

• Like other cheeses, soft cheese such as ricotta is a good source of protein and calcium. Because of its high moisture content, it is lower in fat than many other varieties of soft cheese.

photo, page 57

Each serving provides kcal 310, protein 15 g, fat 11 g (of which saturated fat 5.5 g), carbohydrate 44 g (of which sugars 3 g), fibre 5 g. Excellent source of copper, selenium. Good source of calcium, iron, niacin, vitamin A, vitamin B$_1$, zinc. Useful source of folate, potassium, vitamin B$_2$, vitamin B$_6$, vitamin E.

Pea curry with Indian paneer

Paneer is an Indian cheese, similar to ricotta but drier. It's often combined with peas in a curry. This delicious version uses home-made paneer, which is simple to make. Serve with basmati rice for a well-balanced meal.

Preparation time **15 minutes, plus about 45 minutes draining, 3 hours pressing**
Cooking time **about 20 minutes**   *Serves 4*

Paneer

2.3 litres (4 pints) whole milk

6 tbsp lemon juice

Pea and tomato curry

2 tbsp rapeseed oil

1 large onion, chopped

2 garlic cloves, finely chopped

5 cm (2 in) piece fresh root ginger, finely chopped

1 fresh green chilli, seeded and thinly sliced

1 tbsp coriander seeds, crushed

1 tbsp cumin seeds, crushed

1 tsp turmeric

1 tbsp garam masala

450 g (1 lb) firm tomatoes, quartered

340 g (12 oz) frozen peas

85 g (3 oz) spinach leaves

15 g (½ oz) fresh coriander, roughly chopped

salt

1 First make the paneer. Heat the milk in a large saucepan and bring to the boil. Immediately reduce the heat to low and add the lemon juice. Stir for 1–2 minutes or until the milk separates into curds and whey. Remove the pan from the heat.

2 Line a large sieve or colander with muslin, or a clean, tight-knit dishcloth, and set over a large bowl. Pour in the milk mixture. Leave to drain for 15 minutes or until cool.

3 Bring together the corners of the muslin or cloth to make a bundle containing the drained curds. Squeeze them, then leave to drain for a further 30 minutes or until all the whey has dripped though the sieve into the bowl. Reserve 240 ml (8 fl oz) of the whey.

4 Keeping the curds wrapped in the muslin or cloth, place on a board. Set another board on top and press down to flatten the ball shape into an oblong block. Place cans or weights on top and leave in a cool place for about 3 hours or until firm.

5 Carefully peel off the muslin and cut the cheese into squares about 2 cm (¾ in). Heat 1 tbsp of the oil in a large non-stick frying pan and cook the paneer for 1–2 minutes on each side or until golden. As

the pieces are browned, remove from the pan with a draining spoon and set aside.

6 For the curry, heat the remaining 1 tbsp oil in the pan. Add the onion and cook gently for 5 minutes or until softened. Stir in the garlic and ginger, and cook gently for 1 minute, then stir in the chilli, coriander and cumin seeds, turmeric and garam masala. Cook for 1 more minute, stirring constantly. (Add a little hot water if the mixture begins to stick.)

7 Add the tomatoes, the reserved whey and a pinch of salt, and stir well to mix. Cover and cook gently for 5 minutes.

8 Add the peas and bring back to the boil, then reduce the heat, cover again and simmer for 5 minutes. Add the spinach, stirring it in gently so as not to break up the tomatoes too much. Simmer for 3–4 minutes or until the spinach has just wilted and the peas are hot and tender.

9 Stir in most of the chopped fresh coriander, then transfer the curry to a serving dish and scatter the paneer on top. Spoon the curry gently over the paneer to warm it, then sprinkle with the rest of the coriander and serve.

Each serving provides kcal 275, protein 20 g, fat 12 g (of which saturated fat 4.5 g), carbohydrated 22 g (of which sugars 14 g), fibre 7 g. Excellent source of vitamin A, vitamin C, vitamin E. Good source of calcium, folate, niacin, vitamin B_1, vitamin B_{12}, zinc. Useful source of copper, iron, potassium, vitamin B_2, vitamin B_6.

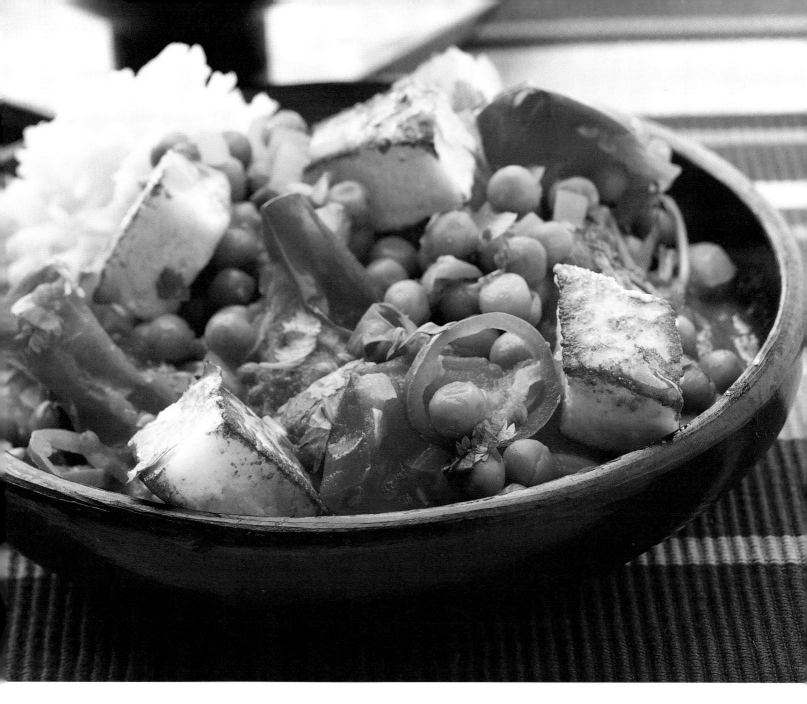

Some more ideas

For a **cottage cheese and vegetable curry**, which is similar but much quicker to make, cook 600 g (1 lb 5 oz) peeled potatoes, cut into large chunks, in a large pan of boiling water for 5 minutes. Add 400 g (14 oz) cauliflower florets and cook for a further 5 minutes. Add 200 g (7 oz) halved fine green beans and cook for a further 3–4 minutes or until all the vegetables are tender. Meanwhile, place 350 g (12½ oz) cottage cheese in a sieve and leave to drain. Cook the onion and spices as in step 6 of the main recipe, then add 300 ml (10 fl oz) vegetable stock and cook gently for a further 5 minutes. Add the drained potatoes, cauliflower and beans to the spiced sauce and stir to coat. Season with salt to taste. Fold in the cottage cheese and heat through gently. Serve hot, with wholewheat parathas or naan bread.

Plus point

● This home-made paneer is lower in fat than bought paneer and very nutritious, providing protein, calcium and vitamins, including vitamins A and D.

Pears grilled with pecorino

Many cuisines have long traditions of combining fruit with cheese. This recipe stems from the Tuscan combination of juicy pears with salty ewe's milk pecorino. With some of the cheese melted over the pears and the rest combined with cool grapes and salad leaves, this makes a stylish first course, or light main dish for two.

Preparation time **15 minutes**   Cooking time **about 2 minutes**   *Serves 4*

55 g (2 oz) pecorino cheese

1 bunch of watercress, about 55 g (2 oz), leaves removed from stalks

115 g (4 oz) rocket leaves

55 g (2 oz) seedless green grapes, halved

2 dessert pears

Balsamic vinaigrette

2 tbsp extra virgin olive oil

1 tbsp best-quality balsamic vinegar

½ tsp Dijon mustard

pinch of caster sugar

salt and pepper

1 First make the dressing. Put the olive oil, balsamic vinegar, mustard, sugar, and salt and pepper to taste into a small screw-top jar. Screw on the lid and shake all the ingredients together until well blended. Keep the dressing in the fridge until needed.

2 Preheat the grill to high. Place a strip of cooking foil on a baking tray and set aside.

3 Using a vegetable peeler, peel the pecorino cheese into fine shavings. Reserve half of these and finely chop the remainder. Put the watercress, rocket leaves and grapes into a salad bowl and toss together.

4 Peel, halve and core the pears. Arrange the pear halves, cut sides down, on the foil strip. Top the pears with the shavings of cheese, slightly overlapping them. Place under the grill, about 15 cm (6 in) from the heat, and grill for 2 minutes or until the cheese just starts to bubble and turn golden.

5 Meanwhile, shake the dressing, pour it over the salad and toss to coat the leaves. Add the chopped pecorino. Divide the salad equally among 4 plates.

6 Using a fish slice, carefully transfer one pear half to each plate, placing it on top of the bed of dressed salad. Serve at once.

Some more ideas

Use diced kiwi fruit instead of grapes.

Parmesan cheese, another Italian firm cheese, is suitable for this recipe and it has less fat.

If you are in a hurry, just chop the pears and toss them in the salad with all the cheese.

Substitute baby spinach leaves for the rocket.

Grill the pear halves cut side up, then sprinkle a blue cheese, such as Shropshire blue, into the cavities and grill until it melts.

A creamy goat's cheese could be used in a fruit and cheese salad instead of high-fat pecorino. Goat's cheese has a natural affinity with fresh raspberries, so for a stylish first course, omit the pears and pecorino cheese from the recipe above and replace the balsamic vinegar in the vinaigrette with raspberry vinegar. Toss 200 g (7 oz) raspberries with the salad. Toast 8 thin slices of baguette on one side under the grill, then turn over and top with slices of goat's cheese. Grill until the cheese is bubbling, then transfer 2 slices to each plate. Dress the salad and arrange next to the cheese-topped toasts.

Each serving provides   kcal 130, protein 4 g, fat 9 g (of which saturated fat 3 g), carbohydrate 9g (of which sugars 9 g), fibre 2 g. Good source of vitamin C. Useful source of calcium, folate, vitamin A, vitamin B$_{12}$.

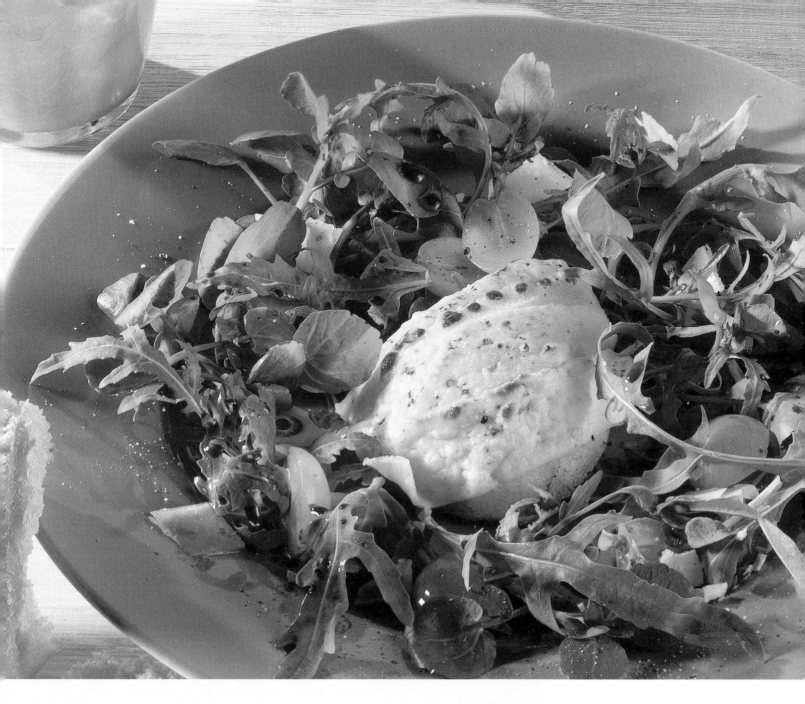

Plus point

* This salad is a useful source of calcium, needed for healthy bones and teeth. The pecorino cheese, watercress and rocket all provide this vital mineral.

Potato and courgette tortilla

Tortilla, Spain's most famous tapa or snack, is made from the simplest of ingredients – eggs, onions and potatoes – cooked like a flat omelette and served warm or cold, cut into wedges. All kinds of extra ingredients can be added, such as the courgette and bacon used here, or asparagus, peas and mushrooms.

Preparation time **15 minutes, plus cooling**   Cooking time **about 15 minutes**   *Serves 8*

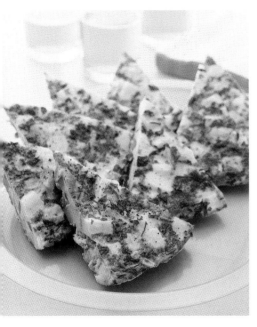

600 g (1 lb 5 oz) waxy potatoes, peeled and cut into 1 cm (½ in) cubes

2 tbsp extra virgin olive oil

1 red onion, finely chopped

1 courgette, about 150 g (5½ oz), diced

2 rashers lean back bacon, derinded and chopped

6 eggs

2 tbsp chopped parsley

pepper

1 Add the potato cubes to a saucepan of boiling water. Bring back to the boil, then lower the heat slightly and cook for 3 minutes. Drain thoroughly.

2 Heat the oil in a heavy-based non-stick frying pan that is about 25 cm (10 in) in diameter. Add the potatoes, onion, courgette and bacon, and cook over a moderate heat for 10 minutes, turning and stirring from time to time, until the potatoes are tender and lightly golden.

3 Preheat the grill to high. In a bowl, beat the eggs with 1 tbsp cold water. Add the parsley and pepper to taste. Pour the egg mixture over the vegetables in the frying pan and cook for 3–4 minutes or until the egg has set on the base, lifting the edges to allow the uncooked egg mixture to run onto the pan.

4 When there is just a little uncooked egg on the top, place the pan under the hot grill and cook for a further 2 minutes to set the top. Slide the tortilla out onto a plate or board and allow to cool for 2–3 minutes. Cut into small wedges or other shapes and serve warm, or leave to cool completely before cutting and serving.

Some more ideas

Instead of courgette, try chopped asparagus, or add chopped tomatoes or cooked peas just before pouring in the eggs. Fresh tarragon, chives or basil can be used in place of parsley.

Make a **potato, mushroom and Parmesan cheese tortilla**. Replace the onion, courgette and bacon with 200 g (7 oz) thinly sliced mushrooms and 1 sliced leek, about 200 g (7 oz). In step 2, cook the potatoes with the leek for 6 minutes, then add the mushrooms and cook for a further 4 minutes or until all the juices from the mushrooms have evaporated. Add 45 g (1½ oz) freshly grated Parmesan cheese to the beaten eggs before pouring them into the pan.

Plus points

• Eggs provide inexpensive protein. Though they contain cholesterol, the health risks this might pose have often been over-stressed. For most people, dietary cholesterol does not raise blood cholesterol levels.

• Courgettes are a good source of vitamin B_6 and niacin. The skins contain the greatest concentration of these vitamins.

Each serving provides   kcal 165, protein 9 g, fat 8 g (of which saturated fat 2 g), carbohydrate 14 g (of which sugars 1 g), fibre 1 g. Good source of vitamin B_{12}. Useful source of copper, folate, niacin, potassium, selenium, vitamin A, vitamin B_1, vitamin B_2, vitamin B_6, zinc.

Spiced couscous tomatoes

Choose ripe, well-flavoured tomatoes for this dish. Hollowed out, they make the perfect container for a spicy aubergine, dried apricot and nut couscous. The vitamin C-rich juices are squeezed out of the scooped-out tomato flesh and seeds, and whisked with a little harissa paste to make a tangy dressing. Serve with sesame breadsticks.

Preparation and cooking time **25 minutes**   *Serves 4*

8 large beefsteak tomatoes, about 170 g (6 oz) each

1½ tbsp extra virgin olive oil

55 g (2 oz) flaked almonds

1 small aubergine, about 170 g (6 oz), cut into 1 cm (½ in) dice

1 tsp ground coriander

½ tsp ground cumin

pinch of ground cinnamon

240 ml (8 fl oz) boiling vegetable stock

125 g (4½ oz) couscous

2 tbsp chopped fresh mint

55 g (2 oz) ready-to-eat dried apricots, chopped

1 tsp harissa paste

salt and pepper

1 Cut the tops off the tomatoes and scoop out the insides using a teaspoon. Place the hollowed-out tomatoes and cut-off tops on one side. Put the seeds and scooped-out flesh in a sieve set over a small jug or bowl and press with the back of a spoon to extract the juices; you will need about 4 tbsp. Leave the jug of juice on one side and discard the seeds and flesh.

2 Sprinkle a little salt over the insides of the hollowed-out tomatoes. Place them upside-down on a plate covered with kitchen paper and leave to drain while making the filling.

3 Heat ½ tbsp of the olive oil in a non-stick saucepan. Add the flaked almonds and cook over a low heat for 2–3 minutes or until golden brown. Remove from the pan with a draining spoon and set aside.

4 Add the remaining 1 tbsp oil to the saucepan. Stir in the aubergine and cook for 5 minutes, turning frequently, until browned and tender. Stir in the coriander, cumin and cinnamon, and cook for a few more seconds, stirring continuously.

5 Pour in the stock and bring to a rapid boil, then add the couscous in a steady stream, stirring constantly. Remove from the heat, cover and leave to stand for 5 minutes.

6 Uncover the pan, return to a low heat and cook for 2–3 minutes, stirring with a fork to separate the couscous grains and fluff them up. Stir in the toasted almonds, mint and dried apricots.

7 Add the harissa paste to the reserved tomato juices and stir to mix, then pour over the couscous. Season with pepper and mix well. Spoon the couscous mixture into the tomatoes, replace the tops and serve.

Another idea
Dried peaches and hazelnuts or pine nuts can be used in place of the dried apricots and almonds.

Plus points
● The presence of vitamin C in a dish – here provided by the tomatoes – improves the body's absorption of iron from grain products such as couscous and from dried apricots.

● Couscous is low in fat and high in starchy carbohydrates and fibre. It has a moderate score on the Glycaemic Index, which means that it is digested and absorbed relatively slowly, releasing glucose gradually into the blood stream. This helps to keep blood sugar levels steady.

Each serving provides kcal 326, protein 11 g, fat 14 g (of which saturated fat 2 g), carbohydrate 40 g (of which sugars 18 g), fibre 6 g. Excellent source of vitamin A, vitamin C, vitamin E. Good source of potassium. Useful source of calcium, copper, folate, iron, niacin, vitamin B$_1$, vitamin B$_6$, zinc.

Polenta and mushroom grills

Cooked and cooled polenta can be cut into shapes and grilled to make an excellent base for a tempting topping. Here the polenta is flavoured with Gruyère cheese, and the topping is a savoury mixture of mushrooms, walnuts and herbs. Serve as a sophisticated starter, with a few mixed salad leaves if you like.

Preparation and cooking time **45 minutes, plus 1 hour cooling**   *Serves 6 (makes 12 polenta grills)*

750 ml (1¼ pints) vegetable stock

170 g (6 oz) instant polenta

85 g (3 oz) Gruyère cheese, grated

15 g (½ oz) dried porcini mushrooms

3 tbsp extra virgin olive oil

225 g (8 oz) chestnut mushrooms, sliced

3 tbsp dry sherry

2 tbsp chopped fresh flat-leaf parsley, plus extra to garnish

2 tsp chopped fresh rosemary

30 g (1 oz) walnuts, finely chopped

salt and pepper

1 Bring the stock to the boil in a large saucepan. Pour in the polenta in a steady stream, stirring with a wooden spoon to prevent lumps from forming. Cook over a low heat, stirring constantly, for about 5 minutes or until the mixture thickens and pulls away from the sides of the pan. Remove from the heat and stir in the Gruyère cheese. Season with salt and pepper to taste.

2 Pour the polenta onto a damp baking tray and spread out into a rectangle measuring about 20 x 18 cm (8 x 7 in) and about 1 cm (½ in) thick. Leave to cool for 1 hour or until set.

3 Meanwhile, put the dried porcini mushrooms in a bowl and cover with boiling water. Leave to soak for 20 minutes. Drain, reserving 2 tbsp of the soaking liquid. Finely chop the mushrooms.

4 Preheat the grill to moderately hot. Lightly brush the polenta rectangle all over with 1 tbsp of the oil. Cut into 12 fingers, each measuring 5 x 6 cm (2 x 2½ in), trimming the edges to straighten them. Place oiled side up on the rack in the grill pan, and grill for 5 minutes or until lightly browned.

5 Turn the polenta slices over and grill for a further 2–3 minutes or until lightly browned. Remove from the grill and keep hot.

6 Heat the remaining 2 tbsp oil in a frying pan. Add the soaked dried mushrooms and the sliced chestnut mushrooms, and sauté over a fairly high heat for 3–4 minutes or until softened.

7 Add the sherry and the reserved mushroom soaking liquid. Cook over a high heat for 1–2 minutes, stirring, until most of the liquid has evaporated. Add the parsley, rosemary, walnuts, and salt and pepper to taste.

8 Spoon the mushroom mixture on top of the warm polenta fingers. Garnish with a little chopped parsley and serve immediately.

Some more ideas

Add 2–3 tbsp half-fat crème fraîche to the mushroom mixture with the herbs and walnuts, and heat.

Replace 150 ml (5 fl oz) of the stock with dry white wine.

Add 1 tsp chilli powder or cayenne pepper to the cooked polenta at the end of step 2.

Each serving provides   (two grills) kcal 203, protein 4 g, fat 9 g (of which saturated fat 1 g), carbohydrate 23.5 g (of which sugars 0.5 g), fibre 3 g. Excellent source of copper. Useful source of selenium.

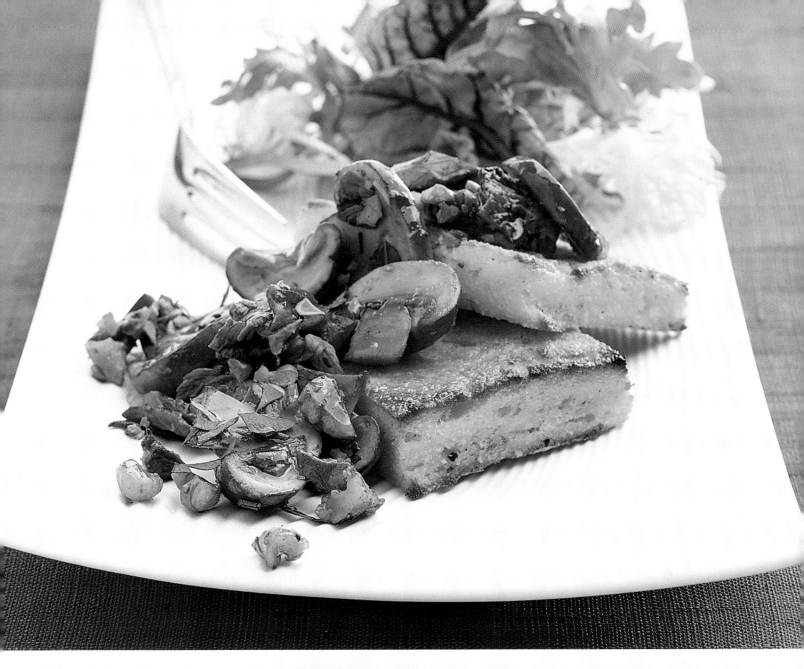

Make **polenta and tapenade squares**. Cut the cooled and set polenta into squares and grill as in the main recipe. For the tapenade topping, blend together 85 g (3 oz) stoned black olives, 2 tbsp capers, 30 g (1 oz) sun-dried tomatoes packed in oil, well drained, 1 crushed garlic clove, 2 tbsp extra virgin olive oil, 2 tbsp chopped fresh flat-leaf parsley, and salt and pepper to taste in a food processor. Alternatively, finely chop the olives, capers and tomatoes, and mix with the garlic, oil, parsley and seasoning.

Plus points

- Polenta is fine corn or maize meal. It provides a starchy carbohydrate alternative for those who need to avoid wheat or gluten in their diet.

- All mushrooms are a good source of copper, a mineral with many functions but particularly needed for the maintenance of healthy bones.

- Walnuts are a good source of many of the antioxidant nutrients, including copper, selenium, vitamin E and zinc.

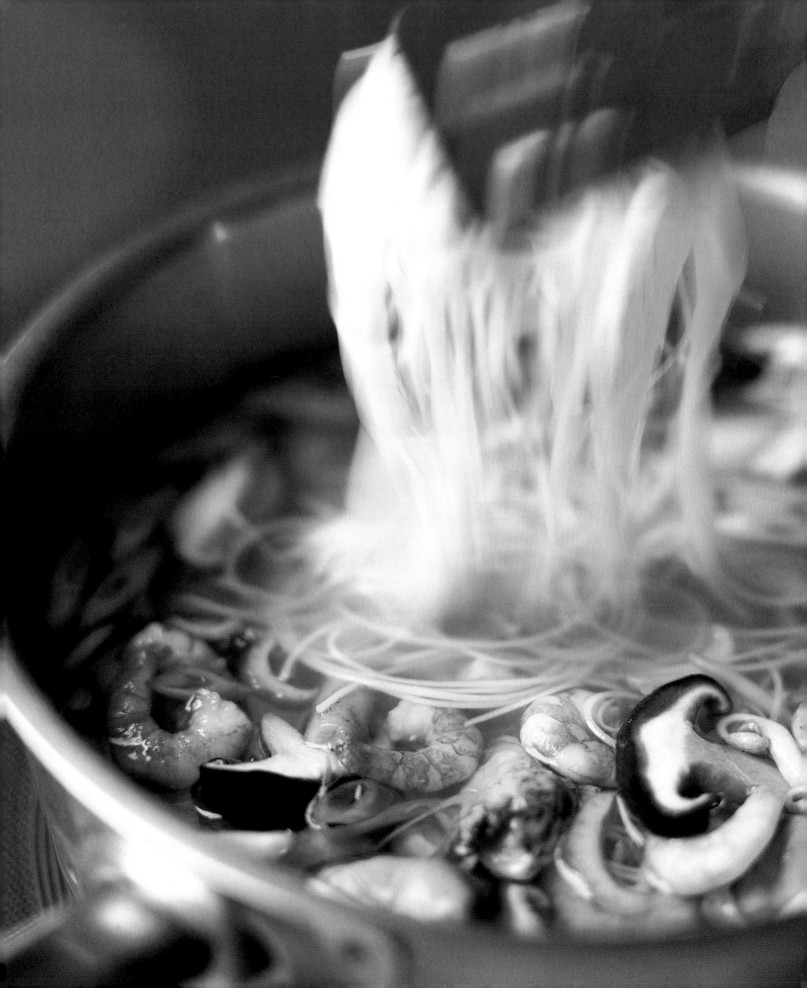

Dinner

(MEAT)

Sirloin Steaks with Port Sauce *70*
Mustardy Beef Fillet Salad *71*
Beef Waldorf *72*
Aromatic Beef Curry *74*
Perfect Pot Roast *75*
New England Simmered Beef *76*
Slow-Braised Beef and Barley *78*
One-Pot Steak and Pasta Casserole *79*
Chilli Con Carne with Cornbread *80*
Goulash Soup *81*
Spinach-Stuffed Meatloaf *82*
Thai Beef Noodle Soup *84*
Thai Beef Salad with Papaya *85*
Veal Escalopes with Herbs *86*
Greek Lamb Kebabs *87*
Lamb Burgers with Fruity Relish *88*
Bulghur Wheat Salad with Lamb *90*
Spring Lamb and Vegetable Stew *91*
Spanish Rabbit and Chickpea Stew *92*
Oriental Pork and Cabbage Rolls *94*
Sesame Pork and Noodle Salad *95*
Sweet and Sour Pork *96*
Pork and Beans *98*
Pork Medallions with Peppers *99*
Five-Spice Pork *100*

(POULTRY)

Japanese Chicken Salad *102*
Creamy Chicken Salad with Ginger *103*
Stir-Fried Chicken and Avocado Salad
   with Hot Balsamic Dressing *104*
Chicken and Artichoke Sauté *106*
Chicken Fajitas with Tomato Salsa *107*
Mexican Tostadas *108*
Chicken and Broccoli Chapatti *109*

Chicken and Vegetable Filo Rolls *110*
Herbed Chicken and Apple Burgers *112*
Chicken Goujons with Mustard Dip *113*
Chicken and Sweet Potatoes *114*
Barbecued Chicken *115*
Spicy Drumsticks with Creole Rice *116*
Chicken and Ham Jambalaya *118*
Indian-style Grilled Chicken Breasts *119*
Chicken and Sweetcorn Chowder *120*
Greek-style Lemon Chicken Soup *121*
French-style Chicken in Wine *122*
Chicken Livers Sautéed with Sage *124*
Marsala Chicken with Fennel *125*
Roasted Herb and Garlic Chicken *126*
Turkey, Chestnut and Barley Broth *128*
Roast Turkey with Lemon Couscous *129*
Turkey Kebabs with Fennel and
   Red Pepper Relish *130*
Turkey and Lentil Pâté *131*
Turkey Sausage and Bean Hotpot *132*
Turkey Drumsticks Braised
   with Baby Vegetables *134*
Pan-fried Turkey Escalopes with
   Citrus Honey Sauce *135*
Turkey Mole *136*
Spiced Stir-Fried Duck *138*

(SEAFOOD)

Piquant Pasta and Tuna Salad *139*
Provençal Tuna and Pepper Salad *140*
Grilled Salmon Salad *141*
Crab and Avocado Salad *142*
Prawn, Melon and Mango Salad *144*
Lobster Salad with Lime Dressing *145*
Italian Seafood Stew *146*
Chunky Fish Soup *147*
Mixed Seafood and Noodle Broth *148*

Seafood Jambalaya *150*
Cod with a Gremolata Crust *151*
Cod with Spicy Puy Lentils *152*
Baked Trout with Cucumber Sauce *154*
Swordfish with Salsa Dressing *155*
Salmon with Tarragon Mayonnaise *156*
Grilled Halibut Steaks with
   Tomato and Red Pepper Salsa *157*
Haddock with Parsley Sauce *158*
Linguine with Pan-Fried Salmon *160*
Spaghetti with Clams *161*
Parmesan-Topped Mussels *162*
Tiger Prawns with Pepper Salsa *163*
Prawn Gumbo *164*
Scampi Provençal *166*
Seafood with Watercress Dressing *167*
Steamed Sea Bass Fillets
   with Spring Vegetables *168*

(VEGETARIAN)

Winter Vegetable Casserole *170*
Caribbean Butternut Squash and
   Sweetcorn Stew *171*
Roast Vegetable and Bean Stew *172*
Mexican Black-Eyed Bean Soup *174*
Chickpea and Pita Salad *175*
Rustic Grilled Vegetable and
   Rigatoni Salad *176*
Tagliatelle with Green Sauce *177*
Penne Rigati with Sesame and
   Orange Dressing *178*
Cheese-Baked Peppers with Linguine *180*
Chickpea and Rice Balls *181*
Dolmades *182*
Minted Barley and Beans *183*
Quinoa with Griddled Aubergines *184*
Rice-Stuffed Squash *186*
Spinach and Potato Frittata *187*

Sirloin steaks with port sauce

Thin sirloin steaks, sometimes sold as minute steaks, can be quickly fried, and the juices left in the pan turned into an instant sauce with the help of a little port. A colourful stir-fry of tiny new potatoes, mushrooms, red pepper and sugarsnap peas is a perfect accompaniment.

Preparation and cooking time **30 minutes**   *Serves 4*

500 g (1 lb 2 oz) miniature new potatoes, scrubbed and any larger ones halved

2 tsp extra virgin olive oil

250 g (8½ oz) large mushrooms, quartered

250 g (8½ oz) sugarsnap peas

1 large red pepper, seeded and cut into thin strips

180 ml (6 fl oz) beef or vegetable stock

1 tbsp Worcestershire sauce

1 tsp Dijon mustard

½ tsp dark brown muscovado sugar

4 thin sirloin steaks, about 140 g (5 oz) each, trimmed of fat

1 tsp butter

1 shallot, finely chopped

2 garlic cloves, crushed

4 tbsp port

salt and pepper

1 Put the potatoes in a saucepan and cover with boiling water. Bring back to the boil, then reduce the heat and simmer for 10–12 minutes.

2 Meanwhile, heat the oil in a wok or large frying pan (preferably non-stick), add the mushrooms, peas and pepper strips, and stir-fry for 1 minute. Mix 120 ml (4 fl oz) of the stock with the Worcestershire sauce, mustard and sugar, and stir into the vegetables. Reduce the heat and simmer gently for 3 minutes or until the vegetables are just tender, stirring frequently.

3 Season the steaks on both sides with coarsely ground black pepper and set aside. Heat a ridged cast-iron grill pan. Meanwhile, drain the cooked potatoes and add to the vegetables. Stir gently, then cover and leave over a very low heat until ready to serve.

4 Put the butter into the hot grill pan and turn up the heat to high. As soon as the butter sizzles and starts to foam, add the steaks. The cooking time depends on the thickness of the meat and whether you like your steaks rare, medium or well done. For steaks 1 cm (½ in) thick, allow 1 minute on each side for rare (it will feel springy when pressed), 1½–2 minutes on each side for medium (it will feel slightly resistant when pressed), and 2½–3 minutes on each side for well done (the meat will feel firm when pressed). Lift the steaks onto warmed dinner plates, and keep warm while making the sauce.

5 Add the shallot and garlic to the cooking juices in the pan and cook, stirring, over a low heat for 1 minute. Pour in the port and increase the heat so the sauce is bubbling. Cook for about 1 minute, stirring. Pour in the remaining stock and let it bubble for a minute. Check the seasoning. Spoon the sauce over the steaks and serve immediately, with the vegetables.

Plus point

• New potatoes are rich in vitamin C and the B vitamin folate. The preparation method makes a big difference to the amount of dietary fibre provided: new potatoes cooked in their skins offer a third more fibre than peeled potatoes do. Cooking potatoes in their skins also preserves the nutrients found just under the skin.

photo, page 73

Each serving provides   kcal 386, protein 38 g, fat 11 g (of which saturated fat 4 g), carbohydrate 31 g (of which sugars 11 g), fibre 4.5 g. Excellent source of vitamin A, vitamin B_6, vitamin B_{12}, vitamin C, zinc. Good source of copper, folate, iron, niacin, potassium, vitamin B_1, vitamin B_2. Useful source of selenium.

Mustardy beef fillet salad

Lean roasted fillet of beef makes a very special salad for entertaining. Here it is combined with new potatoes and green vegetables and tossed in a mustard-flavoured vinaigrette. Serve with French bread.

Preparation time **35–40 minutes, plus cooling and chilling**   *Serves 4*

1 piece of beef fillet, from the tail end, about 450 g (1 lb)

1½ tsp extra virgin olive oil

340 g (12 oz) new potatoes, scrubbed

140 g (5 oz) thin green beans, halved

100 g (3½ oz) shelled fresh or frozen peas

85 g (3 oz) leeks, finely shredded

2 tbsp snipped fresh chives

Mustard vinaigrette

1½ tbsp extra virgin olive oil

2 tsp red wine vinegar

1 tsp Dijon mustard

pinch of caster sugar

salt and pepper

1 Preheat the oven to 230ºC (450ºF, gas mark 8). Rub the fillet with the olive oil and set on a rack in a roasting tin. Roast for 15 minutes for rare beef or up to 25 minutes for well done.

2 Meanwhile, whisk together the ingredients for the vinaigrette in a large mixing bowl.

3 Remove the beef from the oven and leave to stand for 5 minutes, then cut into thin slices against the grain. Add to the dressing and leave to cool.

4 Cook the potatoes in a saucepan of boiling water for 15 minutes or until tender. Drain well. When cool enough to handle, cut in half or into thick slices and add to the beef.

5 Drop the green beans into another pan of boiling water and cook for 1 minute. Add the peas and continue cooking for 3 minutes or until the vegetables are tender. Drain and refresh briefly under cold running water, then add to the beef and potatoes. Toss well. Cover and chill.

6 About 15 minutes before serving, remove the salad from the fridge and stir in the leeks and chives.

Another idea

For a **spicy pork fillet salad**, mix 2 tbsp demerara sugar, 1 tsp celery salt, 1 tsp garlic granules, 1 tsp cider vinegar and ½ tsp each ground ginger, ground allspice and paprika to a thick, grainy paste. Spread this over 450 g (1 lb) pork fillet (tenderloin), then leave to marinate for up to 8 hours. Roast the pork in a preheated 200ºC (400ºF, gas mark 6) oven for 30 minutes or until cooked through. Leave to cool. Rinse 250 g (8½ oz) basmati rice and cook in boiling water for 10–12 minutes or until tender. Drain and leave to cool. Cut the pork into cubes and mix with the rice and 100 g (3½ oz) pineapple chunks, 1 diced mango and 100 g (3½ oz) diced celery. Garnish with chopped parsley and paprika.

Plus points

• Beef is a useful source of vitamin D, which is found in relatively few foods. This vitamin is essential for the absorption of calcium, and thus helps in forming and maintaining healthy bones

• Peas supply good amounts of vitamins B_1, B_6 and niacin, and dietary fibre, particularly the soluble variety. They also provide useful amounts of folate and vitamin C.

photo, page 73

Each serving provides   kcal 305, protein 28 g, fat 13 g (of which saturated fat 4.5 g), carbohydrate 17 g (of which sugars 4 g), fibre 3 g. Excellent source of niacin, vitamin B_1, vitamin B_6, vitamin B_{12}, vitamin C, vitamin E, zinc. Good source of folate, iron, vitamin B_2. Useful source of potassium, selenium.

Beef Waldorf

Raw vegetables and fruits are one of the richest sources of essential vitamins and minerals. This tasty main-dish salad offers plenty of these vital nutrients and it's made extra delicious with a creamy mustard dressing. Serve with lots of crusty fresh bread for a satisfying and healthy meal.

Preparation time **25–30 minutes, plus 15 minutes cooling**   *Serves 4*

2 fillet steaks, about 140 g (5 oz) each, trimmed of fat

¼ tsp extra virgin olive oil

250 g (8½ oz) radishes, thinly sliced

3 carrots, grated

1 small yellow pepper, seeded and cut into thin rings

3 celery sticks, sliced diagonally

3 spring onions, sliced diagonally

30 g (1 oz) walnuts

55 g (2 oz) raisins or sultanas

2 small dessert apples

2 tsp lemon juice

100 g (3½ oz) rocket or watercress

salt and pepper

Mustard dressing

2 tbsp wholegrain mustard

3 tbsp reduced-fat mayonnaise

3 tbsp 0% fat Greek-style yogurt

1 Brush the steaks with the oil and season with pepper. Heat a ridged cast-iron grill pan or non-stick frying pan over a moderately high heat until hot. Put in the steaks and cook for 3 minutes on each side for medium rare or 4 minutes on each side for medium. These cooking times are for 2 cm (¾ in) steaks; adjust slightly for more or less than this thickness. Remove the steaks from the pan and leave to cool for at least 15 minutes.

2 Meanwhile, make the dressing. Put the mustard, mayonnaise and yogurt in a small bowl and stir together until well combined.

3 Put the radishes, carrots, yellow pepper, celery, spring onions, walnuts and raisins or sultanas in a large bowl. Quarter and core the apples, then cut them into 2 cm (¾ in) chunks and toss in the lemon juice. Add to the bowl with half of the dressing and turn to coat everything well. Season with salt and pepper to taste.

4 To serve, pile the rocket or watercress on 4 plates and spoon the apple and vegetable salad alongside. Cut the steak into thin slices and arrange on top. Spoon over the remaining dressing or hand it round separately in a jug.

Some more ideas

Instead of fillet steak, use a 280 g (10 oz) lean sirloin steak, cut about 2 cm (¾ in) thick.

Use the large white radish called mooli or daikon instead of red radishes. It is easy to grate by hand or in a food processor.

For a **roast beef and rice Waldorf**, mix 300 g (10½ oz) cubed leftover roast beef and 250 g (8½ oz) brown rice, cooked and cooled, into the apple and vegetable salad. This Waldorf salad is also good made with cooked chicken.

Plus points

● Apples provide good amounts of vitamin C as well as soluble fibre in the form of pectin. Eating apples with their skin offers the maximum amount of fibre.

● All the sugars in this dish are in the 'intrinsic' form, which means they are natural sugars found in fruit (the raisins and apples) and vegetables (the radishes, carrots, yellow pepper, celery, spring onions and watercress). Fibre in the fruit and vegetables influences the rate at which these sugars are absorbed into the blood.

Each serving provides   kcal 250, protein 18 g, fat 9 g (of which saturated fat 1.5 g), carbohydrate 25 g (of which sugars 25 g), fibre 5 g. Excellent source of niacin, vitamin A, vitamin B$_1$, vitamin B$_6$, vitamin B$_{12}$, vitamin E. Good source of folate, iron, potassium, vitamin B$_2$, zinc. Useful source of calcium, selenium.

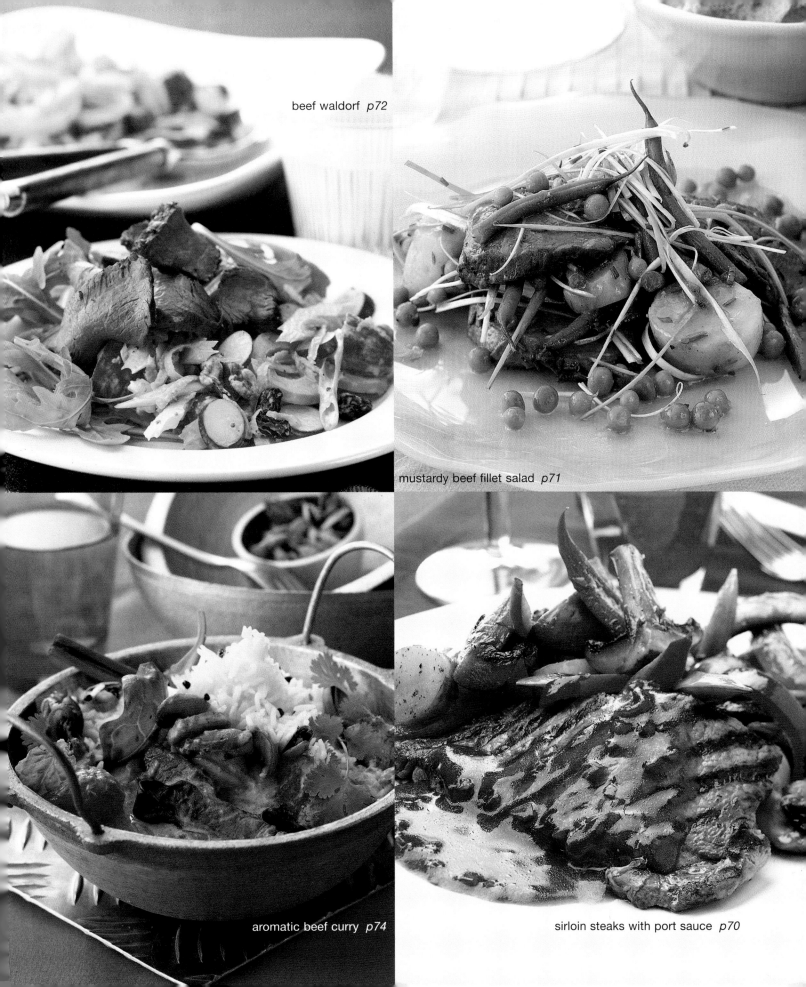

beef waldorf *p72*

mustardy beef fillet salad *p71*

aromatic beef curry *p74*

sirloin steaks with port sauce *p70*

Aromatic beef curry

This will satisfy even the most demanding curry addict. Lean and tender sirloin steak is quickly cooked with lots of spices, tomatoes, mushrooms and spinach, with yogurt added to give a luxurious feel. Served with cardamom-spiced rice, it makes a really healthy and nutritious meal.

Preparation time **10 minutes**   Cooking time **20 minutes**   *Serves 4*

1 tbsp sunflower oil

1 large onion, thinly sliced

150 g (5½ oz) button mushrooms, sliced

400 g (14 oz) sirloin steak, trimmed of fat and cut into thin strips

1½ tsp bottled chopped root ginger in oil, drained

2 garlic cloves, crushed

½ tsp crushed dried chillies

2 tsp ground coriander

¼ tsp ground cardamom

½ tsp turmeric

¼ tsp grated nutmeg

1 can chopped tomatoes, about 400 g

1 tsp cornflour mixed with 1 tbsp water

300 g (10½ oz) plain low-fat yogurt

1 tbsp clear honey

125 g (4½ oz) young spinach leaves

juice of ½ lime

2 tbsp chopped fresh coriander, plus extra leaves to garnish

Cardamom rice

340 g (12 oz) basmati rice, well rinsed

1 cinnamon stick

8 whole green cardamom pods, cracked

juice of ½ lemon

salt

1 Heat the oil in a large saucepan and add the onion and mushrooms. Cook over a high heat for 2 minutes or until the onion slices begin to colour.

2 Add the beef together with the ginger, garlic, chillies, ground coriander, cardamom, turmeric and nutmeg. Cook for 2 minutes, stirring well, then add the tomatoes with their juice and the cornflour mixture. Bring to the boil, stirring. Stir in the yogurt and honey. Bring back to the boil, then reduce the heat, cover and simmer gently for 20 minutes.

3 Meanwhile, prepare the cardamom rice. Put 450 ml (15 fl oz) cold water in a saucepan and bring to the boil. Add the rice, cinnamon stick and cardamom pods. Bring back to the boil, then cover tightly and cook for 10 minutes or until the rice is tender. Drain and return the rice to the saucepan.

Stir in the lemon juice and keep covered until the curry is ready to serve.

4 Stir the spinach, lime juice and chopped coriander into the curry and allow the leaves to wilt down into the sauce. To serve, spoon the curry over the rice and garnish with fresh coriander leaves.

Another idea

If you like a hot curry, add a halved fresh red chilli to the sauce towards the end of the cooking time. The chilli can be left in the sauce or discarded before serving.

Plus points

• Cardamom is believed to be helpful for digestive problems, such as indigestion, flatulence and stomach cramps.

• Mushrooms are low in fat and calories and provide useful amounts of the B vitamins niacin, B_6 and folate. They are also a good source of copper.

• Along with its many other nutritional benefits, beef provides vitamins from the B group and is a useful source of vitamin D, which is found in relatively few foods.

photo, page 73

Each serving provides kcal 570, protein 36 g, fat 9 g (of which saturated fat 3 g), carbohydrate 86 g (of which sugars 16 g), fibre 2 g. Excellent source of iron, zinc. Good source of calcium, copper, potassium, vitamin A, vitamin B_6, vitamin B_{12}, vitamin C. Useful source of folate, selenium, vitamin B_1, vitamin B_2, vitamin E.

Perfect pot roast

This long-simmered, one-pot meal is wonderfully satisfying. It can be prepared ahead, so it's perfect for family dinners as well as informal entertaining. Serve with a crunchy mixed salad and seeded bread.

Preparation and cooking time **4 hours**   *Serves 6*

1 tsp extra virgin olive oil

1 kg (2¼ lb) piece boneless beef chuck, about 7.5 cm (3 in) thick, trimmed of fat and tied

2 large onions, finely chopped

1 celery stick, finely chopped

3 garlic cloves, crushed

250 ml (8½ fl oz) dry red or white wine

1 can chopped tomatoes, about 225 g

1 large carrot, grated

1 tsp chopped fresh thyme

450 ml (15 fl oz) beef stock

600 g (1 lb 5 oz) new potatoes, scrubbed and quartered

340 g (12 oz) celeriac, cut into 2.5 cm (1 in) cubes

340 g (12 oz) swede, cut into 2.5 cm (1 in) cubes

4 carrots, about 280 g (10 oz) in total, sliced

salt and pepper

3 tbsp chopped parsley to garnish

1 Preheat the oven to 160°C (325°F, gas mark 3). Heat the oil in a large flameproof casserole. Add the beef and brown it over a moderately high heat for 6–8 minutes or until it is well coloured on all sides. Remove the meat to a plate.

2 Reduce the heat to moderate. Add the onions, celery and garlic and cook, stirring frequently, for 3 minutes or until the onions begin to soften. Add the wine and let it bubble for about 1 minute, then add the tomatoes with their juice and the grated carrot. Cook for a further 2 minutes.

3 Return the beef to the casserole together with any juices that have collected on the plate and the chopped thyme. Tuck a piece of greaseproof paper or foil around the top of the meat, turning back the corners so that it doesn't touch the liquid, then cover with a tight-fitting lid. Transfer the casserole to the oven and cook for 2½ hours.

4 About 20 minutes before the end of the cooking time, bring the stock to the boil in a deep saucepan with a lid. Add the potatoes, celeriac, swede and sliced carrots. Cover and simmer gently for 12–15 minutes or until they are starting to become tender.

5 Meanwhile, remove the beef from the casserole and set aside. Remove any fat from the cooking liquid, either by spooning it off or by using a bulb baster, then purée the casseroled vegetables and liquid in a blender or food processor until smooth. Season to taste.

6 Drain the potatoes and other root vegetables, reserving the liquid. Make a layer of the vegetables in the casserole, put the beef on top and add the remaining root vegetables and their cooking liquid. Pour over the sauce. Cover the casserole and return to the oven to cook for 20 minutes or until the root vegetables are tender.

7 Remove the beef to a carving board, cover and leave to rest for 10 minutes. Keep the vegetables and sauce in the oven turned down to low.

8 Carve the beef and arrange on warmed plates with the vegetables and sauce. Sprinkle with the parsley and serve immediately.

Plus point
• Swede is a member of the cruciferous family of vegetables. It is a useful source of vitamin C and beta-carotene and rich in phytochemicals that are believed to help protect against cancer.

photo, page 77

Each serving provides kcal 399, protein 43 g, fat 12 g (of which saturated fat 4 g), carbohydrate 33 g (of which sugars 15 g), fibre 8 g. Excellent source of folate, niacin, vitamin A, vitamin B$_1$, vitamin B$_6$, vitamin B$_{12}$, zinc. Good source of iron, vitamin B$_2$. Useful source of selenium.

New England simmered beef

This traditional American dish is a one-pot meal of succulent beef and tender-crisp vegetables in a nutritious and tasty broth. The tangy beetroot and onion relish cuts through the richness of the meat and is an inspired finishing touch. Serve with crusty bread to mop up the juices.

Preparation time **25 minutes**   Cooking time **about 2½ hours**   *Serves 4*

675 g (1½ lb) piece lean chuck steak, trimmed of fat

3 sprigs of fresh thyme

3 sprigs of parsley

1 large bay leaf

2 large garlic cloves, sliced

10 black peppercorns, lightly crushed

250 g (8½ oz) leek, sliced

1 celery stick, cut into 7.5 cm (3 in) pieces

300 g (10½ oz) baby new potatoes, scrubbed

12 small shallots

300 g (10½ oz) baby turnips

300 g (10½ oz) baby carrots

150 g (5½ oz) Savoy cabbage, cored and finely shredded

salt and pepper

finely chopped parsley to garnish

Beetroot and onion relish

340 g (12 oz) cooked beetroot, peeled and finely diced

6 spring onions, finely chopped

3 tbsp finely chopped parsley

1 Place the beef in a flameproof casserole. Add about 1.5 litres (2¾ pints) water to cover the meat very generously. Bring to the boil over a high heat, skimming the surface as necessary to remove all the grey foam.

2 As soon as the liquid comes to the boil, reduce the heat to very low. Tie the thyme, parsley, bay leaf, garlic and peppercorns in a little muslin bag and add to the pan with the leek and celery. Half cover the pan and simmer gently, skimming the surface when necessary, for 1¾–2 hours or until the beef is very tender when pierced with the tip of a sharp knife.

3 Meanwhile, make the beetroot relish. Place the beetroot in a bowl with the spring onions and parsley. Season with salt and pepper to taste and gently stir together. Cover and chill.

4 Preheat the oven on a low setting. When the meat is tender, use 2 large spoons to transfer it to an ovenproof dish. Spoon over enough of the cooking liquid to cover the meat, then tightly cover the dish with foil. Place in the oven to keep warm.

5 Remove the muslin bag from the casserole and discard. Add the potatoes and shallots to the casserole with ½ tsp salt,

increase the heat and cook for 5 minutes. Add the turnips and carrots and simmer for a further 15 minutes or until the vegetables are tender. With a draining spoon transfer them to the dish with the meat.

6 Add the cabbage to the broth in the casserole and simmer for 3 minutes or until it is tender. Remove with a draining spoon and add to the other vegetables.

7 To serve, slice the beef against the grain and place the slices in soup plates or plates with rims. Top with a selection of vegetables and spoon over some of the broth. Sprinkle with parsley and serve with the relish.

Plus point

• Traditionally, beetroot was believed to be good for the health of the blood – probably because of its deep red colour. It does contain folate, an essential vitamin for healthy cells and the prevention of anaemia, and is also believed to contain anti-carcinogens.

Each serving provides kcal 391, protein 45 g, fat 8 g (of which saturated fat 3 g), carbohydrate 36 g (of which sugars 23 g), fibre 10 g. Excellent source of niacin, vitamin A, vitamin B$_1$, vitamin B$_2$, vitamin B$_6$, vitamin B$_{12}$, vitamin C, vitamin E, zinc. Good source of iron, selenium. Useful source of calcium.

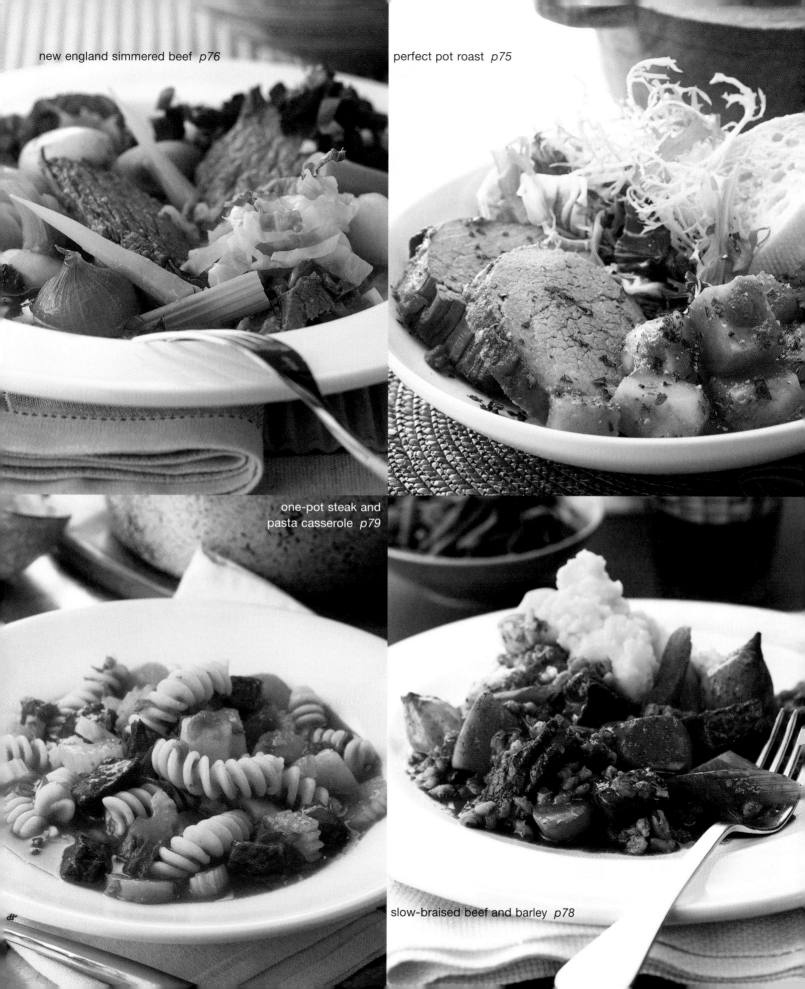

new england simmered beef *p76*

perfect pot roast *p75*

one-pot steak and
pasta casserole *p79*

slow-braised beef and barley *p78*

Slow-braised beef and barley

Juniper berries give this dish a distinctive flavour. The beef is slowly simmered until meltingly tender, while nourishing pot barley soaks up some of the juices and thickens the rich gravy to make a hearty casserole. Serve with mashed potatoes and a green vegetable such as French beans or spring greens.

Preparation time **20 minutes, plus 8 hours marinating**   Cooking time **2–2¼ hours**   *Serves 4*

500 g (1 lb 2 oz) beef chuck or lean braising steak, trimmed and cut into 5 cm (2 in) cubes

2 garlic cloves, halved

3 bay leaves

6 juniper berries, lightly crushed

1 sprig of fresh thyme

250 ml (8½ fl oz) full-bodied red wine

12 button onions, about 400 g (14 oz) in total

1 tbsp extra virgin olive oil

55 g (2 oz) pot barley

400 ml (14 fl oz) beef stock

3 large carrots, cut into large chunks, about 425 g (15 oz) in total

2 celery sticks, sliced

300 g (10½ oz) swede, cut into 4 cm (1½ in) chunks

salt and pepper

1 Put the beef in a bowl with the garlic, bay leaves, juniper berries and thyme. Pour over the wine, then cover and leave to marinate in the fridge for 8 hours or overnight.

2 The next day, preheat the oven to 160°C (325°F, gas mark 3). Put the button onions in a bowl and pour over enough boiling water to cover. Leave for 2 minutes, then drain. When cool enough to handle, peel off the skins. Set the onions aside.

3 Remove the beef from the marinade and pat dry on kitchen paper. Heat the oil in a large flameproof casserole over a moderately high heat. Add the beef and brown on all sides. Do this in batches, if necessary, so the pan is not overcrowded. Remove the beef from the casserole and set aside on a plate.

4 Add the onions to the casserole and cook gently for 3–4 minutes or until lightly coloured all over. Add the barley and cook for 1 minute, stirring, then return the beef and any beefy juices to the casserole. Pour in the stock and bring to a simmer.

5 Strain the marinade into the casserole, and add the bay leaves and sprig of thyme. Season with salt and pepper to taste. Cover with a tight-fitting lid, transfer to the oven and braise for 45 minutes.

6 Add the carrots, celery and swede, and stir to mix. Cover again and braise for a further 1–1¼ hours or until the beef, barley and vegetables are tender. Remove the bay leaves and thyme stalk before serving.

Another idea

The gravy will be quite thick. If you prefer it slightly thinner, stir in an extra 120 ml (4 fl oz) beef stock 20 minutes before the end of the cooking time.

Plus points

• Pot barley retains the outer layers of the grain (these are removed in the milling of pearl barley), and it therefore contains all the nutrients of the whole grain.

• The barley grain contains gummy fibres called beta-glucans, which appear to have significant cholesterol-lowering properties. It also boasts a very low Glycaemic Index.

• Beef is an excellent source of iron, both in terms of the quantity that is present and the efficient way it is absorbed by the body.

photo, page 77

Each serving provides   kcal 367, protein 31 g, fat 10 g (of which saturated fat 3 g), carbohydrate 29 g (of which sugars 18 g), fibre 8 g. Excellent source of vitamin A. Good source of vitamin C. Useful source of calcium, copper, folate, iron, niacin, potassium, vitamin B$_1$, vitamin B$_6$, vitamin E, zinc.

One-pot steak and pasta casserole

Slim pasta spirals called fusilli are delicious cooked in a casserole of beef and vegetables. The dried, uncooked pasta is added towards the end of the cooking time so that it retains its al dente texture while still absorbing the savoury flavours of the meat, vegetables and oregano in the rich stew.

Preparation time **15 minutes**   Cooking time **about 1½ hours**   *Serves 4*

1 tbsp extra virgin olive oil

340 g (12 oz) lean braising steak, cut into 1 cm (½ in) cubes

1 onion, chopped

1 can chopped tomatoes, about 400 g

2 tbsp tomato purée

2 garlic cloves, crushed

1 litre (1¾ pints) beef or vegetable stock

3 large carrots, sliced

4 celery sticks, sliced

1 small swede, about 400 g (14 oz), chopped

225 g (8 oz) fusilli (pasta spirals)

1 tbsp chopped fresh oregano or 1 tsp dried oregano

salt and pepper

1 Heat the oil in a large flameproof casserole and add the beef. Brown the meat all over, stirring frequently. Use a draining spoon to remove the meat from the pan.

2 Add the onion to the casserole and cook for about 5 minutes, stirring often, until it is softened. Then add the tomatoes with their juice, the tomato purée, garlic and 600 ml (1 pint) of the stock. Stir well and bring to the boil.

3 Return the beef to the casserole. Add the carrots, celery and swede, and season to taste. Cover and simmer gently for 1 hour or until the meat is tender.

4 Add the pasta and oregano with the remaining stock. Bring to simmering point, then reduce the heat and cover the casserole. Cook for 20–25 minutes or until the pasta is tender. Serve immediately.

Some more ideas

For a Mediterranean flavour, replace the carrots and swede with 1 red pepper and 1 yellow or green pepper, seeded and chopped. Add the peppers with the onion. Also add 170 g (6 oz) button mushrooms with the pasta.

Try venison steak instead of the beef, and use whole baby carrots and turnips instead of the sliced carrots and chopped swede. Venison is particularly rich in iron.

Plus points

• Beef is an excellent source of iron and zinc. Iron from red meat is far more easily absorbed by the body than iron from vegetable sources.

• Swede is a member of the cruciferous family of vegetables, all of which have an important role to play in cancer prevention.

• Adding pasta and starchy root vegetables to a meat casserole increases its fibre content as well as the carbohydrate. Fusilli pasta has a low to medium Glycaemic Index.

photo, page 77

Each serving provides   kcal 400, protein 27.5 g, fat 8.5 g (of which saturated fat 2 g), carbohydrate 57 g (of which sugars 14 g), fibre 6 g. Excellent source of niacin, vitamin A, vitamin B$_{12}$, vitamin C. Good source of copper, iron, potassium, vitamin B$_1$, vitamin B$_6$, zinc. Useful source of calcium, folate, selenium, vitamin B$_2$, vitamin E.

Chilli con carne with cornbread

Slow-cooked beef and beans in a rich tomato sauce spiced with chillies and cumin makes an inviting meal on a wintry day, and warm, crumbly cornbread studded with sweetcorn kernels and mild green chilli is the perfect accompaniment. Serve with a crisp salad for a hearty, well-balanced meal.

Preparation time **25 minutes**   Cooking time **1–1½ hours**   *Serves 6*

1 tbsp extra virgin olive oil

340 g (12 oz) lean stewing beef, trimmed of fat and cut into small cubes

1 large onion, finely chopped

2 garlic cloves, crushed

½ tsp cumin seeds

1 tsp crushed dried chillies

1 tbsp tomato purée

1 can chopped tomatoes, about 400 g

2 cans red kidney beans, about 400 g each, drained and rinsed

300 ml (10 fl oz) beef stock

salt and pepper

Cornbread

140 g (5 oz) cornmeal

115 g (4 oz) plain flour

2 tsp baking powder

½ tsp salt

1 large egg

225 ml (7½ fl oz) semi-skimmed milk

140 g (5 oz) sweetcorn kernels, either fresh or thawed frozen

1 small mild fresh green chilli, seeded and finely chopped

1 Heat the oil in a large flameproof casserole, add the beef and fry over a high heat, stirring occasionally, for 3–4 minutes or until well browned. Remove the meat with a draining spoon.

2 Reduce the heat to low and add the onion to the pan. Stir well and cook gently for 10 minutes. Add the garlic, cumin seeds and chillies and cook, stirring, for 1 minute, then return the meat to the pan. Add the tomato purée, the tomatoes with their juice, the beans and stock. Stir well and bring to the boil. Reduce the heat so the chilli is simmering gently, then cover with a lid and cook for 1–1½ hours or until the meat is tender, stirring occasionally.

3 Meanwhile, make the cornbread. Preheat the oven to 200°C (400°F, gas mark 6) and grease a shallow 20 cm (8 in) square cake tin with a little melted butter. Mix the cornmeal, flour, baking powder and salt in a bowl. Combine the egg with the milk and stir in to make a thick, rough-looking batter (do not overmix or the bread will be tough). Fold in the sweetcorn and chilli. Spoon into the prepared tin and bake for 20–25 minutes until firm to the touch.

4 Turn the cornbread out of its tin and cut into large squares. Serve the chilli in warmed bowls, with the warm cornbread.

Another idea

Replace the beef with diced boneless lean lamb (leg or neck fillet). Replace the crushed chillies with 1 seeded and finely chopped medium-hot fresh green chilli, ½ tsp ground coriander and 1 cinnamon stick. Instead of kidney beans, use 2 cans chickpeas, about 400 g each, drained and rinsed, adding them to the casserole after the chilli has been cooking for 15 minutes. Also add 2 medium-sized aubergines, cut into 1 cm (½ in) dice. Stir occasionally and add more stock if the mixture looks dry. At the end of the cooking time, stir in 3 tbsp chopped fresh coriander.

Plus points

• Red kidney beans are low in fat and rich in carbohydrate. They provide good amounts of niacin and vitamins B$_1$ and B$_6$, and useful amounts of iron. They are also a good source of soluble fibre, which can help to reduce high cholesterol levels in the blood.

• Sweetcorn is a good source of complex (starchy) carbohydrates and has roughly the same Glycaemic Index as an orange.

photo, page 83

Each serving provides   kcal 408, protein 28 g, fat 8 g (of which saturated fat 2 g), carbohydrate 59 g (of which sugars 10 g), fibre 8 g. Excellent source of niacin, vitamin B$_1$, vitamin B$_6$, vitamin B$_{12}$, zinc. Good source of calcium, folate, iron, selenium, viatmin B$_2$, vitamin C. Useful source of vitamin A.

Goulash soup

This rich meal-in-a-bowl combines beef with vegetables and dumplings and the three essential ingredients of an authentic goulash – paprika, onions and caraway seeds. Serve with boiled or steamed potatoes.

Preparation time **30 minutes**   Cooking time **1½ hours**   *Serves 4*

2 tsp rapeseed oil

2 large onions, sliced

2 garlic cloves, finely chopped

500 g (1 lb 2 oz) lean chuck steak, trimmed of fat and cut into 2 cm (¾ in) cubes

2 large carrots, diced

1 tbsp paprika

¼ tsp caraway seeds

1 can chopped tomatoes, about 400 g

750 ml (1¼ pints) beef stock, preferably home-made

170 g (6 oz) white cabbage, finely shredded

salt and pepper

chopped parsley to garnish

Parsley and onion dumplings

2 tsp rapeseed oil

1 onion, finely chopped

1 egg

3 tbsp skimmed milk

3 tbsp chopped parsley

120 g (4¼ oz) fresh white breadcrumbs

1 Heat the oil in a large saucepan, add the onions and garlic and cook over a moderately low heat, stirring frequently, for 10 minutes or until beginning to brown.

2 Add the cubes of beef and cook, stirring, for 5 minutes or until browned all over. Add the carrots, paprika, caraway seeds, tomatoes with their juice and stock. Season with salt and pepper to taste. Stir well and bring to the boil, then cover and simmer gently for 1 hour or until the beef is just tender.

3 Meanwhile, make the dumplings. Heat the oil in a frying pan, add the onion and cook over a low heat, stirring frequently, for about 10 minutes or until softened but not coloured. In a bowl, beat the egg and milk together, then add the onion, parsley and breadcrumbs. Season with salt and pepper to taste and mix well.

4 Add the cabbage to the saucepan and stir to mix with the beef and other vegetables. With wet hands, shape the dumpling mixture into 12 walnut-sized balls. Add to the pan, cover and cook for a further 15 minutes or until the dumplings are cooked. Taste for seasoning and serve hot in warmed deep soup plates, sprinkled with chopped parsley.

Some more ideas

Replace the beef with 340 g (12 oz) stewing veal and add 100 g (3½ oz) diced smoked pork sausage with the cabbage.

Use 1 seeded and thinly sliced red pepper instead of the cabbage.

For a spicy soup, add 1 seeded and finely chopped fresh red chilli with the paprika.

Plus points

• Cabbage belongs to the brassica group of cruciferous vegetables. These contain glucosinolates and other sulphur compounds associated with lowering the risk of cancer. These vegetables are also good sources of vitamin C and among the richest vegetable sources of folate.

• Dumplings are a nutritious addition to soups or stews, being filling and providing starchy carbohydrate.

photo, page 83

Each serving provides   kcal 450, protein 38 g, fat 15 g (of which saturated fat 4.5 g), carbohydrate 46 g (of which sugars 19 g), fibre 6 g. Excellent source of folate, niacin, vitamin A, vitamin B_1, vitamin B_6, vitamin B_{12}, vitamin C, vitamin E, zinc. Good source of iron, selenium, vitamin B_2.

Spinach-stuffed meatloaf

Vegetables and oats make this meatloaf wonderfully moist and light. When sliced, the creamy spinach layer is revealed in a pretty spiral. Serve with roasted mixed vegetables such as new potatoes in their skins, courgettes and red onions.

Preparation time **45 minutes, plus 10 minutes standing**   Cooking time **50 minutes**   *Serves 6*

1 tbsp extra virgin olive oil

2 large onions, finely chopped

6 garlic cloves, crushed, or to taste

1 can chopped tomatoes, about 400 g

150 ml (5 fl oz) chicken stock

1 tsp dried mixed herbs

500 g (1 lb 2 oz) young spinach leaves

2 tbsp crème fraîche

½ tsp freshly grated nutmeg

450 g (1 lb) lean minced beef

450 g (1 lb) lean minced pork

1 celery stick, finely chopped

1 large carrot, grated

50 g (1¾ oz) porridge oats

2 tsp chopped fresh thyme

5 tbsp semi-skimmed milk

1 egg, beaten

2 tsp Dijon mustard

salt and pepper

1 Heat the oil in a saucepan over a moderate heat. Add the onions and garlic and cook, stirring often, for about 5 minutes or until the onions are soft and golden.

2 Transfer half of the onion mixture to a large bowl and set aside. Stir the tomatoes with their juice, the stock and mixed herbs into the onions remaining in the pan. Season to taste. Bring to the boil, then cover and leave to simmer very gently, stirring occasionally, while preparing the meatloaf.

3 Preheat the oven to 180°C (350°F, gas mark 4). Wash the spinach and put it in a large saucepan. Cover and cook over a high heat for 2–3 minutes, shaking the pan often, until the leaves are wilted.

4 Tip the spinach into a colander to drain. When it is cool enough to handle, squeeze it dry with your hands, then chop it roughly and put it into a bowl. Stir in the crème fraîche and season with half of the nutmeg and salt and pepper to taste.

5 Add the meat to the reserved onion, with the celery, carrot, porridge oats, thyme, milk, egg, mustard and remaining nutmeg. Season to taste. Mix the ingredients well.

6 Lay a large sheet of cling film on the work surface and place the meat mixture in the centre. With a palette knife, spread the meat into a 23 x 18 cm (9 x 7 in) rectangle. Spread the spinach mixture evenly over the meat,

leaving a 1 cm (½ in) border all round. Starting at a short end, carefully roll up the meat and spinach like a Swiss roll, using the cling film to help. Pat the sides into a neat shape and place the roll on a non-stick baking tray, discarding the cling film.

7 Place the meatloaf in the centre of the oven and cook for 45 minutes, then remove from the oven and brush lightly all over with a little of the tomato sauce. Return to the oven and cook for 5 minutes to set the glaze and brown it slightly. To check if the meatloaf is cooked right through, insert a skewer into the centre and remove after a few seconds – it should feel very hot when lightly placed on the back of your hand.

8 When the meatloaf is ready, remove it from the oven, cover loosely with foil and leave to stand for 10 minutes. Serve cut into slices, with the rest of the tomato sauce.

Plus points

• Spinach provides good amounts of carotenoid compounds and several antioxidants, including vitamins C and E, and substantial amounts of the B vitamins.

• Porridge oats are an excellent source of soluble fibre, which can help to reduce high blood cholesterol levels.

Each serving provides kcal 340, protein 40 g, fat 14 g (of which saturated fat 4 g), carbohydrate 19 g (of which sugars 11 g), fibre 5 g. Excellent source of niacin, vitamin A, vitamin B₁, vitamin B₆, vitamin B₁₂, vitamin C, vitamin E, zinc. Good source of calcium, selenium, vitamin B₂. Useful source of iron.

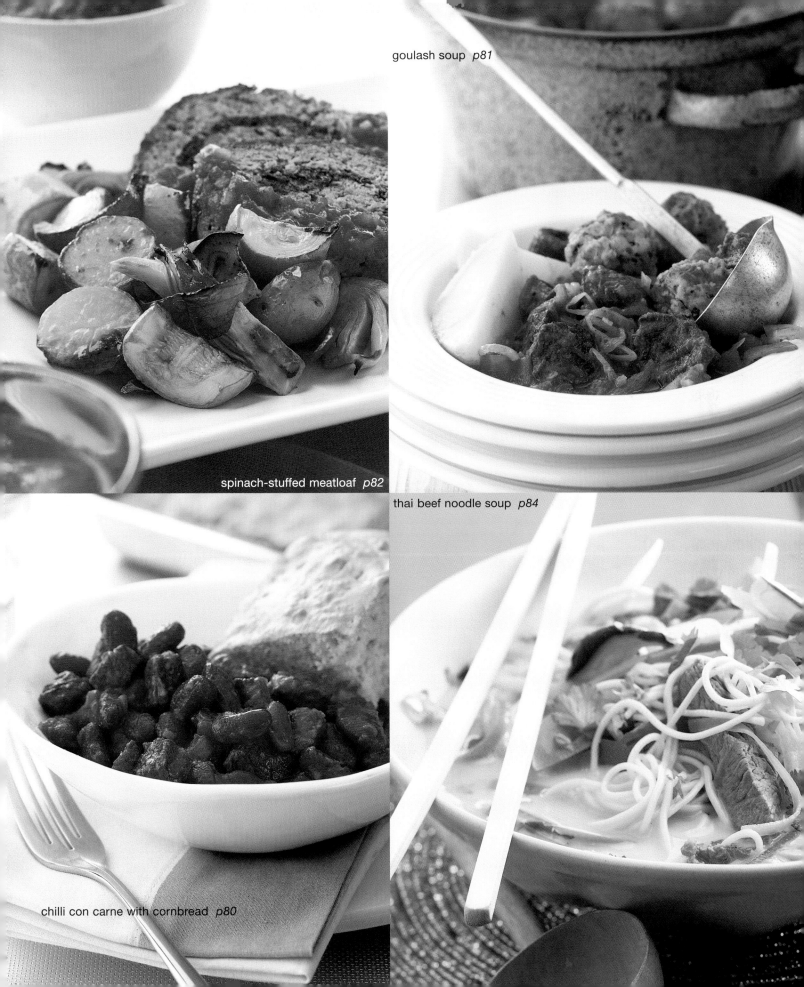

goulash soup *p81*

spinach-stuffed meatloaf *p82*

thai beef noodle soup *p84*

chilli con carne with cornbread *p80*

Thai beef noodle soup

Bursting with flavour, this main-course beef soup is packed with vegetables and noodles. You can eat the noodles, beef and vegetables with chopsticks, then enjoy the soup with a spoon.

Preparation and cooking time **about 50 minutes**   *Serves 4*

15 g (½ oz) dried shiitake mushrooms

100 ml (3½ fl oz) boiling water

1 litre (1¾ pints) beef stock

4 fresh lime leaves, torn

1 lemongrass stalk, cut into 3 pieces

1 garlic clove, crushed

1 fresh red chilli, seeded and chopped

2.5 cm (1 in) piece fresh root ginger, grated

15 g (½ oz) fresh coriander

150 g (5½ oz) carrot

100 g (3½ oz) leek

2 celery sticks, about 100 g (3½ oz) in total

100 g (3½ oz) sugarsnap peas

100 g (3½ oz) Chinese leaves

340 g (12 oz) lean rump steak, trimmed of fat

100 ml (3½ fl oz) low-fat coconut milk

3 sheets dried medium Chinese egg noodles, about 260 g (9 oz) in total

finely grated zest and juice of 1 lime

4 tsp fish sauce, or to taste

1 Put the mushrooms into a small bowl, add the boiling water and leave to soak for 20 minutes.

2 Meanwhile, pour the stock into a large saucepan and add the lime leaves, lemongrass, garlic, chilli and ginger. Separate the coriander leaves from the stalks and set the leaves aside. Chop the stalks and add them to the stock. Cover the pan and bring the stock just to the boil, then reduce the heat to very low. Let the stock simmer gently for 10 minutes while you prepare the vegetables and beef.

3 Drain the mushrooms, pouring the soaking liquid into the simmering stock. Cut each mushroom in half lengthways. Chop the carrot, leek and celery into fine strips about 5 cm (2 in) long. Slice the sugarsnap peas in half lengthways, and finely shred the Chinese leaves. Slice the beef into thin strips about 1 cm (½ in) wide.

4 Remove the lemongrass and lime leaves from the stock. Bring the stock back to the boil, then add the carrot, leek and celery. Cover and simmer for 3 minutes. Pour in the coconut milk and increase the heat. Just as the liquid comes to the boil, add the noodles, crushing them in your hands as you drop them into the pan. Stir in the mushrooms and beef, bring back to a

simmer and cook, uncovered, for 1 minute. Stir well, then add the sugarsnap peas and Chinese leaves. Simmer for a further 3 minutes or until the beef, noodles and vegetables are just tender. Add the lime zest and juice and the fish sauce and stir well. Taste and add more fish sauce if you like.

5 To serve, transfer the noodles, beef and vegetables to bowls using a draining spoon. Ladle the coconut stock over, sprinkle with the coriander leaves and serve immediately.

Plus points

• Celery provides potassium, a mineral that is important for the regulation of fluid balance in the body, thus helping to prevent high blood pressure.

• Coconut milk is a typical ingredient of Thai cooking. The low-fat version (88% fat-free) has 12 g fat per 100 g (3½ oz) compared with 17 g in ordinary full-fat coconut milk.

• Sugarsnap peas are a good source of soluble fibre and vitamin C.

photo, page 83

Each serving provides   kcal 357, protein 23 g, fat 7 g (of which saturated fat 3 g), carbohydrate 25 g (of which sugars 7 g), fibre 3 g. Excellent source of niacin, vitamin A, vitamin B_1, vitamin B_6, vitamin B_{12}, vitamin C, vitamin E. Good source of vitamin B_2, zinc. Useful source of calcium, iron.

Thai beef salad with papaya

Sweet juicy papaya, crisp leaves and aromatic herbs are a sensational combination in this Thai-inspired salad. Thai fragrant rice – jasmine rice simmered in stock and scented with lime leaves – is the perfect complement.

Preparation time 35 minutes   *Serves 4*

2 thick-cut lean sirloin steaks, about 450 g (1 lb) in total, trimmed of fat

250 g (8½ oz) jasmine rice

1.2 litres (2 pints) chicken stock

4 fresh lime leaves, crushed

2 tsp sunflower oil

2 firm, ripe papayas, peeled, seeded and sliced

½ small cucumber, halved lengthways, seeded and sliced across

20 fresh mint leaves, shredded

15 g (½ oz) fresh coriander, chopped

1 red onion, thinly sliced

2 Little Gem lettuces, separated into leaves

Thai lime dressing

2 tbsp sunflower oil

1 tbsp clear honey

grated zest and juice of 1 lime

2 tbsp Thai fish sauce

2 tbsp light soy sauce

1 fresh red chilli, or to taste, seeded and finely chopped

2 garlic cloves, crushed

To garnish

4 tbsp roasted peanuts, roughly chopped

sprigs of fresh mint

1 First make the dressing. Mix all the ingredients together in a small bowl. Spoon 3 tbsp over the steaks and set aside to marinate while you cook the rice. Reserve the remaining dressing.

2 Put the rice in a saucepan with the stock and lime leaves. Bring to the boil, then cover and leave to simmer for 10 minutes, or according to the packet instructions, until tender.

3 While the rice is cooking, pat the steaks dry with kitchen paper. Heat a ridged cast-iron grill pan or non-stick frying pan over a high heat until hot. Brush with the oil, then add the steaks and cook for 2½ minutes on each side. The meat will be rare. Cook longer if you prefer it medium or well done. Remove the steaks to a chopping board and leave to rest for a few minutes.

4 Place the papayas, cucumber, mint, coriander and red onion in a bowl. Add all but 2 tbsp of the remaining dressing and toss gently to mix.

5 Drain the rice well and divide among individual plates. Arrange the lettuce leaves on the plates and top with the papaya salad. Slice the beef into strips, arrange on top of the salad and spoon over the remaining dressing. Garnish with the peanuts and mint sprigs. Serve at room temperature.

Another idea

For a **Thai red curry and orange dressing**, mix together 2 tbsp sunflower oil, 2 tbsp light soy sauce, 1 tbsp light soft brown sugar, 1 tsp Thai red curry paste, ½ tsp grated orange zest and 3 tbsp orange juice.

Plus points

• Beef is an excellent source of zinc and a useful source of iron. Iron from red meat is far more easily absorbed by the body than iron from vegetable sources. Choose lean varieties.

• Papaya is a useful source of vitamin A (from the beta-carotene it provides), which is needed for good vision. This tropical fruit plays a vital role in preventing blindness in many parts of the world where those foods that provide most vitamin A in the UK (full-fat milk, cheese, butter, egg yolks) are not part of the average diet. Papaya also provides good amounts of vitamin C and useful amounts of the micromineral magnesium.

photo, page 89

Each serving provides kcal 563, protein 44 g, fat 13 g (of which saturated fat 5 g), carbohydrate 67 g (of which sugars 14 g), fibre 3 g. Excellent source of niacin, vitamin B₁, vitamin B₆, vitamin B₁₂, vitamin C, vitamin E, zinc. Good source of iron. Useful source of folate, potassium, selenium, vitamin A.

Veal escalopes with herbs

In this light summery dish, ultra-thin and tender veal escalopes are in and out of the pan in less than 5 minutes, after which the pan is quickly deglazed with wine to make a sauce and fresh herbs are added to pep up the flavour. New potatoes and spinach are excellent accompaniments.

Preparation and cooking time **about 45 minutes**   *Serves 4*

900 g (2 lb) baby new potatoes, scrubbed

4 veal escalopes, about 140 g (5 oz) each, beaten to 5 mm (¼ in) thickness

2 tbsp plain flour

1 tbsp extra virgin olive oil

2 tsp unsalted butter

400 g (14 oz) baby leaf spinach

grated zest and juice of 1 lemon

75 ml (2½ fl oz) dry white wine

4 tbsp chopped mixed fresh herbs, such as parsley, chervil, chives and tarragon

salt and pepper

To serve

lemon wedges

1 First cook the potatoes. Place them in a large saucepan of boiling water and boil for 15 minutes or until tender.

2 Meanwhile, pat the escalopes dry with kitchen paper. Season the flour with a little salt and pepper, then toss the escalopes in the flour to coat them lightly and evenly all over. Shake off any excess flour.

3 Heat half of the oil in a large non-stick frying pan over a moderate heat. Add half of the butter and heat until it starts to foam, then add the escalopes. Fry for 2–3 minutes on each side or until the juices run clear and not pink when the meat is pierced with a skewer or fork. You may need to cook the meat in 2 batches. Remove the escalopes from the pan with a draining spoon, place on a warmed serving dish and keep hot.

4 Drain the potatoes in a colander. Add the remaining 1 tbsp oil to the hot saucepan in which you cooked the potatoes and set over a low heat. Add the potatoes and toss gently until they are coated with oil. Add the spinach to the pan in 4 batches, gently tossing and stirring so that it wilts in the heat from the potatoes. Add the lemon juice, and season with salt and pepper to taste. Stir gently to mix. Cover and keep warm while you make the sauce.

5 Return the frying pan to the heat and add the wine. Increase the heat so the liquid bubbles, then stir vigorously to dislodge any bits of sediment in the pan. Boil for 1 minute or until reduced and syrupy, then season lightly. Remove the pan from the heat and add the rest of the butter. Stir until it has melted.

6 Scatter the mixed herbs over the escalopes, then drizzle with the wine sauce. Sprinkle the lemon zest over the potatoes and spinach. Serve the vegetables alongside the escalopes, with lemon wedges for squeezing.

Plus points

• This dish is especially rich in B vitamins. There is B_6 in the veal and the new potatoes, B_3 and B_{12} in the veal. The veal, spinach and new potatoes together provide an excellent source of folate.

• New potatoes in their skins and lemon juice are both good sources of vitamin C, which helps to provide resistance to infection from the common cold.

photo, page 89

Each serving provides kcal 400, protein 39 g, fat 10 g (of which saturated fat 3 g), carbohydrate 42 g (of which sugars 5 g), fibre 5 g. Excellent source of folate, niacin, vitamin A, vitamin B_1, vitamin B_6, vitamin B_{12}, vitamin E, zinc. Good source of calcium, iron, selenium, vitamin B_2.

Greek lamb kebabs

Cubes of lamb flavoured with a mixture of garlic, lemon and fresh oregano are cooked on skewers and served with a Greek-style tomato and cabbage salad and pitta bread for a deliciously aromatic main dish.

Preparation and cooking time **30 minutes**   *Serves 4*

1 tbsp extra virgin olive oil

2 large garlic cloves, crushed

juice of ½ lemon

1 tbsp chopped fresh oregano

450 g (1 lb) boneless leg of lamb, trimmed of all fat and cut into 2.5 cm (1 in) cubes

salt and pepper

Greek-style salad

6 tomatoes, thickly sliced

1 red onion, finely chopped

1 baby white cabbage, about 225 g (8 oz), core removed and thinly shredded

4 tbsp chopped fresh mint

¼ cucumber, halved and thinly sliced

juice of ½ lemon

1 tbsp extra virgin olive oil

To serve

4 pitta breads, cut into triangles

0% fat Greek-style yogurt (optional)

1 Preheat the grill or heat a ridged cast-iron grill pan. Put the olive oil, garlic, lemon juice and chopped oregano in a bowl and stir to mix together. Add the cubes of lamb and turn until very well coated. Thread the cubes onto 4 skewers.

2 Cook the lamb under the grill or on the grill pan for 7–8 minutes or until tender, turning frequently. Towards the end of cooking, warm the pitta bread under the grill or on the grill pan.

3 Meanwhile, make the salad. Put all the ingredients in a salad bowl and season with salt and pepper to taste. Toss together gently.

4 Serve the kebabs with the salad, pitta bread and yogurt.

Another idea

To make **chilli beef kebabs**, use 4 beef fillet or sirloin steaks, about 400 g (14 oz) in total, cut into 2.5 cm (1 in) cubes. Mix together 1 tsp chilli powder, ¼ tsp ground cumin, 1 tbsp extra virgin olive oil, 2 large garlic cloves, crushed, the juice of ½ lime and seasoning to taste. Coat the steak cubes on all sides with the spice mixture, then thread onto 4 skewers. Cook with 1 large sliced onion under the grill or on the ridged grill pan for 4–6 minutes or until tender, turning frequently. Take the skewers from the pan and continue cooking the onion until tender. Meanwhile, make the salad as in the main recipe. Remove the steak from the skewers and divide with the onion among 8 warmed flour tortillas. Add 1 tbsp bottled Caesar salad dressing and some of the salad to each tortilla, and roll up into wraps. Serve with the rest of the salad.

Plus points

• Lamb is a rich source of B vitamins, needed for a healthy nervous system. It is also a good source of zinc and iron.

• Cabbage contains a number of different phytochemicals that may help to protect against breast cancer. It is also a good source of vitamin C and among the richest vegetable sources of folate.

• Onions, along with chicory, leeks, garlic, Jerusalem artichokes, asparagus, barley and bananas, contain a type of dietary fibre called fructoligosaccarides (FOS). This is believed to stimulate the growth of friendly bacteria in the gut while inhibiting the growth of bad bacteria.

photo, page 89

Each serving provides kcal 470, protein 32 g, fat 16 g (of which saturated fat 5 g), carbohydrate 52 g (of which sugars 10 g), fibre 5 g. Excellent source of vitamin B_{12}, vitamin C. Good source of iron, vitamin A, vitamin B_6, vitamin E, zinc. Useful source of folate, niacin, potassium, vitamin B_1.

Lamb burgers with fruity relish

The advantage of making your own burgers is that you know exactly what's in them – and they can look and taste better than any takeaway while being a really healthy meal. An orange and raspberry relish adds a lovely fresh flavour to these juicy lamb burgers as well as lots of vitamins. Serve with a green or mixed salad.

Preparation and cooking time **30 minutes**   *Serves 4*

400 g (14 oz) lean minced lamb

1 carrot, about 125 g (4½ oz), grated

1 small onion, finely chopped

50 g (1¾ oz) fresh wholemeal breadcrumbs

pinch of freshly grated nutmeg

2 tsp fresh thyme leaves or 1 tsp dried thyme

1 large egg, beaten

2 tsp extra virgin olive oil

4 granary baps, weighing about 55 g (2 oz) each

salt and pepper

shredded lettuce to garnish

Orange and raspberry relish

1 orange

100 g (3½ oz) fresh or thawed frozen raspberries

2 tsp demerara sugar

1 Preheat the grill. Put the lamb into a large bowl. Add the carrot, onion, breadcrumbs, nutmeg and thyme, and season with salt and pepper to taste. Mix roughly with a spoon. Add the egg and use your hands to mix the ingredients together thoroughly.

2 Divide the mixture into 4 and shape each portion into a burger about 10–12 cm (4–5 in) in diameter, or about 2.5 cm (1 in) bigger than the diameter of the baps. Brush both sides of the burgers with oil, then put them in the grill pan. Cook for 4–5 minutes on each side, depending on thickness.

3 Meanwhile, make the relish. Cut the peel and pith from the orange with a sharp knife and, holding it over a bowl to catch the juice, cut between the membrane to release the segments. Roughly chop the segments and add them to the juice. Add the raspberries and sugar, lightly crushing the fruit with a fork to mix it together.

4 Split the baps and toast them briefly under the grill. Put a lamb burger in each bap and add some lettuce to garnish and a good spoonful of relish. Serve with the remaining relish.

Another idea

Make **turkey burgers with an orange and summer fruit relish**. Use minced turkey instead of lamb, and flavour with the zest of ½ lemon and 4 tbsp chopped parsley in place of the nutmeg and thyme; omit the breadcrumbs. Serve in toasted sesame buns, with rocket leaves and a relish made by simmering 100 g (3½ oz) frozen summer fruits until thawed, and mixing with 1 tbsp caster sugar and the chopped orange.

Plus points

• Although lamb still tends to contain more fat than other meats, changes in breeding, feeding and butchery techniques mean that lean cuts only contain about a hird of the fat that they would have 20 years ago. More of the fat is monounsaturated, which is good news for healthy hearts.

• Using granary baps instead of white ones doubles the amount of fibre. The bread also provides B-complex vitamins, iron and calcium. The seeds also help to reduce the rise in blood glucose.

• A fruity relish gives a huge bonus of protective antioxidants, and provides useful amounts of potassium and fibre.

Each serving provides kcal 390, protein 29 g, fat 13 g (of which saturated fat 5 g), carbohydrate 40 g (of which sugars 12 g), fibre 6 g. Excellent source of vitamin A, vitamin B$_{12}$. Good source of copper, iron, niacin, selenium, vitamin B$_1$, vitamin B$_6$, vitamin C, zinc. Useful source of calcium, folate, potassium, vitamin B$_2$.

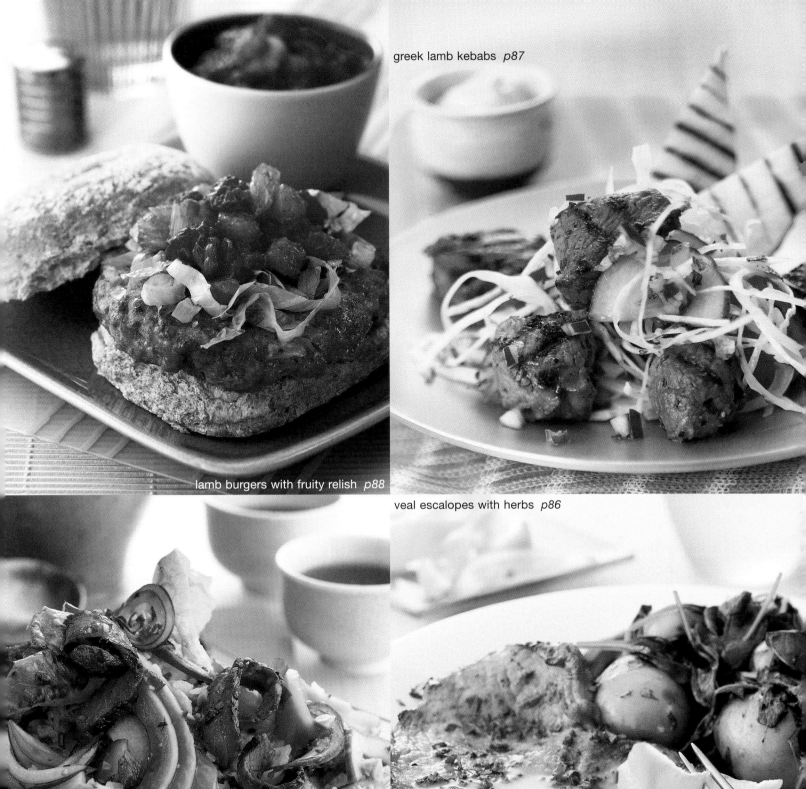

greek lamb kebabs *p87*

lamb burgers with fruity relish *p88*

veal escalopes with herbs *p86*

thai beef salad with papaya *p85*

Bulghur wheat salad with lamb

For this tasty dish, tender lamb fillet is quickly cooked under the grill, then cut up and mixed into a salad of bulghur wheat, red pepper, green olives and fresh mint. No oil is used to dress the salad, just fresh lemon and orange juices, so the fat content is kept healthily low.

Preparation and cooking time **about 40 minutes**   *Serves 4*

200 g (7 oz) bulghur wheat

400 g (14 oz) lamb neck fillet, trimmed of fat and cut in half lengthways

4 shallots, finely chopped

1 large red pepper, seeded and chopped

100 g (3½ oz) stoned green olives

½ cucumber, chopped

4 tbsp chopped fresh mint

juice of 1 lemon

grated zest and juice of 1 orange

2 Little Gem lettuces, sliced across into shreds

salt and pepper

1 Preheat the grill. Put the bulghur wheat in a mixing bowl, pour over enough boiling water to cover and stir well. Leave to soak for 15–20 minutes.

2 Meanwhile, grill the lamb pieces for 6–7 minutes on each side or until browned on the outside but still slightly pink inside. Remove from the heat and leave to rest in a warm place for 5–10 minutes, then slice into chunky pieces.

3 Put the shallots, red pepper, olives, cucumber and chopped mint in a salad bowl.

4 Drain the bulghur wheat in a sieve, pressing out excess water. Add to the salad bowl, together with the lemon and orange juices, the orange zest, and salt and pepper to taste. Toss to mix everything well.

5 Add the lamb and lettuce, and toss again. Serve immediately.

Another idea

Make a **spicy pork and bulghur wheat salad** with pineapple. Preheat the oven to 220ºC (425ºF, gas mark 7). Mix together the grated zest of ½ orange, the juice of 1 orange, 1 tbsp sunflower oil, 1 tbsp dark rum or soy sauce, 2 tbsp muscovado sugar, 1 large crushed garlic clove, and ½ tsp each ground cinnamon, ground allspice and pepper in a shallow ovenproof dish. Add 400 g (14 oz) pork fillet (tenderloin) and turn to coat with the mixture. Roast for 25 minutes or until tender but still moist. Meanwhile, soak the bulghur wheat as in the main recipe, then mix with ½ sweet ripe pineapple, peeled, cored and chopped, 1 large red pepper, seeded and chopped, 4 shallots, thinly sliced, the juice of 1 orange, 55 g (2 oz) watercress sprigs and 1 tbsp chopped fresh coriander. Season to taste. Spoon onto 4 plates. Slice the pork and arrange on top of the salad. Spoon over the cooking juices and serve immediately.

Plus points

• Lamb is an excellent source of zinc, which is necessary for healing wounds. Lamb also provides useful amounts of iron.

• Olives contain about 18 per cent fat by weight, and most of this is healthy monounsaturated fat.

• Bulghur wheat makes a refreshing alternative to potatoes, and it has a relatively lower Glycaemic Index.

photo, page 93

Each serving provides   kcal 395, protein 27 g, fat 12 g (of which saturated fat 4 g), carbohydrate 45 g (of which sugars 6 g), fibre 3 g. Excellent source of niacin, viatamin A, vitamin B$_1$, vitamin B$_6$, vitamin B$_{12}$, vitamin C, vitamin E, zinc. Good source of copper, folate, iron, vitamin B$_2$. Useful source of potassium.

Spring lamb and vegetable stew

Based on a classic French dish called *navarin*, this is a delectable stew. In France it is made in spring, as a celebration of the new season's lamb and the delicate young vegetables. Serve with a dish of freshly cooked spring greens, and hand round a basket of crusty French bread.

Preparation time **30 minutes**   Cooking time **1¾–2 hours**   *Serves 4*

2 tbsp extra virgin olive oil

1 large onion, chopped

1 garlic clove, finely chopped

450 g (1 lb) lean boneless leg of lamb, trimmed of fat and cut into cubes

150 ml (5 fl oz) dry white wine

450 ml (15 fl oz) lamb or chicken stock

1 bay leaf

1 sprig of fresh thyme

900 g (2 lb) baby new potatoes, scrubbed

225 g (8 oz) baby carrots

150 g (5½ oz) button onions

200 g (7 oz) small turnips, diced

250 g (8½ oz) shelled fresh peas or 125 g (4½ oz) frozen peas

2 tbsp chopped parsley

salt and pepper

1 Preheat the oven to 180°C (350°F, gas mark 4). Heat the oil in a large flameproof casserole, add the chopped onion and garlic and cook, stirring, for 5 minutes or until softened. Add the cubes of lamb and cook for 5 minutes or until browned on all sides, stirring so they colour evenly.

2 Add the wine, stock, bay leaf, thyme, potatoes, carrots and button onions. Season with salt and pepper to taste. Bring to the boil, then cover with a tight-fitting lid and transfer to the oven. Cook for 1 hour.

3 Add the turnips and stir. Cover the casserole again and continue cooking for 30–45 minutes or until the meat and vegetables are tender, adding the peas 10 minutes before the end of the cooking time.

4 Add the parsley and stir well. Taste and add more salt and pepper if needed. Serve hot.

Some more ideas

For a lamb stew with a Provençal flavour, use red wine instead of white. Omit the stock and add 1 can chopped tomatoes, about 400 g, with the juice, and a large sprig of fresh rosemary. When you add the peas, also stir in 50 g (1¾ oz) stoned black olives.

Mange-tout or French beans can be used instead of the peas.

Plus points

• Peas provide good amounts of the B vitamins B_1, B_6 and niacin. They also provide dietary fibre, particularly the soluble variety, some folate and vitamin C. Frozen vegetables are just as nutritious as fresh, and in many cases they have been shown to contain higher levels of vitamin C.

• In addition to providing fibre, turnips contain the B vitamins niacin and B_6, and are a useful source of vitamin C.

photo, page 93

Each serving provides   kcal 495, protein 31 g, fat 16 g (of which saturated fat 5 g), carbohydrate 52 g (of which sugars 14 g), fibre 8 g. Excellent source of folate, niacin, vitamin A, vitamin B_1, vitamin B_6, vitamin B_{12}, vitamin C, vitamin E, zinc. Good source of iron. Useful source of selenium, vitamin B_2.

Spanish rabbit and chickpea stew

In Spain, the home of this spicy dish, chickpeas are very popular and are often stewed with a small amount of meat and a vegetable or two to make hearty one-pot feasts. Serve this with chunks of rustic sourdough bread on the side, so that you can dip it in to enjoy every drop of the delicious gravy.

Preparation time **20 minutes**   Cooking time **about 1½ hours**   *Serves 4*

2 tbsp extra virgin olive oil

340 g (12 oz) boneless rabbit, cut into large chunks

2 onions, roughly chopped

3 garlic cloves, chopped

1 large red pepper, seeded and roughly chopped

1 tbsp paprika, preferably smoked

½ tsp mild chilli powder

½ tsp ground cumin

large pinch of ground cinnamon

2 bay leaves

250 ml (8½ fl oz) dry white wine

250 ml (8½ fl oz) chicken stock

1 can chopped tomatoes, about 225 g

2 tbsp tomato purée

3 tbsp chopped fresh flat-leaf parsley

2 pinches of saffron threads

4 tbsp hot water

1 can chickpeas, about 400 g, drained and rinsed

225 g (8 oz) new potatoes, scrubbed and halved

2 sprigs of fresh oregano or marjoram, leaves coarsely chopped

grated zest and juice of 1 small orange, preferably a blood orange

salt and pepper

1 Heat the oil in a flameproof casserole, add the chunks of rabbit and sauté until browned on all sides. Add the onions, garlic and red pepper and fry, stirring frequently, for 5 minutes or until the onions have softened. Add the paprika, chilli powder, cumin, cinnamon and bay leaves, stir well and fry for 1 minute.

2 Add the wine, stock, tomatoes with their juice, tomato purée and half of the parsley. Cover and bring to the boil, then reduce the heat to very low and simmer for about 40 minutes or until the rabbit is very tender. Meanwhile, crumble the saffron into a small bowl and add the hot water. Stir, then leave to soak for 15–20 minutes.

3 Add the chickpeas and potatoes to the stew, together with the saffron and its soaking water, the oregano or marjoram, and orange zest and juice. Stir, then simmer for 25–30 minutes or until the gravy has thickened and is not too soupy. Taste and add seasoning if needed, and remove the bay leaves if you prefer. Serve hot, sprinkled with the remaining parsley.

Another idea

Instead of rabbit, use lean pork fillet (tenderloin) or lamb fillet or boneless leg, trimmed of fat and cut into bite-sized chunks.

Plus points

● Chickpeas are an important source of vegetable protein in many parts of the world, and they are a good source of soluble dietary fibre. In this recipe the chickpeas provide a greater amount of iron per portion than the rabbit (1.5 mg compared with 0.9 mg). The absorption of the iron is helped by the generous amounts of vitamin C provided by the vegetables, in particular red pepper.

● Rabbit is an excellent low-fat source of protein. It can be substituted for chicken breast in many recipes because its pale-coloured meat looks and tastes quite similar. Nutritionally, it contains twice as much iron as chicken breast.

Each serving provides   kcal 417, protein 33 g, fat 15 g (of which saturated fat 3 g), carbohydrate 41 g (of which sugars 14 g), fibre 9 g. Excellent source of niacin, vitamin A, vitamin B$_1$, vitamin B$_6$, vitamin B$_{12}$, vitamin C, vitamin E. Good source of folate, iron, selenium, vitamin B$_2$, zinc.

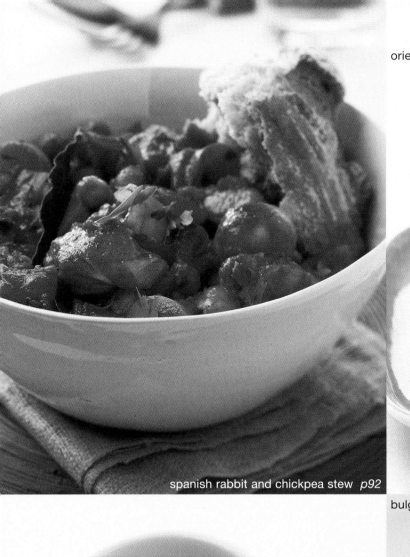

spanish rabbit and chickpea stew *p92*

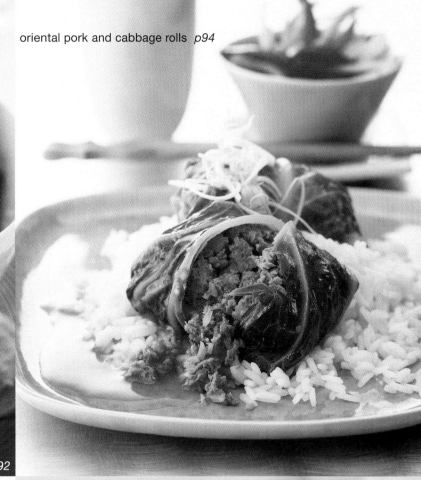

oriental pork and cabbage rolls *p94*

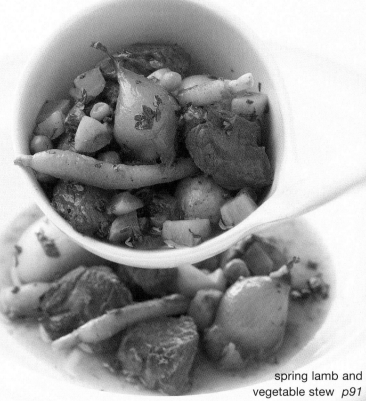

spring lamb and
vegetable stew *p91*

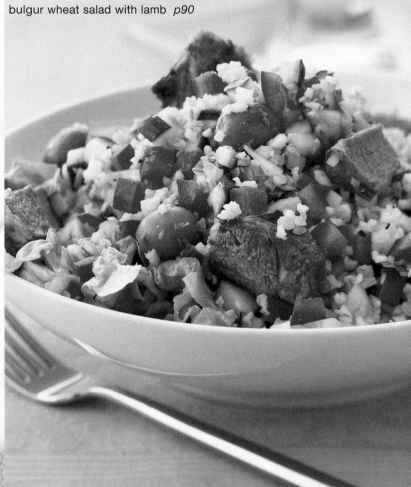

bulgur wheat salad with lamb *p90*

Oriental pork and cabbage rolls

Crunchy water chestnuts are combined with minced pork, soy sauce, fresh ginger and five-spice powder to make a flavoursome, Oriental-style filling for fresh green cabbage leaves. Serve with steamed white rice and a simple red pepper, chicory and onion salad for a quick-and-easy family meal.

Preparation time **10 minutes**   Cooking time **15 minutes**   *Serves 4*

500 g (1 lb 2 oz) extra-lean minced pork

1 can water chestnuts, about 220 g, drained and finely chopped

2 tsp five-spice powder

1 tbsp finely grated fresh root ginger

2 spring onions, finely chopped

2 tbsp dark soy sauce

2 garlic cloves, crushed

1 egg, beaten

8 large green cabbage leaves

450 ml (15 fl oz) hot chicken stock

2 tsp cornflour

1 tsp sweet chilli sauce, or to taste

curled strips of spring onion garnish

1 Place the pork in a bowl and add the water chestnuts, five-spice powder, ginger, spring onions, soy sauce, garlic and egg. Mix thoroughly with your hands or a fork until the ingredients are well blended, then divide into 8 equal portions.

2 Cut the tough stalk from the base of each cabbage leaf with a sharp knife. Place a portion of the pork mixture in the centre of each cabbage leaf, then wrap the leaf around the filling to enclose it.

3 Pour the stock into the bottom section of a large steamer. Arrange the cabbage rolls, join side down, in one layer in the top section. Steam for 15 minutes or until the cabbage is tender and the rolls are firm when pressed. Remove the top section from the steamer and keep the cabbage rolls hot.

4 Mix the cornflour with 2 tbsp water, then stir this mixture into the stock in the bottom of the steamer. Bring to the boil and simmer, stirring constantly, until slightly thickened. Add the chilli sauce.

5 Serve the cabbage rolls with the sauce spooned over and sprinkled with curls of spring onion.

Another idea

For **Chinese pork balls with wilted greens**, shape the pork mixture into 16 balls. Place in the steamer over the pan of stock and steam for 12 minutes. Meanwhile, heat 1 tbsp sunflower oil in a wok and stir-fry 1 sliced bunch of spring onions with 200 g (7 oz) broccoli florets and 200 g (7 oz) sugarsnap peas for 4 minutes. Add 4 tbsp water and 200 g (7 oz) pak choy separated into leaves, and stir-fry for a further 3 minutes. Finally, add 4 tbsp oyster sauce, or to taste. Serve the vegetables topped with the pork balls.

Plus points

• Extra-lean minced pork is lower in fat than minced beef or lamb and only slightly fattier than skinless chicken breast.

• Water chestnuts provide small amounts of potassium, iron and fibre, but their big advantage is that they contain no fat and very few calories.

• Cabbage, like broccoli and cauliflower, contains flavonoids, which research has shown help to suppress cancer-causing cells. It also contains the beneficial anti-cancer antioxidants, vitamins C and E.

photo, page 93

Each serving provides kcal 234, protein 32 g, fat 7 g (of which saturated fat 2 g), carbohydrate 12 g (of which sugars 5 g), fibre 2 g. Excellent source of niacin, vitamin B_1, vitamin B_2, vitamin B_6, vitamin B_{12}, vitamin C. Good source of folate, selenium, zinc. Useful source of copper, iron, vitamin A.

Sesame pork and noodle salad

With its typical Chinese flavours – ginger, sesame, soy sauce and rice vinegar – this salad makes a delectable lunch or supper dish. It is very nutritious as most of the vegetables are raw. For the best effect, cut the pepper, carrot and spring onions about the same thickness as the noodles.

Preparation and cooking time **45 minutes**   *Serves 4*

400 g (14 oz) pork fillet (tenderloin)

2 tsp grated fresh root ginger

1 large garlic clove, finely chopped

1½ tsp toasted sesame oil

3 tbsp light soy sauce

2 tbsp dry sherry

2 tsp rice vinegar

225 g (8 oz) fine Chinese egg noodles

1 red pepper, seeded and cut into matchstick strips

1 large carrot, cut into matchstick strips

6 spring onions, cut into matchstick strips

250 g (8½ oz) bean sprouts

150 g (5½ oz) mange-tout

2 tbsp sesame seeds

1 tbsp sunflower oil

1 Trim all visible fat from the pork fillet. Cut the pork across into slices about 5 cm (2 in) thick, then cut each slice into thin strips.

2 Combine the ginger, garlic, sesame oil, soy sauce, sherry and vinegar in a bowl. Add the pork strips and toss to coat, then leave to marinate while you prepare the other ingredients.

3 Put the noodles in a large mixing bowl and pour over enough boiling water to cover generously. Leave to soak for about 4 minutes, or according to the packet instructions, until tender. Drain well and tip back into the bowl. Add the red pepper, carrot, spring onions and bean sprouts.

4 Drop the mange-tout into a pan of boiling water and cook for about 1 minute or until just tender but still crisp. Drain and refresh under cold running water. Add the mange-tout to the noodle and vegetable mixture and toss to mix. Set aside.

5 Toast the sesame seeds in a large frying pan over a moderate heat for 1–2 minutes or until golden, stirring constantly. Tip the seeds onto a piece of kitchen paper. Heat the sunflower oil in the frying pan, increase the heat slightly and add the pork with its marinade. Stir-fry for 4–5 minutes or until the pork is no longer pink.

6 Add the strips of pork and any cooking juices to the noodle and vegetable mixture, and stir gently to combine. Divide among 4 shallow bowls, sprinkle with the toasted sesame seeds and serve.

Plus points

• In the past, pork has had a reputation for being rather fatty, but this is certainly no longer the case. Over the past 20 years, in response to consumer demands, farmers have been breeding leaner pigs. Pork now contains considerably less fat, and it also contains higher levels of the 'good' polyunsaturated fats. The average fat content of lean pork is less than 3 per cent, much the same as that contained in skinless chicken breast.

• The vegetables in this dish provide a good variety of different nutrients, in particular vitamin C and beta-carotene.

photo, page 97

Each serving provides   kcal 454, protein 33 g, fat 13 g (of which saturated fat 3 g), carbohydrate 51 g (of which sugars 9 g), fibre 5 g. Excellent source of niacin, vitamin A, vitamin B$_1$, vitamin B$_6$, vitamin B$_{12}$, vitamin C, vitamin E. Good source of copper, folate, iron, vitamin B$_2$, zinc. Useful source of potassium, selenium.

Sweet and sour pork

Sweet and sour sauce doesn't have to be thick, gloopy and bright orange. This modern, light version allows the succulence of the meat and the fresh flavours and different textures of a colourful variety of vegetables and noodles to shine through. Some plainly cooked rice is all that is needed to complete the meal.

Preparation time **35 minutes**   Cooking time **15 minutes**   *Serves 4*

340 g (12 oz) pork fillet (tenderloin), trimmed of fat and cut into 5 x 1 cm (2 x ½ in) strips

1 tbsp light soy sauce

2 tsp cornflour

2 sheets medium Chinese egg noodles, about 125 g (4½ oz) in total

2 tbsp sunflower oil

8 baby corn, about 75 g (2½ oz) in total, quartered lengthways

170 g (6 oz) carrots, cut into fine shreds about 5 cm (2 in) long

1 large garlic clove, finely chopped

1 tbsp finely diced fresh root ginger

300 g (10½ oz) bean sprouts

4 spring onions, sliced diagonally

1 tsp toasted sesame oil

pepper

Sweet and sour sauce

1 tbsp cornflour

1 tbsp demerara sugar

1 tbsp rice wine vinegar

2 tbsp rice wine or dry sherry

2 tbsp tomato ketchup

3 tbsp light soy sauce

1 can pineapple slices in natural juice, about 425 g, drained and chopped, with juice reserved

1 Place the pork strips in a bowl, sprinkle over the soy sauce and pepper to taste and stir to coat the meat. Sprinkle over the cornflour and stir again. Cover and set aside.

2 To make the sauce, mix together the cornflour, sugar, vinegar, rice wine or sherry, ketchup, soy sauce and reserved pineapple juice in a small bowl. Set aside.

3 Cook the noodles in a saucepan of boiling water for 3 minutes, or cook or soak them according to the packet instructions. Drain well and set aside.

4 Heat a wok or heavy-based frying pan until really hot, then add 1 tbsp of the oil and swirl to coat the wok. Add the pork and leave for 1 minute to brown, then stir-fry over a high heat for 3–4 minutes. Remove the pork with a draining spoon and set aside.

5 Heat the remaining oil in the wok, then add the corn and stir-fry for 1 minute. Add the carrots, garlic and ginger and stir-fry for another minute. Sprinkle over 5 tbsp water and let the vegetables steam for 2–3 minutes.

6 Pour in the sauce mixture, stir well and bring to the boil. Put the meat back in the wok and add the noodles, pineapple and bean sprouts. Heat through, stirring and tossing. Add the spring onions and sesame oil and serve.

Some more ideas

For a hotter sauce, add 1 small fresh red chilli, seeded and finely chopped.

Use boneless pork shoulder instead of fillet.

Plus points

• Over the past 20 years, farmers have been breeding leaner pigs, and pork now contains considerably less fat than it did in the past. The average fat content is much the same as skinless chicken breast.

• Bean sprouts are rich in vitamin C and several of the B vitamins; they also provide some potassium. Adding them at the last minute preserves as much of their vitamin C content as possible.

Each serving provides kcal 369, protein 25 g, fat 11 g (of which saturated fat 2 g), carbohydrate 45 g (of which sugars 2 g), fibre 4 g. Excellent source of folate, niacin, vitamin A, vitamin B_1, vitamin B_6, vitamin B_{12}, vitamin C, vitamin E. Good source of iron, vitamin B_2, zinc. Useful source of selenium.

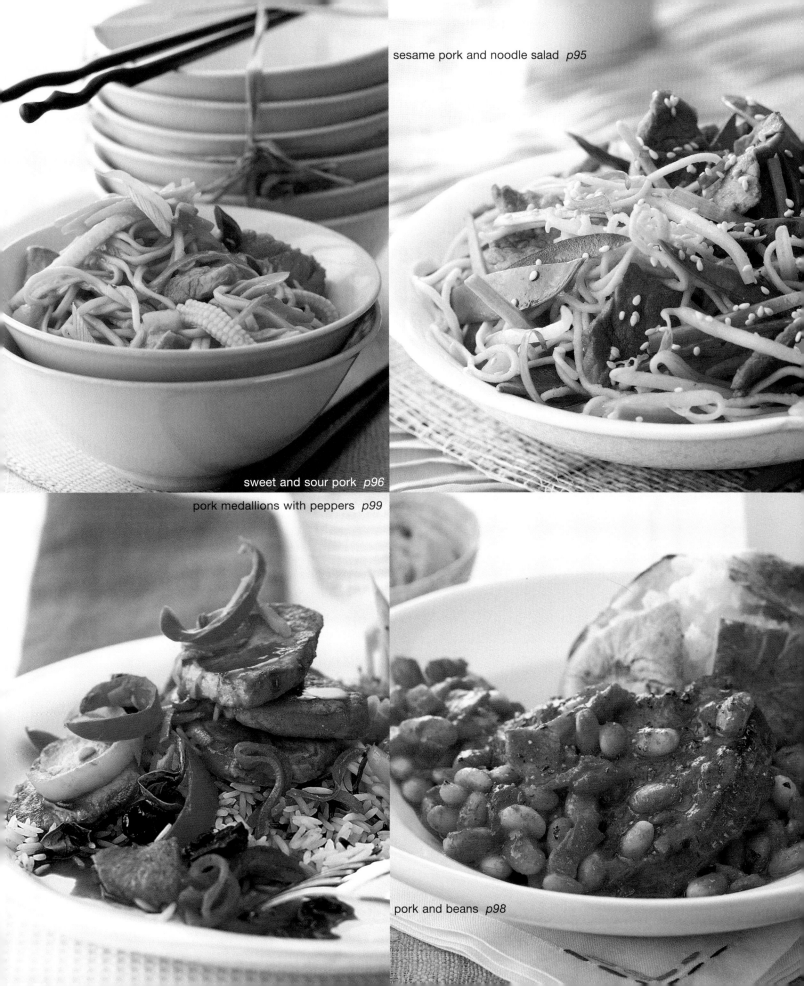

sesame pork and noodle salad *p95*

sweet and sour pork *p96*

pork medallions with peppers *p99*

pork and beans *p98*

Pork and beans

This is a dish from the Eastern seaboard of America, where the pork and beans are traditionally simmered slowly in an earthenware casserole. It is the kind of dish that you can prepare ahead and leave to bubble away while you tend to other things. Baked jacket potatoes and crusty bread are perfect for soaking up the delicious sauce.

Preparation time **25 minutes, plus overnight soaking**   Cooking time **about 2 hours**   *Serves 4*

250 g (8½ oz) dried white haricot beans, soaked overnight in cold water

1 tbsp sunflower oil

4 thin lean pork chump chops, about 625 g (1 lb 6 oz) in total, trimmed of fat

1 onion, chopped

250 ml (8½ fl oz) beer, such as dark ale, or lager or cider

1 can chopped tomatoes, about 400 g

2 tsp Worcestershire sauce, or to taste

2 tbsp dark soft brown sugar

3 allspice berries

2 tbsp mild American or French mustard

2 smoked lean back bacon rashers, rinded and cut into bite-sized pieces

1 tsp cider vinegar, or to taste

1 Drain and rinse the beans, then place them in a large saucepan and pour over enough cold water to come up to about twice the depth of the beans. Cover the pan with its lid and bring to the boil. Skim off any scum, then reduce the heat to low, cover the pan again and cook the beans for 45–60 minutes or until they are just tender.

2 Meanwhile, heat the oil in a deep flameproof casserole, add the pork chops and onion, and fry until the chops are browned on both sides. Pour in the beer and tomatoes with their juice, then add the Worcestershire sauce, sugar and allspice. Reduce the heat, cover and cook for about 1 hour or until the meat is very tender.

3 Drain the beans and add to the pork chops. Add the mustard, bacon and vinegar and stir well to mix. Cook, covered, over a low heat for a further hour or until the beans and the pork are meltingly tender.

4 Before serving, taste for seasoning and add a dash or two more Worcestershire sauce or vinegar if liked.

Some more ideas

Instead of soaking and cooking dried beans, add a can of cannellini beans, about 400 g, drained and rinsed, at the beginning of step 3.

Make **Tuscan-style beans with sausages**. Use 500 g (1 lb 2 oz) high-meat-content sausages, cut into bite-sized pieces, instead of the pork chops. Brown the sausages with the onion in a deep, non-stick frying pan; set aside. Pour off fat from the pan (do not add fat), then add 125 ml (4½ fl oz) red wine, 200 ml (7 fl oz) vegetable stock, 1 can chopped tomatoes, about 400 g, with the juice, 8 chopped fresh sage leaves, 2 bay leaves, 2 crushed garlic cloves and pepper to taste. Cook uncovered over a low heat for 30 minutes. Add the sausages and onion together with 1 can cannellini beans, about 400 g, drained and rinsed, and simmer for 15 minutes.

Plus points

• Tomatoes contain lycopene, a carotenoid compound and a valuable antioxidant that is thought to protect against prostate, bladder and pancreatic cancers. Lycopene is enhanced by cooking and so is most readily available in processed tomato products, such as canned tomatoes, tomato purée and passata, and tomato ketchup.

photo, page 97

Each serving provides   kcal 490, protein 51 g, fat 11 g (of which saturated fat 3 g), carbohydrate 46 g (of which sugars 16 g), fibre 12 g. Excellent source of iron, niacin, vitamin B_1, vitamin B_2, vitamin B_6, vitamin B_{12}, vitamin E, zinc. Good source of calcium, vitamin C. Useful source of folate.

Pork medallions with peppers

This quick sauté makes an excellent dinner party dish, with its well-balanced sweet and sour elements coming from balsamic vinegar, oranges and olives. It is especially good – and extra nutritious – served with broccoli.

Preparation and cooking time **about 50 minutes**   *Serves 4*

340 g (12 oz) mixed basmati and wild rice

600 ml (1 pint) boiling water

2 oranges

1 tbsp extra virgin olive oil

340 g (12 oz) pork fillet (tenderloin), sliced across into medallions 1 cm (½ in) thick

1 large sweet onion, such as Vidalia, Spanish or red, halved lengthways and thinly sliced into half rings

1 red pepper, seeded and sliced into strips

1 yellow pepper, seeded and sliced into strips

1 large carrot, grated

1 garlic clove, finely chopped

90 ml (3 fl oz) orange juice

3 tbsp balsamic vinegar

30 g (1 oz) stoned black olives, chopped or sliced

30 g (1 oz) fresh basil leaves

salt and pepper

1 Put the rice in a saucepan and pour over the boiling water. Bring back to the boil, then reduce the heat to low. Cover and simmer for about 15 minutes, or according to the packet instructions, until the rice is tender and all the water has been absorbed.

2 Meanwhile, peel the oranges and cut them crossways into slices about 1 cm (½ in) thick. Stack the slices 3 or 4 at a time and cut into quarters. (If possible, use a chopping board with a well to catch the juices.) Set the orange slices and juice aside.

3 Heat the oil in a large non-stick frying pan over a moderately high heat. Cook the pork medallions, in batches, for 2–3 minutes on each side. Remove the meat with a draining spoon and set aside.

4 Reduce the heat to moderate and add the onion, pepper strips, carrot and garlic to the pan. Cover and cook, stirring frequently, for 5–6 minutes or until the vegetables start to soften. Add 2 tbsp water, then the measured orange juice and the balsamic vinegar. Stir well to mix. Cover and cook for 3–4 minutes or until the vegetables are tender.

5 Return the pork to the pan. Add the olives, orange slices and their juice and the basil leaves. Cook for 1 minute to reheat the pork, stirring well. Taste and add salt and pepper, if needed.

6 To serve, divide the rice among 4 warmed plates and place the pork medallions and vegetables on top. Drizzle over any juices in the pan and serve.

Another idea

For **lamb with peppers and Puy lentils**, use lean lamb neck fillets or boneless lean lamb leg steaks, beaten thin, instead of pork fillet, and substitute 250 g (8½ oz) Puy lentils, cooked according to the packet instructions, for the rice. Omit the basil and flavour the lamb with ½ tsp chopped fresh rosemary.

Plus points

● Wild rice comes from North America. It is not a true rice, but the seeds of a wild aquatic grass. It is gluten-free, like the basmati rice it is mixed with here, and contains useful amounts of B vitamins, particularly niacin, as well as dietary fibre.

photo, page 97

Each serving provides   kcal 539, protein 27 g, fat 8 g (of which saturated fat 2 g), carbohydrate 89 g (of which sugars 19 g), fibre 5 g. Excellent source of niacin, vitamin A, vitamin B$_1$, vitamin B$_6$, vitamin B$_{12}$. Good source of folate, vitamin B$_2$. Useful source of iron, potassium, selenium, zinc.

Five-spice pork

The simple Oriental technique of stir-frying is perfect for preparing meals in a hurry. It is also a great healthy cooking method because it uses just a small amount of oil and cooks vegetables quickly so that most of their beneficial vitamins and minerals are preserved.

Preparation and cooking time **30 minutes**   *Serves 4*

400 g (14 oz) pork fillet (tenderloin), trimmed of fat

250 g (8½ oz) medium Chinese egg noodles

1 tbsp sunflower oil

1 large onion, finely chopped

1 large garlic clove, crushed

1 tbsp five-spice powder

300 g (10½ oz) mange-tout or sugarsnap peas

2 large red peppers (or 1 red and 1 yellow or orange), seeded and thinly sliced

120 ml (4 fl oz) hot vegetable stock

salt and pepper

fresh coriander leaves to garnish

1 Cut the pork fillet across into 5 mm (¼ in) slices, then cut each slice into 5 mm (¼ in) strips. Cover and set aside.

2 Cook the noodles in a saucepan of boiling water for 4 minutes, or cook or soak them according to the packet instructions. Drain the noodles well and set aside.

3 While the noodles are cooking, heat a wok or a large heavy-based frying pan until hot. Add the oil and swirl to coat the wok, then add the onion and garlic and stir-fry for 1 minute. Add the five-spice powder and stir-fry for another minute.

4 Add the pork strips to the wok and stir-fry for 3 minutes. Add the mange-tout or sugarsnap peas and the peppers and stir-fry for a further 2 minutes. Pour in the stock, stir well and bring to the boil.

5 Add the noodles to the wok and stir and toss for 2–3 minutes or until all the ingredients are well combined. Season to taste and serve immediately, sprinkled with coriander leaves.

Some more ideas

To reduce the fat content of this dish even further, use just 250 g (8½ oz) pork and add 250 g (8½ oz) firm tofu. Drain the tofu well and

cut it into 2.5 cm (1 in) cubes, then add in step 5 with the mange-tout and peppers. Add 2 tbsp light soy sauce with the stock.

For a vegetarian dish, replace the pork with 450 g (1 lb) drained and diced firm tofu and add 140 g (5 oz) broccoli florets. Add the tofu and broccoli with the mange-tout and peppers in step 5, and add 75 g (2½ oz) bean sprouts with the noodles in step 6.

Plus points

• Peppers have a naturally waxy skin that helps to protect them against oxidisation and prevents loss of vitamin C during storage. As a result, their vitamin C content remains high even several weeks after harvesting.

• Heating the pan until hot before adding any oil not only helps to prevent ingredients sticking, it also means less oil is needed.

• Chinese egg noodles are a low-fat source of starchy carbohydrate as well as offering some protein. When they are eaten with ingredients high in vitamin C, such as the peppers in this recipe, the body is better able to absorb the iron they contain.

Each serving provides kcal 467, protein 34 g, fat 13 g (of which saturated fat 3 g), carbohydrate 58 g (of which sugars 12 g), fibre 6 g. Excellent source of niacin, vitamin A, vitamin B$_1$, vitamin B$_6$, vitamin B$_{12}$, vitamin C, vitamin E. Good source of folate, potassium, vitamin B$_2$. Useful source of calcium, folate, selenium.

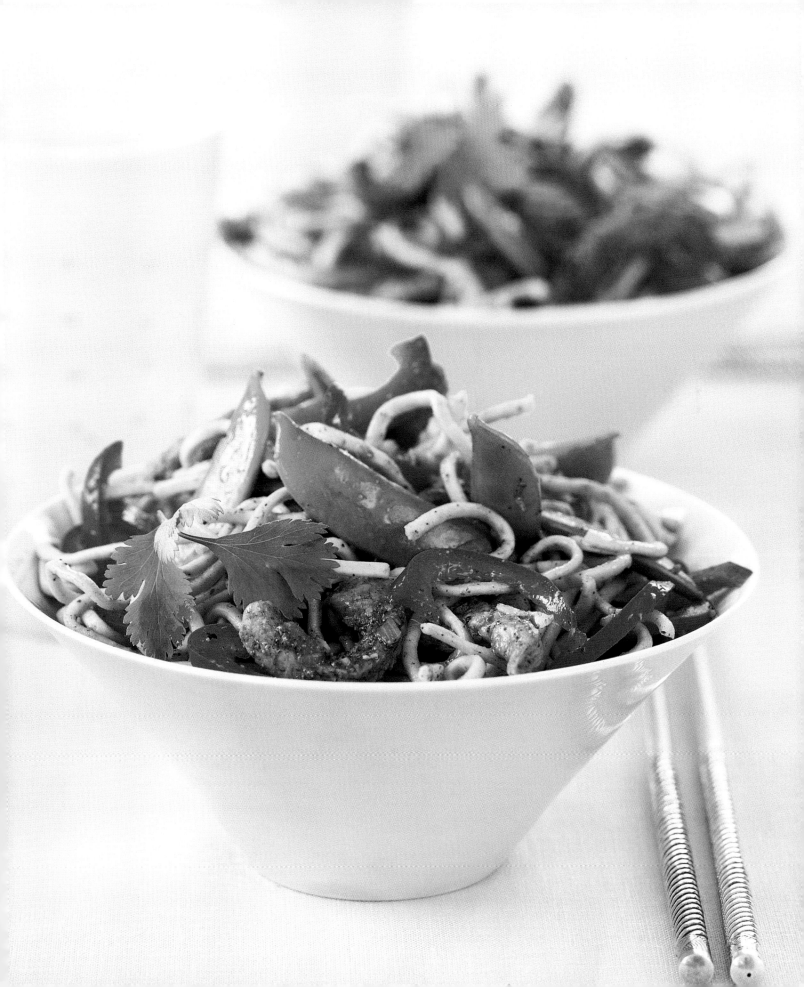

Japanese chicken salad

The ingredients for this salad are presented individually on a platter rather than being mixed together, with a simple tahini-based dressing so everyone can help themselves. Typical of Japanese cooking, there is a fairly small amount of meat per person, but plenty of raw vegetables to crunch through and fill you up.

Preparation time **25–30 minutes, plus cooling**   Cooking time **10 minutes**   *Serves 4*

2 skinless boneless chicken breasts (fillets), about 300 g (10½ oz) in total

1 tbsp mirin or sake

salt and pepper

Tahini dressing

2 tbsp tahini

1 small garlic clove, crushed

1 tbsp soy sauce

2 tsp lemon juice, or to taste

chilli powder to garnish

Salad

10 cm (4 in) piece cucumber

2 carrots

1 red pepper, seeded

2 Little Gem lettuces, separated into leaves

handful of fresh basil leaves, finely shredded

handful of fresh mint leaves, finely shredded

8 spring onions, halved lengthways

115 g (4 oz) button mushrooms, thinly sliced

1 Place the chicken breasts on a heatproof plate in a steamer set over gently boiling water. Sprinkle with the mirin or sake and a little seasoning. Cover and steam for 10–12 minutes or until cooked. Set aside to cool.

2 To make the dressing, mix all the ingredients, except the chilli powder, in a bowl. Drain the cooking juices from the chicken and make up to 4 tbsp with water. Add to the dressing. Taste and add more lemon juice, if necessary. Pour into a serving bowl and sprinkle with a pinch of chilli powder.

3 For the salad, cut the cucumber, carrots and red pepper into fine strips of similar length, about 5 cm (2 in). Arrange the lettuce leaves at one end of a large platter. Scatter over the shredded basil and mint. Cut the chicken into strips and place on the lettuce. Arrange all the other salad ingredients attractively on the platter. Serve with the dressing in a separate bowl for people to help themselves.

Some more ideas

Make a **Chinese-style salad** by halving the amount of carrot, cucumber and red pepper and add instead ½ can of bamboo shoots,

well drained, about 12 canned water chestnuts, thinly sliced, 125 g (4½ oz) fresh bean sprouts, and a few baby sweetcorn, cooked and sliced lengthways. Mix the salad ingredients together and pile them high in a large bowl. Make a dressing from 4 tbsp bottled plum sauce, 2 tbsp soy sauce, 2 tbsp toasted sesame oil and 1–2 tsp lemon juice with a pinch of caster sugar. Sprinkle a few toasted sesame seeds on top.

For a **vegetarian salad**, use 250 g (9 oz) marinated or smoked tofu, sliced or diced, instead of the steamed chicken.

Plus points

• Because all the vegetables are eaten raw, this salad offers lots of vitamin C. The vegetables are also an excellent source of fibre and of beta-carotene, which with vitamin C plays a role in protecting against cancer.

• Mushrooms provide useful amounts of some of the B vitamins as well as good quantities of the trace mineral copper. Copper is a component of many enzymes and is needed for bone growth and the formation of connective tissues.

photo, page 105

Each serving provides   kcal 170, protein 20 g, fat 7.5 g (of which saturated fat 1.5 g), carbohydrate 6 g (of which sugars 5.5 g), fibre 3 g. Excellent source of vitamin A, vitamin B$_6$, vitamin C. Good source of copper, folate, iron, niacin. Useful source of potassium, selenium, vitamin B$_1$, vitamin B$_2$, zinc.

Creamy chicken salad with ginger

This creamy yet light chicken salad is ideal for serving as a luncheon or cold buffet dish. Basing the dressing on low-fat Greek-style yogurt mixed with reduced-fat mayonnaise makes it lower in fat than many other creamy dressings while still keeping the richness. Don't be tempted to omit the stem ginger – its subtle flavour makes all the difference.

Preparation time **20–25 minutes**   *Serves 6*

1 cold roasted chicken, about 1.5 kg (3 lb 3 oz), or 675 g (1½ lb) cooked chicken meat

1 tbsp lime juice

2 crisp, green-skinned dessert apples such as Granny Smith

4 celery sticks, thinly sliced

115 g (4 oz) ready-to-eat dried apricots, quartered

5 tbsp 0% fat Greek-style yogurt

2 tbsp reduced-fat mayonnaise

2 pieces stem ginger, finely diced

30 g (1 oz) broken walnuts

pepper

sprigs of watercress to garnish

1 If using a whole roast chicken, remove the meat from the carcass, discarding the skin. Cut the chicken meat into bite-sized pieces and place in a large serving bowl.

2 Put the lime juice in a small bowl. Core and chop the apples, then add them to the lime juice and toss well to coat the apple pieces (this will prevent them from turning brown). Add the apples, celery and apricots to the chicken and mix together.

3 Next, combine the yogurt and mayonnaise in another small bowl and season with pepper. Stir in the stem ginger. Spoon this dressing over the chicken salad and toss until all the pieces are coated. Sprinkle over the walnuts and serve garnished with watercress.

Some more ideas

Serve this at Christmas time, using leftover turkey instead of chicken.

Substitute ready-to-eat dried pears for the dried apricots.

Add 85 g (3 oz) seedless green grapes, halved, or 2 slices of fresh pineapple, cut into wedges.

Use toasted hazelnuts or pecan nuts instead of the walnuts.

Serve the salad on a bed of baby spinach leaves or on a mixture of spinach and watercress. Alternatively, use your favourite salad leaves.

Plus points

• This recipe offers useful amounts of dietary fibre, from the dried apricots, apples with their skins and celery. Fibre is essential to keep the digestive tract healthy.

• Dried apricots provide useful quantities of vitamin A (from beta-carotene), and are one of the richest fruit sources of iron.

• Some studies indicate that eating a small quantity of walnuts daily, as part of a low-fat diet, can help to reduce high blood cholesterol levels. Also, when nuts are added to a meal, they help to maintain satiety due to their high fat content.

photo, page 105

Each serving provides kcal 310, protein 36 g, fat 14 g (of which saturated fat 2 g), carbohydrate 11 g (of which sugars 11 g), fibre 2 g. Excellent source of niacin, vitamin B_6. Good source of copper, vitamin E. Useful source of iron, potassium, selenium, vitamin A, vitamin B_2, zinc.

Stir-fried chicken and avocado salad with hot balsamic dressing

This excellent salad combines stir-fried chicken and turkey rashers in a hot piquant dressing with creamy avocado and sweet cherry tomatoes. Turkey rashers are a great low-fat alternative to bacon, giving a similar savoury flavour.

Preparation time **15 minutes**   Cooking time **10 minutes**   Serves 4

1½ tbsp olive oil

2 garlic cloves, cut into slivers

300 g (10½ oz) skinless bone-less chicken breasts (fillets), cut into strips

2 tbsp clear honey

1 tbsp balsamic vinegar

1 tbsp wholegrain mustard

100 g (3½ oz) turkey rashers, diced

salt and pepper

Tomato and avocado salad

2 Little Gem lettuces, separated into leaves

55 g (2 oz) watercress sprigs

2 ripe avocados

juice of ½ lemon

250 g (9 oz) cherry tomatoes, halved

1 small red onion, thinly sliced

1 First prepare the salad. Put the lettuce and watercress in a large wide salad bowl. Peel and thickly slice the avocados and toss with the lemon juice to prevent discoloration. Then scatter the avocados, tomatoes and red onion on top of the lettuce and watercress. Set the salad aside.

2 Heat the oil in a large frying pan, add the garlic and stir round the pan for just 30 seconds or so until softened. Toss in the strips of chicken and stir-fry for 2–3 minutes or until they change colour.

3 Add the honey, vinegar and mustard, and stir to mix well. Add the diced turkey rashers and stir-fry for 1 minute more or until they are cooked, but still tender and moist (take care not to overcook or they will be dry). Season to taste.

4 Spoon the chicken mixture over the salad. Toss together, then serve immediately with crusty bread.

Some more ideas

For a **turkey and artichoke salad with a lemon dressing**, replace the chicken with 2 small skinless turkey breast steaks, about 300 g (10½ oz) in total, and use 2 lean rashers of back bacon instead of the turkey rashers. Stir-fry the turkey with the bacon and garlic for 5–6 minutes or until lightly golden, then add the grated zest and juice of 1 lemon to the pan with the honey and balsamic vinegar. Instead of the tomato and avocado salad, serve the turkey stir-fry spooned over an artichoke salad made with 100 g (3½ oz) baby spinach leaves, 55 g (2 oz) rocket and a 285 g jar of well-drained antipasto artichokes.

For a milder flavour, 2 shallots can be used instead of the small red onion.

Plus points

• Turkey rashers, which are widely available in large supermarkets, contain a fraction of the fat of bacon and are lower in calories: 100 g (3½ oz) contains just 1.6 g fat and 99 kcal, compared with 21 g fat and 249 kcal in the same weight of back bacon.

• Although avocados are high in fat, most of it is the healthier mono-unsaturated fat. They are also a rich source of vitamin B_6 – one avocado provides half the recommended daily intake of this vitamin.

Each serving provides kcal 335, protein 28 g, fat 19 g (of which saturated fat 3.5 g), carbohydrate 14 g (of which sugars 13 g), fibre 4 g. Excellent source of vitamin B_6. Good source of niacin, potassium, vitamin C, vitamin E. Useful source of copper, folate, iron, selenium, vitamin A, vitamin B_1, vitamin B_6, vitamin B_{12}, zinc.

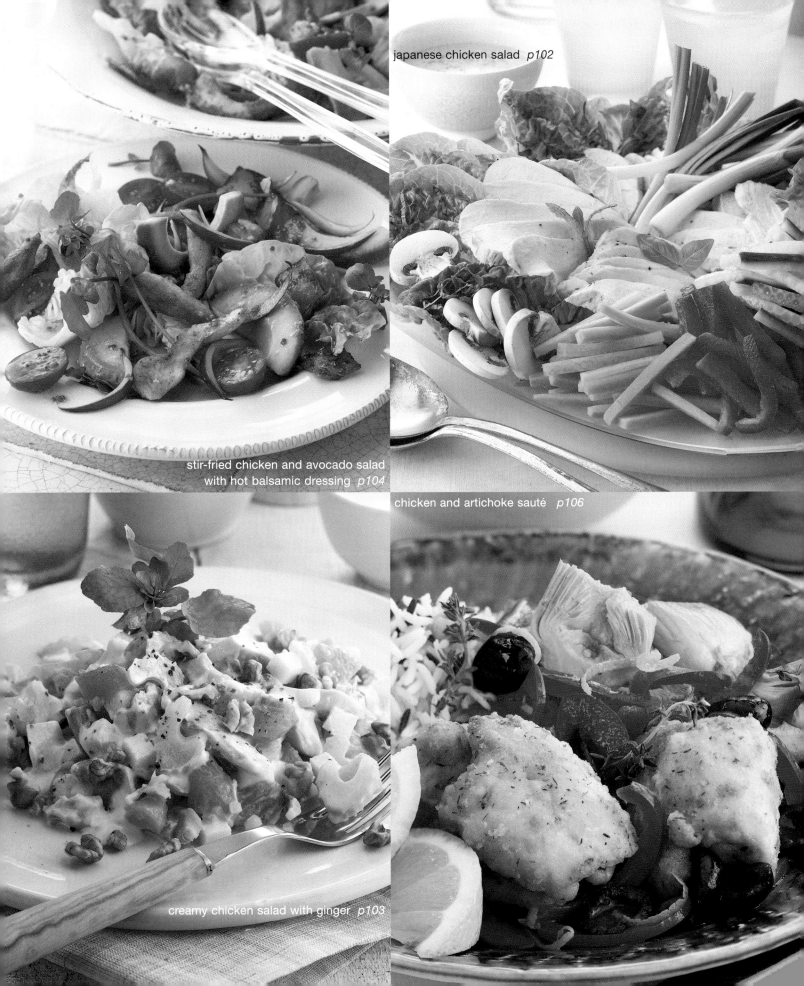

japanese chicken salad *p102*

stir-fried chicken and avocado salad
with hot balsamic dressing *p104*

chicken and artichoke sauté *p106*

creamy chicken salad with ginger *p103*

Chicken and artichoke sauté

Chicken with artichokes is a classic flavour combination, here given a Mediterranean touch with thin slices of red pepper, black olives, thyme and a hint of lemon. Boiled rice or new potatoes are ideal accompaniments for this vitamin-packed dish that is healthily low in calories and saturated fat.

Preparation time **about 5 minutes**   Cooking time **20 minutes**   *Serves 4*

4 tbsp plain flour

1 tbsp dried thyme

8 skinless boneless chicken thighs, about 450 g (1 lb) in total

3 tbsp sunflower oil

1 garlic clove, crushed

1 can artichokes (canned in water), about 400 g, drained and halved

2 red peppers, seeded and thinly sliced

85 g (3 oz) stoned black olives, halved

4 tbsp dry white wine

125 ml (4½ fl oz) chicken stock, preferably home-made (see page 212)

finely grated zest of 1 lemon

salt and pepper

To garnish

sprigs of fresh thyme

lemon wedges

1 Place the flour, thyme, salt and pepper in a large polythene bag and shake well. Add the chicken thighs to the bag and shake until they are lightly and evenly coated. Remove the chicken to a plate, shaking off any excess flour. Preheat the oven to its lowest setting.

2 Heat the oil in a large, heavy-based frying pan over a moderate heat. Add the thighs and sauté for about 3 minutes on each side, moving around occasionally, until golden brown. If they stick, add a little hot water.

3 Turn the thighs over and cook for a further 8 minutes or until the juices run clear when they are pierced. Transfer to a heatproof platter and keep warm in the oven.

4 Pour off excess oil from the pan, leaving just a film, then add the garlic and cook for 10 seconds, stirring. Add the artichokes and red peppers, and sauté for 3–5 minutes, stirring frequently, until the peppers are tender. Stir in the black olives.

5 Add the wine and allow to bubble, stirring, until it has evaporated. Stir in the stock and lemon zest, bring to the boil and cook until reduced by about half. Season.

6 Transfer the chicken thighs to serving plates and spoon the artichoke and pepper mixture alongside. Garnish with thyme sprigs and lemon wedges, and serve.

Some more ideas

You can prepare 4 skinless turkey breast fillets in the same way.

For a colourful variation, replace the red peppers with yellow or orange peppers, the olives with 200 g (7 oz) sliced courgettes and the artichokes with 100 g (3½ oz) sliced meaty mushrooms, such as shiitake. Sauté the mushrooms with the garlic until they give off their juices, then add the peppers and courgettes and sauté for 3–5 minutes or until the courgettes are just tender but not too soft.

Plus points

• As well as being low in calories and fat, globe artichokes provide calcium and vitamins A and C.

• Although olives have a high fat content, most of this fat is unsaturated, the type of fat thought to help lower blood cholesterol levels.

• Invest in a good-quality non-stick frying pan if you want to keep fat consumption low. This will allow you to sauté poultry and vegetables using very little oil. If you heat the pan well you don't need to add as much oil because the food is less likely to stick to a hot pan.

photo, page 105

Each serving provides kcal 350, protein 25 g, fat 17 g (of which saturated fat 3.5 g), carbohydrate 21.5 g (of which sugars 6 g), fibre 2.5 g. Excellent source of vitamin A, vitamin B_6, vitamin B_{12}, vitamin C. Good source of copper, iron, niacin, vitamin E. Useful source of potassium, selenium, vitamin B_1, vitamin B_2, zinc.

Chicken fajitas with tomato salsa

Although in northern Mexico 'fajitas' refers to a specific cut of beef, elsewhere in the world the term has come to describe a combination of sizzling pan-grilled chicken strips with peppers and onions, wrapped in a flour tortilla. The dish has very little fat, but lots and lots of fresh flavours.

Preparation time **30 minutes**   Cooking time **25–30 minutes**   *Serves 4*

400 g (14 oz) skinless boneless chicken breasts (fillets), cut in strips

2 garlic cloves, chopped

1 tsp ground cumin

1 tsp mild chilli powder

1 tsp paprika

¼ tsp dried oregano

grated zest and juice of ½ orange

juice of ½ lemon

2 tbsp sunflower oil

30 g (1 oz) fresh coriander, chopped

2 green peppers, thinly sliced

2 onions, thinly sliced lengthways

8 flour tortillas

120 ml (4 fl oz) plain low-fat yogurt

salt and pepper

Tomato salsa

4 spring onions, thinly sliced

125 g (4½ oz) ripe tomatoes, diced

1 medium-hot fresh green chilli, seeded and chopped, or to taste

2 tbsp tomato passata

2 garlic cloves, chopped

½ tsp ground cumin

lemon juice to taste

1 In a bowl combine the chicken strips with the garlic, cumin, chilli, paprika, oregano, orange zest and juice, lemon juice, 1 tbsp of the oil and 3 tbsp of the coriander. Mix well so that all the chicken strips are coated, then leave to marinate for at least 15 minutes.

2 To make the salsa, combine all the ingredients. Add the remaining chopped coriander. Season with ¼–½ tsp lemon juice and some salt and pepper to taste. Set aside.

3 Preheat the oven to 180°C (350°F, gas mark 4) and preheat the grill to high. Heat a ridged cast-iron grill pan or heavy-based frying pan until it is very hot. Brush with the remaining 1 tbsp of oil. Put in the green peppers and onions and cook for 6–8 minutes or until lightly charred. Remove from the pan and set aside.

4 Wrap the tortillas, stacked up, in foil and put into the oven to warm for 10 minutes. Meanwhile, spread out the chicken in a shallow layer in the grill pan. Grill close to the heat, turning once or twice, for about 5 minutes or until thoroughly cooked.

5 To serve, divide the chicken, onions and peppers among the warm tortillas and roll up. Serve with the fresh salsa and

yogurt. Alternatively, present the ingredients separately, with the tortillas wrapped in a cloth to keep them warm, and let your guests make their own fajitas.

Another idea

For **quesadillas**, use only 170 g (6 oz) chicken. Allow 1 tortilla per person. Sprinkle one half of each tortilla with 15 g (½ oz) grated Cheddar cheese and add a spoonful or two of the hot cooked chicken strips and green peppers and onions. Fold into a half-moon shape, pressing the edges together, and fry until lightly golden on each side.

Plus points

● Onions and garlic are not just valuable assets in the kitchen, they have been used throughout history as a cure-all. Recent research suggests that garlic can help to reduce the risk of heart disease. Both are thought to prevent blood clotting and act as natural decongestants. Include them in your cooking as much as possible.

● Substituting the traditional soured cream with low-fat yogurt helps to keep the fat content down.

photo, page 111

Each serving provides   kcal 450, protein 29 g, fat 11 g (of which saturated fat 2 g), carbohydrate 60 g (of which sugars 10 g), fibre 5 g. Excellent source of vitamin B_6, vitamin C. Good source of copper, iron, niacin, vitamin E. Useful source of calcium, folate, potassium, selenium, vitamin A, vitamin B_1, vitamin B_2, zinc.

Mexican tostadas

Tostadas comes from the Spanish word for toasted – in Mexico it refers to flat, crisply toasted corn tortillas, topped with all sorts of savoury things. Chicken with beans and salad is a favourite. A base layer of a thick mixture – often refried beans, but here a spicy pepper and tomato mixture – keeps everything together.

Preparation time **35 minutes**   Cooking time **20 minutes**   *Serves 4*

2 chicken breasts, about 500 g (1 lb 2 oz) in total, skinned

2 tbsp extra virgin olive oil

2 red peppers, seeded and coarsely chopped

1 onion, coarsely chopped

2 garlic cloves, thinly sliced

1 tbsp mild chilli powder

2 tsp paprika

1 tsp ground cumin

1 can chopped tomatoes, about 400 g

pinch of sugar

8 corn tortillas

1 can borlotti or pinto beans, about 425 g

salt and pepper

To serve

1 tomato, diced

pickled jalapeño chillies (optional)

125 g (4½ oz) iceberg lettuce, shredded

8 radishes, sliced

4 tbsp plain low-fat yogurt

Tabasco or other hot chilli sauce

1 Place the chicken in a saucepan with cold water to cover. Bring to the boil, then reduce the heat and simmer for 10–15 minutes. Remove from the heat and leave to cool. When cool enough to handle, drain and take the meat from the bones. Shred the meat and set aside.

2 Heat the olive oil in a frying pan and add the peppers, onion and garlic. Sauté over a moderate heat for 5 minutes or until softened. Add the chilli powder, paprika and cumin, stir well, and cook for a few more minutes. Stir in the tomatoes with their juice and the sugar. Simmer for 5–8 minutes or until thick. Season to taste. Remove from the heat and keep warm.

3 Heat a heavy-based frying pan. Toast the tortillas, one at a time, for about 15 seconds on each side or until slightly crisp and lightly browned. As they are done, keep them warm stacked in a tea towel. Meanwhile, warm the beans in the can liquid. Drain well.

4 To assemble the tostadas, place 2 toasted tortillas on each plate. Spread each one with the tomato mixture, then spoon on the beans and chicken. Sprinkle with the diced tomato, pickled jalapeños, if using, lettuce and radishes, piling up these toppings. Top with a spoonful of yogurt. Serve with Tabasco sauce, to be added to taste.

Another idea

Instead of beans, use a mixture of sweetcorn and courgette. Cook 1 corn on the cob and 1 whole courgette in separate pans of boiling water until tender, about 5 minutes for the corn and 10 minutes for the courgette. Drain. Dice the courgette, and cut the kernels of corn off the cob. Scatter the vegetables over each sauce-spread tortilla, then add the chicken.

Plus points

- Pulses such as borlotti and pinto beans are a good source of soluble fibre and an excellent source of protein – even better when they are eaten with grains such as wheat or maize (in corn tortillas).

- Radishes are low in fat and calories, and provide useful amounts of vitamin C. They contain phytochemicals that may help to protect against cancer.

photo, page 111

Each serving provides   kcal 425, protein 31 g, fat 11 g (of which saturated fat 3 g), carbohydrate 53 g (of which sugars 14 g), fibre 10 g. Excellent source of niacin, vitamin A, vitamin B$_6$, vitamin C. Good source of calcium, folate, iron, potassium, selenium, vitamin B$_1$, vitamin E. Useful source of copper, vitamin B$_2$, zinc.

Chicken and broccoli chapatti

These mouth-watering Indian-style snacks are very quick to make. Chapattis are the healthiest of Indian breads, as they are often made with wholemeal flour and are usually cooked on a dry griddle or pan without any fat. A yogurt-based raita, containing cucumber and tomato, is the perfect accompaniment.

Preparation time **about 10 minutes**   Cooking time **about 10 minutes**   *Serves 4*

Chapattis

200 g (7 oz) cooked chicken breast

2 tbsp sunflower oil

250 g (9 oz) broccoli florets, finely chopped

45 g (1½ oz) unsalted cashew nuts, coarsely chopped

2 tsp grated fresh root ginger

1 garlic clove, finely chopped

4 tbsp mango chutney

4 chapattis

pepper

Raita

340 g (12 oz) plain low-fat yogurt

1 cucumber, about 300 g (10½ oz), cut into quarters lengthways and seeded

100 g (3½ oz) tomato, very finely chopped

½ tsp ground coriander

½ tsp ground cumin

pinch of cayenne pepper

pinch of salt

1 Combine all the ingredients for the raita in a serving bowl. Cover and refrigerate.

2 Preheat the grill. Then cut the chicken into small bite-sized pieces, discarding any skin.

3 Heat the oil in a large frying pan, add the broccoli, cashews, ginger and garlic, and cook for 5 minutes, stirring, until the broccoli is tender.

4 Add the chicken, mango chutney and pepper to taste to the broccoli mixture and stir to mix. Then cook for a further 2 minutes, stirring constantly, until the chicken is hot.

5 Meanwhile, place the chapattis on the rack in the grill pan and sprinkle with water. Grill for 2 minutes, turning once.

6 Put the chicken mixture on top of the chapattis and roll them up. Serve hot, with the raita as an accompaniment.

Another idea

For **Mexican-style chicken and broccoli tortillas**, use 8 flour tortillas instead of chapattis. Heat the tortillas, one at a time, in a dry frying pan for 20 seconds, turning once. Make a fresh tomato salsa by mixing together 4 ripe tomatoes, skinned and finely diced,

1 small onion, finely chopped, 1–2 tbsp finely chopped fresh coriander, a squeeze of lemon juice, a few drops of Tabasco sauce, and pepper to taste. Prepare the chicken and broccoli mixture as above, omitting the chutney and using pine nuts instead of cashews. Divide the mixture among the hot tortillas, add a spoonful of salsa and roll up.

Plus points

• Broccoli is packed with vitamins. It is an excellent source of the antioxidants beta-carotene and vitamin C as well as vitamin E. Just 1 serving of cooked broccoli (about 85 g/3 oz) provides nearly 50 per cent of the recommended daily intake of vitamin C. It also provides good amounts of the B vitamins niacin and B_6.

• In common with other members of the Cruciferae family of vegetables, such as cauliflower, Brussels sprouts, cabbage and kale, broccoli contains a number of different phytochemicals. One of these, indoles, may help to protect against breast cancer by inhibiting the action of the oestrogens that trigger the growth of tumours.

photo, page 111

Each serving provides   kcal 386, protein 26 g, fat 17 g (of which saturated fat 3.5 g), carbohydrate 43 g (of which sugars 18 g), fibre 3 g. Excellent source of vitamin C. Good source of copper, folate, iron, vitamin B_6, vitamin E. Useful source of calcium, niacin, potassium, vitamin B_1, zinc.

Chicken and vegetable filo rolls

These filo pastry rolls make an excellent starter, or you could serve two rolls each for a light meal. The filling is a colourful mixture of low-fat minced chicken and plenty of vegetables, with a little smoked ham and fresh herbs to add to the flavour. The rolls are served with a piquant cranberry relish.

Preparation time **40 minutes**   Cooking time **30 minutes**   *Serves 8 (makes 8)*

1 large carrot, about 100 g (3½ oz), cut into very fine matchsticks

75 g (2½ oz) savoy cabbage, finely shredded

2 spring onions, cut in fine strips

225 g (8 oz) minced chicken

55 g (2 oz) lean smoked ham, finely chopped

½ small onion, finely chopped

2 tbsp fresh white breadcrumbs

2 tsp chopped fresh sage

2 tsp chopped fresh thyme

4 large sheets filo pastry, each about 46 x 28 cm (18 x 11 in)

2 tbsp extra virgin olive oil

10 g (¼ oz) butter, melted

1 tsp sesame seeds

salt and pepper

Cranberry relish

3 tbsp cranberry sauce

2 tsp extra virgin olive oil

1 tbsp red wine vinegar

1 tsp made English mustard

To serve

115 g (4 oz) mixed salad leaves

1 Blanch the carrot, cabbage and spring onions in boiling water for 1 minute. Drain, then plunge into a bowl of cold water to refresh. Drain again and pat dry with kitchen paper. Put the vegetables in a large mixing bowl with the chicken, ham, onion, breadcrumbs, herbs and seasoning. Mix together well, then set aside.

2 Preheat the oven to 190°C (375°F, gas mark 5). Halve each filo pastry sheet lengthways and then trim to a strip measuring 36 x 12 cm (15 x 5 in). Mix the oil and butter together.

3 Brush one pastry strip lightly with the butter mixture. Place an eighth of the filling at one end, shaping it into a sausage. Roll up the filling inside the pastry, folding in the long sides as you go, to make a spring roll-shaped parcel. Place on a baking sheet and brush with a little of the butter and oil mixture. Repeat to make another 7 parcels.

4 Score 3 diagonal slashes on top of each parcel. Sprinkle the sesame seeds. Bake for 30 minutes or until the pastry is golden.

5 Meanwhile, put all the relish ingredients in a screw-top jar, season and shake well.

6 Arrange the mixed salad leaves on serving plates, place a filo roll on each and drizzle around the relish.

Another idea

For **Greek-style chicken parcels**, cook 30 g (1 oz) long-grain rice for 12 minutes or until just tender; drain and rinse. Meanwhile, soften 1 finely chopped onion in 1 tsp extra virgin olive oil for 5 minutes, then set aside. Put the rice and onion in a bowl with 225 g (8 oz) minced chicken or turkey, 2 tbsp toasted pine nuts, 2 tbsp raisins, 2 tbsp chopped fresh mint and 2 tbsp chopped fresh dill. Season to taste. Mix together well and divide into 8 equal portions. Cut the sheets of filo pastry into 8 strips as before. Brush each strip lightly with the olive oil and butter mixture, and put one portion of the filling at one end. Fold the pastry over the filling into a triangle. Continue folding down the pastry strip to make a triangular-shaped parcel. Brush all the parcels with the butter and oil mixture, and scatter over 1 tsp poppy seeds. Bake for 30 minutes.

Plus points

* Unlike most other types of pastry, filo contains very little fat – in 100 g (3½ oz) filo there are 2 g fat and 300 kcal. The same weight of shortcrust pastry contains 29 g fat and 449 kcal.

Each serving provides   (one filo roll) kcal 120, protein 8.5 g, fat 6.5 g (of which saturated fat 1.5 g), carbohydrate 7 g (of which sugars 4 g), fibre 1 g. Useful source of vitamin A, vitamin B$_6$.

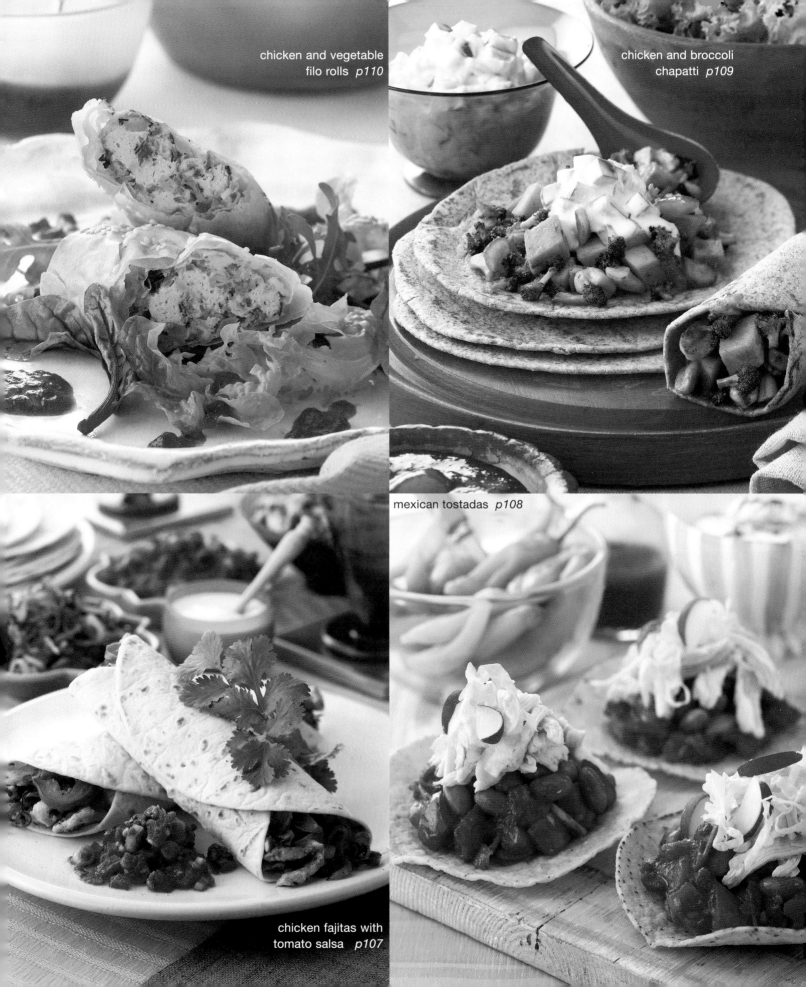

chicken and vegetable
filo rolls *p110*

chicken and broccoli
chapatti *p109*

mexican tostadas *p108*

chicken fajitas with
tomato salsa *p107*

Herbed chicken and apple burgers

Adding diced apple – tart or sweet fruit, to your taste – to chicken burgers not only gives a fruity flavour that complements the meat and herbs, but also lightens up the meaty patties and provides fibre. Served in baps or buns, with honey mustard and crisp fresh watercress, these are a great alternative to beefburgers.

Preparation time **20 minutes, plus 1 hour chilling**   Cooking time **20 minutes**   *Serves 4*

340 g (12 oz) minced chicken

1 red onion, finely chopped

4 tbsp fresh breadcrumbs

2 green-skinned apples, such as Granny Smith (for a tart taste) or Golden Delicious (for a sweet taste), coarsely grated

1 tbsp chopped fresh sage

2 tsp fresh thyme leaves

sunflower oil, for brushing

salt and pepper

To serve

1 tbsp clear honey

3 tbsp Dijon mustard

4 floury baps or burger buns, split open

55 g (2 oz) watercress sprigs, large stalks discarded

1 Put the minced chicken, onion, breadcrumbs, apples, herbs and some seasoning in a bowl. Mix together with your hands. Wet your hands, then divide the mixture into 4 portions and shape each into a burger. Chill for 1 hour to firm up.

2 Brush the chicken burgers with a little oil and cook over a moderate heat in a non-stick frying pan until browned on both sides, then reduce the heat a little and continue cooking until the burgers are completely cooked through – this should take about 20 minutes altogether. Turn from time to time to ensure cooking is even.

3 Meanwhile, mix together the honey and mustard. Spread over the top cut surface of each bap or bun. Divide the watercress among the baps, piling it on the bottom cut side.

4 When the chicken burgers have finished cooking, transfer them to the baps, placing them on the watercress. Put on the tops and serve.

Some more ideas

Minced turkey will make burgers that are even lower in fat than those made with chicken.

Use baby spinach leaves instead of watercress.

For a creamy, more savoury alternative to honey mustard, mix 2 tbsp Dijon mustard with reduced-fat mayonnaise.

Use wholemeal breadcrumbs and wholemeal baps to increase the fibre content.

Plus points

- Apples provide good amounts of vitamin C as well as soluble fibre in the form of pectin. If you eat apples with their skin on you get even more fibre – a third more, to be exact.

- Minced chicken has much less fat than lean minced beef.

- Small amounts of honey are perfectly acceptable for those with diabetes. The Glycaemic Index of honey is about half that of glucose (see box on page 8).

photo, page 117

Each serving provides (one burger) kcal 400, protein 25 g, fat 7 g (of which saturated fat 2 g), carbohydrate 59 g (of which sugars 12 g), fibre 3 g. Good source of copper, iron, selenium, vitamin B_6, vitamin B_{12}, vitamin E. Useful source of calcium, folate, niacin, potassium, vitamin B_1, vitamin B_2, vitamin C, zinc.

Chicken goujons with mustard dip

A favourite with both adults and children, this is a simple healthy version of the popular deep-fried take-away snack. Served hot, with 5 per cent fat oven chips and fresh vegetables, it makes a good family meal. Served cold, the goujons are ideal for a picnic or a packed lunch.

Preparation time **25 minutes, plus 30 minutes chilling**   Cooking time **30–40 minutes**   *Serves 4*

150 ml (5 fl oz) 0% fat Greek-style yogurt

7 tbsp wholegrain mustard

1 tbsp snipped fresh chives

550 g (1¼ lb) skinless boneless chicken breasts (fillets)

2 tbsp plain flour

200 g (7 oz) fresh wholemeal breadcrumbs

1 garlic clove, crushed (optional)

1 tbsp paprika

2 eggs

pepper

lemon or lime wedges to serve

1 To make the mustard dip, mix together the yogurt, 1 tbsp of the mustard, the chives and pepper to taste. Spoon into a small serving bowl. Cover and chill until required.

2 Meanwhile, split open each chicken breast horizontally, then cut lengthways into thin strips. Put the flour in a large polythene bag, add the chicken and shake until all the strips are coated in flour.

3 Put the breadcrumbs, garlic, if using, the remaining 6 tbsp of mustard and the paprika in a large bowl, and mix together until well blended. Tip the mixture onto a large plate. Break the eggs onto a deep plate and lightly beat with a fork.

4 Remove the chicken strips, one at a time, from the bag of flour, shaking off any excess, and dip first into the beaten egg and then into the breadcrumb mixture, pressing the breadcrumbs evenly over them. Arrange the goujons on a large non-stick baking tray and chill for about 30 minutes.

5 Preheat the oven to 200°C (400°F, gas mark 6).

6 Bake the goujons for 30–40 minutes or until they are golden brown and crisp. Serve hot or cold, with the mustard dip and with lemon or lime wedges.

Some more ideas

For **curry-flavoured goujons**, replace the mustard in both the chicken coating and dip with curry paste (mild or medium, to taste).

For **spicy goujons**, omit the mustard and add ½ tsp ground cardamom, ½ tsp ground cinnamon, 1 tsp ground cumin and 2 tsp ground coriander to the breadcrumbs.

To make **oven chips**, scrub 675 g (1½ lb) baking potatoes and cut into chips. Toss in a polythene bag with 1 tbsp sunflower oil and seasoning. Heat a baking tray in an oven preheated to 200°C (400°F, gas mark 6). Bake for 20 minutes. Turn them over, then bake for a further 40 minutes until crisp and browned.

Plus points

• Greek yogurt contains only half the fat of soured cream, which forms the basis of a classic soured cream and chive dip. In this recipe, the fat content is cut even further by using 0% fat Greek yogurt.

• Wholemeal breadcrumbs offer considerably more fibre than white breadcrumbs. They contain 5.8 g fibre per 100 g/3½ oz as compared to 1.5 g.

photo, page 117

| Each serving provides | kcal 400, protein 45 g, fat 12 g (of which saturated fat 2 g), carbohydrate 31 g (of which sugars 3.5 g), fibre 4.5 g. Excellent source of niacin, vitamin B$_6$. Good source of copper, iron, selenium, vitamin A, vitamin B$_{12}$, zinc. Useful source of calcium, folate, potassium, vitamin B$_1$, vitamin B$_2$. |

Chicken and sweet potatoes

This salad is a riot of tastes, perfect when you are craving wholesome yet interesting food. Slices of chicken and sweet potatoes are served on a bed of leafy greens and vegetables, with a chunky pineapple salsa to spoon over.

Preparation time **40–45 minutes, plus cooling**   *Serves 4*

900 g (2 lb) sweet potatoes, scrubbed and cut into 1 cm (½ in) slices

4 skinless boneless chicken breasts (fillets), about 140 g (5 oz) each

pinch each of ground cinnamon and cumin

200 g (7 oz) mixed salad leaves

¼ cucumber, thinly sliced

4 tomatoes, cut into thin wedges

2 tbsp chopped fresh coriander

2 tbsp toasted sunflower seeds

2 spring onions, finely shredded

Pineapple salsa

½ ripe pineapple, about 340 g (12 oz), peeled and chopped

½ small red onion, chopped

½ red pepper, seeded and finely diced

2 tbsp chopped fresh mint

¼ tsp mild chilli powder, or to taste

pinch each of ground cinnamon and cumin

juice of ½ lime

Lime and soy dressing

1 tsp caster sugar

juice of ½ lime

1 tbsp olive oil

dash of soy sauce, or to taste

1 Cook the sweet potato slices in boiling water for 6–8 minutes or until tender. Drain and leave to cool.

2 Poach the chicken breasts in simmering water (use the water from the sweet potatoes, if liked) for 4–6 minutes or until cooked through. Drain and leave to cool, then cut into 1 cm (½ in) slices.

3 Put the chicken and sweet potato slices in a bowl and sprinkle with the cinnamon and cumin.

4 To make the salsa, combine the pineapple, red onion, red pepper, mint, chilli powder, cinnamon, cumin and lime juice in a mixing bowl.

5 Mix the dressing ingredients in a large shallow salad bowl. Add the salad leaves and toss to coat with the dressing. Arrange the chicken and sweet potato slices, the cucumber slices and tomato wedges on top of the leaves, and scatter over the chopped coriander, sunflower seeds and spring onions. Serve with the pineapple salsa, to be added to taste.

Another idea

For a **smoked chicken and papaya salad**, use 350 g (12½ oz) sliced smoked chicken. Make the dressing with 1 tbsp olive oil, the juice of 1 lime, a dash of wine vinegar and 1 chopped garlic clove. Arrange the chicken, sweet potatoes and tomatoes on the dressed salad leaves, together with 1 papaya and 1 avocado, peeled and sliced, and ½ bulb of fennel, cut into thin strips. Scatter over the coriander, sunflower seeds and spring onions.

Plus point

* The sweet potato is native to central America – Columbus was believed to have brought it to Europe after his first voyage to the New World. Sweet potatoes contain slightly more calories than white potatoes, but they provide more vitamin E. They also supply good amounts of vitamin C, potassium and dietary fibre. The orange-fleshed variety is an excellent source of beta-carotene.

photo, page 117

Each serving provides   kcal 435, protein 25 g, fat 10 g (of which saturated fat 1.5 g), carbohydrate 65 g (of which sugars 28 g), fibre 9 g. Excellent source of copper, niacin, potassium, vitamin A, vitamin B$_1$, vitamin B$_6$, vitamin C, vitamin E. Good source of folate, iron, selenium, vitamin B$_2$, zinc. Useful source of calcium.

Barbecued chicken

Because the flavour of chicken is quite mild, it benefits from a tasty baste when barbecued or grilled, and this also helps to keep the outside from burning until the chicken is cooked through – especially when cooking over charcoal. This recipe is for a spicy Jamaican jerk baste, and there are four more deliciously different ideas.

Preparation time **20 minutes, plus at least 1 hour marinating**   Cooking time **20-25 minutes**   *Serves 4*

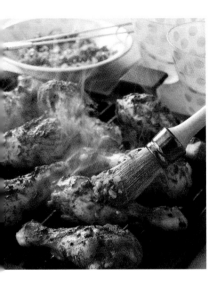

8 chicken drumsticks, skinless

lime wedges to garnish

Jamaican jerk baste

2 tbsp extra virgin olive oil

1 onion, very finely chopped

2 garlic cloves, finely chopped

1 red chilli, seeded and chopped

¼ tsp salt

½ tsp ground allspice

¼ tsp ground cinnamon

grated zest and juice of 1 lime

1 To make the baste, heat the oil in a small frying pan over a moderately low heat. Add the onion, garlic and chilli and cook, stirring frequently, for about 10 minutes or until the onion is softened and starting to brown.

2 Tip into a large shallow bowl. Add the spices and the lime zest and juice, and stir well to mix.

3 Make a few shallow slashes in the meat of each piece, then add to the bowl. Turn the pieces to coat thoroughly with the baste, rubbing it into the slashes in the meat. Cover and leave to marinate at room temperature for 1 hour or in the fridge for up to 24 hours.

4 Prepare a charcoal fire. When it has burned down to coals covered with grey ash, remove the chicken pieces from the marinating baste and barbecue them for 20–25 minutes, turning and brushing frequently with the baste, until cooked all the way through.

5 Alternatively, preheat the grill to moderately high. Arrange the chicken on the grill rack and grill for 20–25 minutes, turning and basting frequently.

6 Serve the chicken hot, garnished with lime wedges.

Some more ideas

For an **American barbecue baste**, fry the onion and garlic, then add 4 tbsp tomato ketchup, 2 tbsp Worcestershire sauce, 2 tbsp red wine vinegar and 2 tbsp treacle.

For a **New Orleans baste**, fry the onion and garlic, then add the lime zest and juice, 150 g (5½ oz) plain low-fat yogurt, 3 tbsp chopped parsley and 2 tbsp Cajun seasoning.

For a **red wine and thyme baste**, fry the onion and garlic with 2 fresh bay leaves and 1 tbsp fresh thyme. Add 175 ml (6 fl oz) red wine and ½ tsp coarse black pepper.

Plus points

• Shop-bought barbecue sauce is often high in sugar. This homemade version is extremely flavoursome due to the onions, garlic and fresh lime juice, and is much lower in calories.

• The Mediterranean diet is thought to be much healthier than the average UK diet. One of the reasons for this is the use of olive oil, a monounsaturated fat, rather than butter and other saturated fats.

Each serving provides kcal 235, protein 33 g, fat 10 g (of which saturated fat 2.5 g), carbohydrate 3 g (of which sugars 2 g), fibre 0.5 g. Excellent source of niacin, vitamin B_{12}. Useful source of copper, iron, potassium, selenium, zinc.

Spicy drumsticks with Creole rice

These chicken drumsticks, coated in a mixture of dried herbs and spices, can be cooked under the grill in next to no time. They are served with Creole-style red beans and rice.

Preparation and cooking time **30 minutes**   *Serves 4*

1 tbsp plain flour

1 tsp paprika

1 tsp ground black pepper

1 tsp garlic granules

½ tsp crushed dried chillies

1 tsp dried thyme

8 chicken drumsticks, about 675 g (1½ lb) in total, skinned

1 tbsp extra virgin olive oil

salt and pepper

sprigs of fresh parsley to garnish

Creole rice

1 tbsp extra virgin olive oil

1 onion, chopped

1 red pepper, seeded and diced

2 celery sticks, diced

170 g (6 oz) long-grain rice

600 ml (1 pint) vegetable stock

1 can red kidney beans, about 410 g, drained and rinsed

2 tbsp chopped parsley

1 Preheat the grill to moderate. Put the flour, paprika, pepper, garlic granules, chillies, thyme and a pinch of salt in a polythene bag and shake to mix. Make 2 slashes in each chicken drumstick and rub with the olive oil. Toss them one at a time in the bag to coat with the spice mixture. Shake off any excess mixture and place the chicken on the grill rack. Grill for 20–25 minutes or until golden and cooked through, turning frequently.

2 Meanwhile, make the Creole rice. Heat the oil in a large saucepan, add the onion, pepper and celery, and cook for 2 minutes or until softened. Stir in the rice, then add the stock and kidney beans. Bring to the boil. Cover and simmer gently for 15–20 minutes or until all the stock has been absorbed and the rice is tender.

3 Stir the chopped parsley into the rice and season with salt and pepper to taste. Spoon the rice onto 4 plates and place 2 drumsticks on top of each portion. Serve hot, garnished with sprigs of parsley.

Another idea

For **sticky chilli drumsticks**, mix 2 tbsp tomato ketchup with 1 tbsp soy sauce and 2 tbsp sweet chilli sauce or paste. Rub onto the chicken drumsticks and grill as in the main recipe. Meanwhile, put 125 g (4½ oz) bulghur wheat in a heatproof bowl, cover with boiling water and soak for 15–20 minutes. Squeeze out any excess water, then mix with 1 can borlotti beans, drained, ¼ diced cucumber, 2 chopped tomatoes, 2 tbsp chopped fresh mint and 2 tbsp chopped parsley. Add 1 tbsp lemon juice and 1 tbsp extra virgin olive oil and season to taste. Toss to mix. Serve with the sticky chilli drumsticks.

Plus points

• Chicken is an excellent source of protein and provides many B vitamins, in particular niacin. Eaten without the skin, chicken is low in fat and what fat it does contain is mostly unsaturated.

• In diabetes, it is important to maintain an appropriate blood pressure level. Celery contains a compound called phthalide, which is believed to help lower high blood pressure.

Each serving provides   kcal 480, protein 41 g, fat 11 g (of which saturated fat 2 g), carbohydrate 58 g (of which sugars 5 g), fibre 6 g. Good source of iron, niacin, selenium, vitamin B_1, vitamin B_6, zinc. Useful source of calcium, copper, folate, potassium.

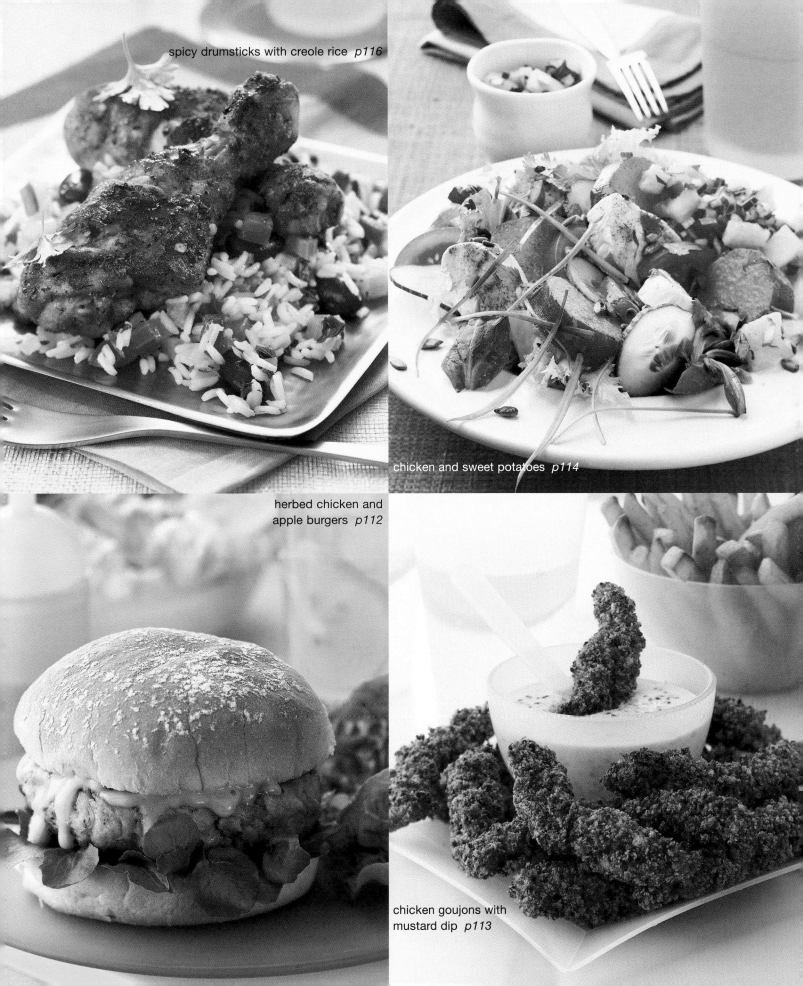

spicy drumsticks with creole rice *p116*

chicken and sweet potatoes *p114*

herbed chicken and
apple burgers *p112*

chicken goujons with
mustard dip *p113*

Chicken and ham jambalaya

A typical Cajun recipe, this is full of spicy, complex flavours. With lots of rice and vegetables, it is a great dish to make a small amount of meat go a long way, and offers a healthy balance of protein and carbohydrate.

Preparation time **15 minutes**   Cooking time **35–40 minutes**   *Serves 6*

300 g (10½ oz) skinless boneless chicken breasts (fillets)

2 tsp Cajun seasoning (see note below)

1 tsp dried sage or marjoram

2 tbsp sunflower oil

1 onion, sliced

1 green pepper, seeded and sliced

2 celery sticks, sliced

2 garlic cloves, crushed

400 g (14 oz) basmati rice

1 litre (1¾ pints) chicken stock, preferably home-made (see page 212)

100 g (3½ oz) cooked smoked ham, cubed

1 can Italian cherry tomatoes, or 1 can chopped tomatoes, about 400 g

Tabasco sauce, salt and pepper

To garnish

4–6 spring onions, trimmed and chopped

coarsely chopped parsley

1 Cut the chicken into 2 cm (¾ in) cubes. Sprinkle with the Cajun seasoning and the sage or marjoram, making sure that the chicken is coated all over. Heat 1 tbsp of the oil in a large flameproof casserole or pan over a moderately high heat, add the chicken and fry for about 5 minutes, stirring frequently, until the cubes are browned on all sides. Remove from the pan with a draining spoon.

2 Add the remaining oil to the pan with the onion, green pepper and celery, and fry for about 2 minutes, stirring. Add the garlic and rice, and fry for another minute.

3 Pour in the stock and stir well. Return the chicken to the pan. Bring to the boil, then reduce the heat, cover and simmer for 15 minutes. Add the ham and canned tomatoes with their juice. Cook, covered, for a further 5–10 minutes or until the rice has absorbed all the liquid.

4 Season to taste with Tabasco sauce and a little salt and pepper. Serve sprinkled with the chopped spring onions and parsley.

Some more ideas

If you cannot find ready-made Cajun seasoning, use a mixture of 1½ tsp paprika and ½ tsp cayenne pepper.

Use brown rice instead of white rice. It will take 5–10 minutes longer to cook and may need more liquid. Brown rice retains the nutritious high-fibre bran coating that is removed from white rice.

For a **chicken and prawn jambalaya**, leave out the smoked ham and add 200 g (7 oz) peeled raw tiger prawns instead. Also add extra vegetables – 100 g (3½ oz) each frozen green beans and frozen peas. Add these 10 minutes before the end of cooking.

Add white wine in place of some of the stock – 150 ml (5 fl oz) will give a good flavour.

Plus points

• Green pepper provides vitamin C and beta-carotene, both of which have strong protective antioxidant functions against cancer, heart disease and stroke.

• The antioxidant lycopene, found in tomatoes, becomes even more potent when the tomatoes are processed. Although using a can of tomatoes in this recipe may seem like a short-cut, be assured that your meal is packed with hidden benefits.

photo, page 123

Each serving provides   kcal 390, protein 18 g, fat 8 g (of which saturated fat 0.5 g), carbohydrate 58 g (of which sugars 4 g), fibre 1.5 g. Excellent source of vitamin C. Good source of iron, vitamin B$_6$, vitamin E. Useful source of copper, niacin, potassium, zinc.

Indian-style grilled chicken breasts

Tandoori dishes are one of the healthiest options in most Indian restaurants because the food is cooked in a tandoor oven without fat. At home, using a hot grill gives similar results. These lean chicken breasts are served with creamy raita. All that is needed to complete the meal is some boiled basmati rice or naan bread.

Preparation time **about 15 minutes**   Cooking time **15 minutes**   *Serves 4*

4 skinless boneless chicken breasts (fillets), about 140 g (5 oz) each

sunflower oil for brushing

lemon or lime wedges to serve

sprigs of fresh coriander to garnish

Yogurt marinade

1 garlic clove, crushed

1 tbsp finely chopped fresh root ginger

1½ tsp tomato purée

1½ tsp garam masala

1½ tsp ground coriander

1½ tsp ground cumin

¼ tsp turmeric

pinch of cayenne pepper, or to taste

100 g (3½ oz) plain low-fat yogurt

Raita

See ingredients list on page 109.

1 Preheat the grill to high. To make the marinade, put the marinade ingredients into a large bowl and whisk together well. If you prefer, put the ingredients in a blender or food processor and process until well blended. Transfer to a bowl large enough to hold all the chicken breasts.

2 Score 2 slits on each side of the chicken breasts. Place them in the marinade, turning to coat and rubbing the marinade into the slits. (If you have time, leave the chicken to marinate in the fridge overnight.)

3 Brush the grill rack with oil, then place the chicken breasts on top. Grill for 12–15 minutes, turning and basting with the remaining marinade, until the juices run clear when the chicken is pierced with a knife, and the marinade is beginning to look slightly charred.

4 Meanwhile, combine all the ingredients for the raita in a bowl. Stir well to mix. Spoon the raita into a serving bowl.

5 Transfer the chicken breasts to a serving plate. Add lemon or lime wedges and garnish with coriander sprigs. Serve with the raita on the side.

Some more ideas

Try this **onion and herb raita**: finely chop 200 g (7 oz) spring onions and place in a bowl. Stir in 4–6 tbsp finely chopped mint, 2 tbsp finely chopped coriander, 1 finely chopped fresh green chilli and 340 g (12 oz) plain low-fat yogurt. Fry 2 tsp cumin seeds over a high heat, stirring constantly, until they start to jump. Sprinkle on top of the raita.

For **Indian-style kebabs**, cut the breasts into cubes before you put them in the marinade. While preheating the grill, soak 8 bamboo skewers in water. Thread the chicken cubes onto the skewers, alternating with chunks of courgette and red and yellow peppers. Grill, basting with the marinade and turning the skewers over often, for 12–15 minutes.

Plus points

• Yogurt is an excellent source of protein and calcium, needed for healthy bones and teeth. It also provides useful amounts of phosphorus and vitamins B_2 and B_{12}, as well as bacteria that are beneficial to gut health.

• Basmati rice is a good accompaniment as it has a low Glycaemic Index.

photo, page 123

Each serving provides   kcal 250, protein 40 g, fat 5 g (of which saturated fat 1.5 g), carbohydrate 11 g (of which sugars 11 g), fibre 1 g. Excellent source of niacin, vitamin B_6. Good source of calcium, potassium, selenium, vitamin B2. Useful source of copper, folate, iron, vitamin B_1, vitamin B_{12}, vitamin C, vitamin E, zinc.

Chicken and sweetcorn chowder

This hearty soup tastes really special, yet despite its creamy texture it doesn't contain any cream. Made with cooked chicken and fresh sweetcorn and potatoes, with a garnish of grilled back bacon, it's substantial enough for a light lunch, served with crusty bread and followed by salad or fruit.

Preparation time **15 minutes**   Cooking time **25 minutes**   *Serves 4*

3 fresh corn-on-the-cob

1 tbsp sunflower oil

1 onion, finely chopped

2 potatoes, about 300 g (10½ oz) in total, peeled and diced

500 ml (17 fl oz) chicken stock, preferably home-made (see page 212)

500 ml (17 fl oz) skimmed milk

250 g (9 oz) cooked chicken meat, without skin, finely chopped

2 tsp chopped fresh tarragon

salt and pepper

To garnish

2 rashers lean smoked back bacon

fresh tarragon leaves

1 Remove the green husks and all the 'silk' from the corn. Holding each cob upright on a chopping board, cut the kernels from the cob. You should end up with 225–250 g (8–9 oz) loose corn kernels. Set aside.

2 Heat the sunflower oil in a large saucepan, add the onion and fry over a moderate heat until softened, but not browned. Add the potatoes and sweetcorn kernels to the pan and cook for a further 5 minutes, stirring frequently. Pour in the chicken stock and bring to the boil. Reduce the heat and simmer gently for 5 minutes or until the potatoes are just tender.

3 Stir in the milk, three-quarters of the chicken and the chopped tarragon. Season to taste. Cook, stirring, for a further 2–3 minutes.

4 Pour half of the mixture into a food processor and process to a coarse texture, not to a purée. Return to the pan. Add the rest of the chicken and stir to mix. Set the chowder over a low heat to warm through.

5 Meanwhile, grill the rashers of bacon until cooked and starting to brown. Drain the bacon on kitchen paper, then finely chop.

6 Ladle the chowder into bowls, scatter on some bacon and a sprinkling of tarragon leaves, and serve.

Another idea

For a **creamy chicken soup with mushrooms**, use 100 g (3½ oz) chestnut mushrooms, finely chopped, instead of the sweetcorn and potato. Add 1 tablespoon Madeira after cooking the mushrooms for 5 minutes and allow most of it to evaporate before pouring in the stock. Blend a little of the milk with 1 heaped tbsp of plain flour until smooth, then stir in the remaining milk and add to the pan with the chicken and tarragon. Cook, stirring, until thickened.

Plus points

• Milk is an excellent source of protein, calcium and many of the B vitamins. Choose skimmed or semi-skimmed in cooking.

• Sweetcorn is a useful source of soluble fibre, which helps to keep blood glucose levels under control.

• Bacon provides iron as well as vitamin B_1, essential for maintaining a healthy nervous system. Choose small amounts of lean bacon to limit salt content.

photo, page 123

Each serving provides   kcal 297, protein 26 g, fat 7.5 g (of which saturated fat 1.5 g), carbohydrate 27 g (of which sugars 7.5 g), fibre 1.5 g. Good source of calcium, vitamin B_6, vitamin E. Useful source of copper, folate, iron, niacin, potassium, vitamin B_1, vitamin B_2, vitamin B_{12}, vitamin C.

Greek-style lemon chicken soup

This delicate yet rich-tasting soup is packed with good things, and makes a warming and sustaining main course. Chicken breasts are poached with vegetables, then rice is cooked in the well-flavoured stock. At the last minute, the soup is enriched with eggs and fresh lemon juice in traditional Greek fashion.

Preparation time **15 minutes**   Cooking time **30 minutes**   *Serves 4*

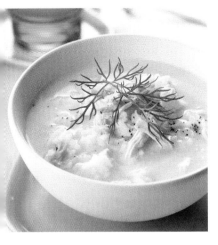

3 small skinless boneless chicken breasts (fillets), about 340 g (12 oz) in total

1 large onion, thinly sliced

2 celery sticks, chopped

1 large carrot, thinly sliced

6 black peppercorns

strip of lemon zest

1 small bunch of fresh dill or flat-leaf parsley

150 g (5½ oz) long-grain white rice

juice of 1 lemon

2 eggs, beaten

salt and pepper

sprigs of fresh dill or flat-leaf parsley to garnish

1 Put the chicken breasts, onion, celery, carrot, black peppercorns, lemon zest and bunch of dill or parsley into a large saucepan. Add 1.4 litres (2½ pints) water. Bring to the boil over a moderate heat, skimming off any foam that comes to the surface. Reduce the heat and half-cover the pan with a lid, so the water just bubbles gently. Simmer for 15 minutes or until the chicken is cooked through.

2 Remove the chicken from the pan with a draining spoon and set aside. Strain the stock through a sieve into a clean pan, discarding the vegetables and flavourings.

3 Reheat the stock until boiling, then stir in the rice. Simmer gently for 8–10 minutes or until the rice is almost tender. Meanwhile, cut or tear the chicken into thin shreds, and mix the lemon juice with the beaten eggs.

4 Add the shredded chicken to the soup. Heat over a moderate heat until the soup almost starts to boil again. Remove the pan from the heat and pour in the lemon juice mixture, stirring constantly. Season with salt and pepper to taste. Serve hot, garnished with sprigs of dill or parsley.

Another idea

For **Chinese-style duck and rice soup**, replace the chicken with 2 medium-sized skinless duck breasts, about 300 g (10½ oz) in total. Instead of lemon zest and dill or parsley, flavour the stock with 4 slices of fresh root ginger and a handful of coriander stalks. Simmer for 20 minutes, then remove the duck and shred. Strain the stock, then reheat with 1 tsp grated fresh root ginger. Add 2 thinly sliced celery sticks and 85 g (3 oz) basmati rice. When the rice is almost cooked, add the shredded duck, 1 tbsp chopped coriander, a pinch of crushed dried chillies and a dash of soy sauce. Bring back to the boil, then serve.

Plus points

• The combination of rice, lean chicken and vegetables keeps this soup low in fat and provides protein and starchy carbohydrate.

• Although eggs contain cholesterol, they are an excellent source of protein and many other nutrients. Also, it is now generally agreed that, for most people, eating them has little effect on blood cholesterol levels. Rather, it is the intake of saturated fat, as well as other factors, that can increase blood cholesterol.

Each serving provides   kcal 305, protein 28 g, fat 5 g (of which saturated fat 1 g), carbohydrate 40 g (of which sugars 6 g), fibre 2 g. Excellent source of niacin, vitamin A. Good source of selenium, vitamin B_6. Useful source of copper, folate, iron, potassium, vitamin B_1, vitamin B_2, vitamin B_{12}, vitamin C.

French-style chicken in wine

Think of a French country-style meal and chances are your mind will conjure up the image of chicken simmering in robust red wine. This up-dated version of a classic bistro dish contains shallots, mushrooms and carrots, so the only accompaniment needed is potatoes – or some warmed seeded bread.

Preparation time **15 minutes**   Cooking time **about 1¼ hours**   *Serves 4*

12 shallots or button onions

1½ tbsp garlic-flavoured olive oil

55 g (2 oz) lean back bacon, cut across into thin strips

12 chestnut or button mushrooms

4 chicken joints such as breasts, about 170 g (6 oz) each, skinless

several sprigs of parsley, stalks bruised

several sprigs of fresh thyme

1 bay leaf

150 ml (5 fl oz) chicken stock, preferably home-made (see page 212)

360 ml (12 fl oz) full-bodied red wine, such as Burgundy

300 g (10½ oz) carrots, cut into chunks

pinch of caster sugar

1 tbsp cornflour

salt and pepper

chopped parsley to garnish

1 Put the shallots or onions in a heatproof bowl and cover with boiling water. Leave for 30 seconds, then drain. When cool enough to handle, peel and set aside.

2 Heat 1 tbsp of the oil in a flameproof casserole. Add the bacon and fry for about 3 minutes, stirring often, until crispy. Remove with a draining spoon and set aside.

3 Add the shallots to the casserole and fry, stirring often, over a moderately high heat for 5 minutes or until browned all over. Remove with a draining spoon and set aside.

4 Add the mushrooms to the casserole, with the remaining ½ tbsp oil if needed, and fry for 3–4 minutes, stirring often, until golden.

5 Return half of the bacon and shallots to the casserole. Place the chicken joints on top and sprinkle with the remaining bacon and shallots. Tie the herbs into a bouquet garni and add to the casserole with the stock and wine. Season generously with pepper.

6 Bring to the boil, then reduce the heat to very low and simmer for 15 minutes. Add the carrots and continue simmering over a low heat for a further 30 minutes or until the chicken is cooked through and the carrots are tender but still crisp.

7 Lift out the chicken and arrange on a warmed platter. Strain the liquid into a saucepan. Add the bacon, mushrooms, shallots and carrots and keep warm.

8 Put the bouquet garni back in the strained liquid, add the sugar and bring to the boil. Boil until the sauce is reduced to about 360 ml (12 fl oz). Mix the cornflour with a little water to make a smooth paste. Add to the sauce, stirring, and simmer until thickened. Adjust the seasoning to taste and discard the bouquet garni. Spoon the sauce over the chicken and vegetables, sprinkle with the parsley and serve.

Another idea

If you cannot find garlic-flavoured olive oil, use extra virgin olive oil and fry 1 garlic clove, crushed, with the mushrooms.

Plus points

• Cooked chicken breast with the skin has about six times more fat than without the skin. If you prefer, you can cook the chicken with the skin on to keep the moisture in and then remove the skin just before serving. Sprinkle a little paprika on top to add colour.

• Red wine contains flavonoid compounds, which may protect against heart disease.

Each serving provides   kcal 300, protein 37 g, fat 6 g (of which saturated fat 1 g), carbohydrate 22 g (of which sugars 7 g), fibre 3 g. Excellent source of copper, niacin, vitamin A, vitamin B_6. Good source of iron, potassium, selenium, vitamin B_1, vitamin B_2, zinc. Useful source of folate, vitamin E.

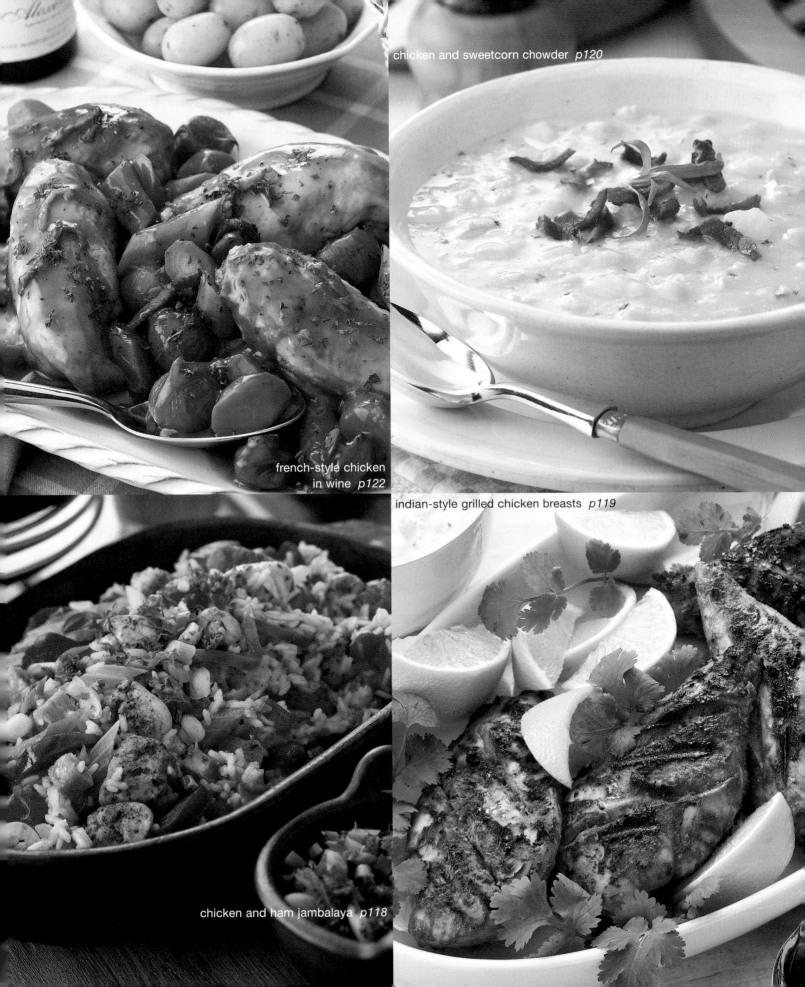

chicken and sweetcorn chowder *p120*

french-style chicken
in wine *p122*

indian-style grilled chicken breasts *p119*

chicken and ham jambalaya *p118*

Chicken livers sautéed with sage

Chicken livers can be found fresh or frozen in most supermarkets and are an extremely economical standby ingredient to have in the freezer. The addition of a few well-chosen flavouring ingredients, like the fresh sage and balsamic vinegar used here, can transform the livers into something rather special.

Preparation time **5 minutes**   Cooking time **12–15 minutes**   *Serves 4*

8 rounds French bread

2 tbsp extra virgin olive oil

1 small red onion, finely chopped

2 garlic cloves, chopped

400 g (14 oz) chicken livers

225 g (8 oz) small chestnut or button mushrooms, quartered

3 tbsp balsamic vinegar

2 tbsp shredded fresh sage

salt and pepper

small sprigs of fresh sage to garnish

1 Preheat the oven to 180°C (350°F, gas mark 4). Arrange the French bread on a baking tray. Using 1 tbsp of the oil, lightly brush the slices of bread on the top side, then bake for 10 minutes or until golden brown.

2 Meanwhile, heat the remaining 1 tbsp of oil in a heavy-based frying pan. Add the onion and garlic, and sauté over a moderately high heat for 2–3 minutes or until softened.

3 Add the chicken livers and mushrooms, and cook, stirring constantly, to brown on all sides. Add a little hot water if the liver begins to stick to the pan. As they cook, break up any large livers into bite-sized pieces, using the side of the spatula.

4 Add the balsamic vinegar, shredded sage and seasoning to taste. Reduce the heat a little and continue cooking for 5–10 minutes or until the livers are just cooked through.

5 Serve the chicken livers on top of the baked French bread rounds, garnished with sprigs of fresh sage.

Some more ideas

Serve on thick slices of wholemeal toast rather than French bread, or with a celeriac and potato purée.

For **Provençal chicken livers**, replace the balsamic vinegar with 4 tbsp red wine and use 1 tsp dried herbes de Provence instead of the fresh sage. Serve with rice.

The chicken livers can be baked instead of sautéed. Put all the ingredients in an ovenproof dish and mix together. (If preparing in advance, cover and refrigerate until ready to cook.) Place in the oven preheated to 220°C (425°F, gas mark 7) and bake for 12–15 minutes.

Plus points

• Like all liver, chicken livers are a rich source of iron, necessary to help prevent anaemia.

• Garlic (along with leeks, onions and chives) contains allicin, which has anti-fungal and antibiotic properties. Garlic also contains other compounds, which in animal studies have been shown to protect against cancer.

photo, page 127

Each serving provides kcal 285, protein 24 g, fat 9.5 g (of which saturated fat 2 g), carbohydrate 29 g (of which sugars 2 g), fibre 1.5 g. Excellent source of copper, folate, iron, vitamin A, vitamin B$_2$, vitamin B$_6$, vitamin B$_{12}$. Good source of niacin, selenium, vitamin B$_1$, vitamin C, zinc. Useful source of vitamin E.

Marsala chicken with fennel

Cooking with a little wine – in this case the famous dessert wine from Sicily – gives great depth to a sauce: nearly all the alcohol and calories burn away, leaving behind only flavour. This sauce is thickened with a mixture of egg and lemon juice, which is typically Mediterranean and less rich than beurre manié or cream.

Preparation time **15 minutes**   Cooking time **45 minutes**   *Serves 4*

1 chicken, about 1.35 kg (3 lb), jointed

2 tbsp plain flour

2 tbsp extra virgin olive oil

1 large leek, coarsely chopped

1 tbsp chopped parsley

1 tsp fennel seeds

90 ml (3 fl oz) Marsala

500 ml (17 fl oz) chicken stock, preferably home-made (see page 212)

2 medium-sized bulbs of fennel, trimmed and cut into chunks

280 g (10 oz) shelled fresh or frozen peas

juice of 1 lemon

1 egg, lightly beaten

salt and pepper

To garnish

chopped parsley

shreds of lemon zest

1 Remove the skin from the chicken joints, except for any small pieces such as the wings. Season the flour and coat the joints.

2 Heat 1 tbsp of the oil in a sauté pan and add the leek, parsley and fennel seeds. Cook over a moderate heat until the leek is softened, stirring frequently. Remove from the pan with a draining spoon and set aside.

3 Add the remaining oil to the pan and sauté the chicken for 6–7 minutes or until golden. Remove the chicken from the pan and set aside. Pour in the Marsala and bubble until it is reduced to about 2 tbsp of glaze. Pour in the stock, and return the leek mixture and dark meat chicken joints and wings to the pan (wait to add the breasts as they can overcook). Add the fennel. Cover and simmer over a low heat for 10–15 minutes, then add the breasts and continue to cook, covered, for 15 minutes or until all the chicken joints are tender. Add the peas for the last 5 minutes of cooking.

4 Using a draining spoon, remove the chicken pieces and vegetables to a platter. Keep warm.

5 In a small bowl, mix the lemon juice into the egg. Slowly add about 4 tbsp of the hot cooking liquid to the lemon and egg mixture, stirring well, then slowly stir this

mixture back into the liquid in the pan. Return the chicken and vegetables to the pan and gently warm on a very low heat so the sauce does not curdle. Season to taste. Serve garnished with parsley and lemon zest.

Another idea

For **chicken with asparagus and fennel seeds**, omit the peas and bulb fennel. Cut 1 bunch of asparagus (about 225 g/8 oz) into bite-sized pieces and add to the simmering chicken at the end of step 3. Thicken with the egg and lemon mixture, as above.

Plus points

• Bulb fennel contains more phytoestrogen than most vegetables. This plant hormone encourages the body to excrete excess oestrogen (a high level of oestrogen is linked with greater risk of breast cancer).

• Peas provide good amounts of the B vitamins B_1, B_6 and niacin. They also offer dietary fibre, particularly the soluble variety, plus some folate and vitamin C.

• The dark meat of chicken contains twice as much iron and zinc as the light meat. It is, however, higher in fat.

photo, page 127

Each serving provides kcal 380, protein 46 g, fat 12 g (of which saturated fat 2.5 g), carbohydrate 18 g (of which sugars 5 g), fibre 5.5 g. Excellent source of niacin, vitamin B_6. Good source of folate, iron, potassium, selenium, vitamin B_1, vitamin B_2, vitamin C, zinc. Useful source of calcium, copper, vitamin A, vitamin B_{12}, vitamin E.

Roast herb and garlic chicken

Rather than rubbing butter over a bird before roasting, here a paste of fresh herbs and fromage frais is pushed under the skin. This keeps the roasting chicken beautifully moist as well as adding a wonderful flavour. The pan juices are used to make a simple sauce.

Preparation time **15 minutes**   Cooking time **1¾–2 hours**   *Serves 4*

1 lemon

1 chicken, about 1.35 kg (3 lb), without giblets

15 g (½ oz) fresh coriander

15 g (½ oz) parsley

2 garlic cloves, peeled

2 tbsp fromage frais

150 ml (5 fl oz) dry white wine

salt and pepper

To garnish

lemon slices

sprigs of fresh coriander or parsley

1 Preheat the oven to 180°C (350°F, gas mark 4). Grate the zest from the lemon, then cut the lemon in half. Squeeze the lemon juice inside the chicken's cavity. Push the lemon halves inside and sprinkle half the zest.

2 Place the chicken in the tin, breast side up. Very carefully ease your fingers under the skin, starting at the neck end. Loosen the skin over the breasts and thighs, without breaking it.

3 Combine the herbs and garlic in a blender or food processor and process until finely chopped. Add the fromage frais, remaining lemon zest and seasoning, and process again briefly to mix. Push the paste under the skin, easing it along so that it covers the breasts and thighs evenly in a thin layer. Secure the end of the neck skin by folding the wing tips under.

4 Cover the chicken with foil and roast for 45 minutes. Remove the foil and roast, uncovered, for a further 1–1¼ hours or until the juices run clear when a knife is inserted into the thickest part of the thigh. Baste once or twice with the juices in the tin.

5 Lift up the chicken, tipping it so that the juices can run out of the cavity into the tin. Set the chicken aside on a carving board to rest. Skim all the fat from the surface of the juices in the tin, then bring to the boil on top of the cooker. Add the white wine and bring back to the boil, scraping up all of the browned bits from the bottom of the tin. Boil the sauce for 1 minute. Season to taste.

6 Carve the chicken into slices. Garnish with lemon slices and sprigs of coriander or parsley, and serve with the pan sauce.

Another idea

For a very **simple roast chicken**, just squeeze the lemon juice into the cavity and push in the lemon halves; omit the herb and fromage frais paste. Make the pan sauce with chicken stock, vegetable cooking water or even just with plain water, instead of wine.

Plus points

• The latest research has found that moderate alcohol consumption is associated with a lower risk of death from coronary heart disease. Moderate means avoiding binges and taking no more than 3–4 units a day for men and 2–3 units a day for women.

• Some studies suggest that garlic may help to reduce high blood cholesterol levels and inhibit blood clotting, thereby reducing the risk of heart attack and stroke.

Each serving provides kcal 229, protein 37 g, fat 6 g (of which saturated fat 2 g), carbohydrate 1 g (of which sugars 1 g), fibre 0 g. Excellent source of niacin, vitamin B_6, vitamin B_{12}. Good source of copper. Useful source of iron, potassium, selenium, vitamin B_1, vitamin B_2, zinc.

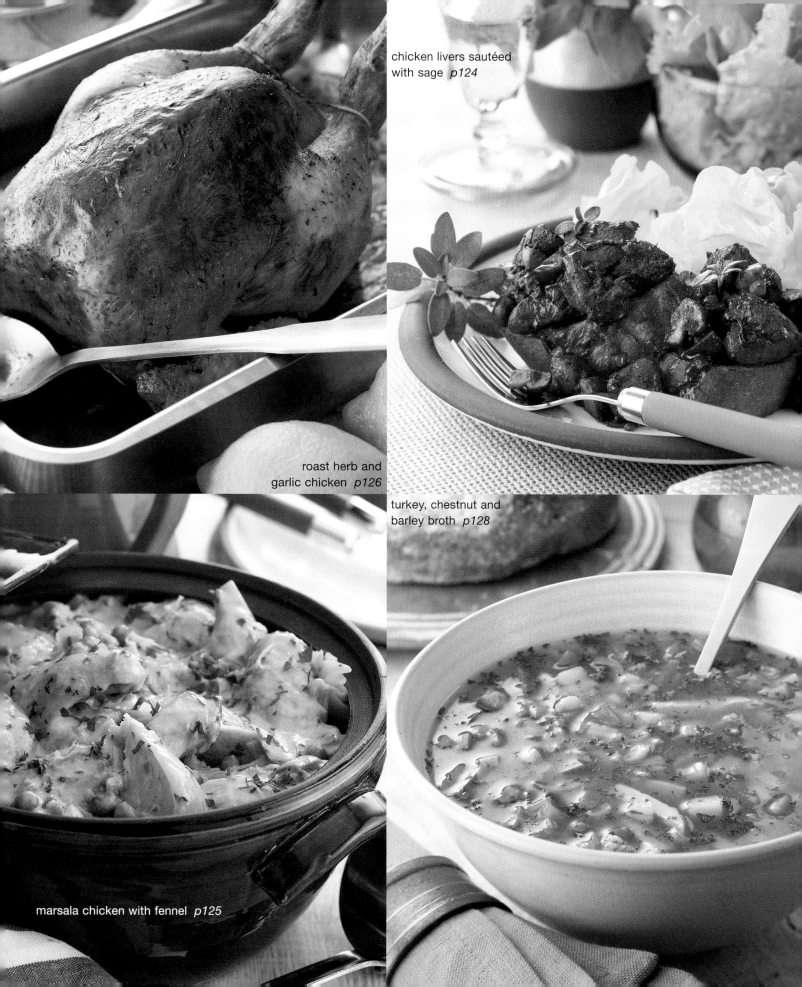

chicken livers sautéed
with sage *p124*

roast herb and
garlic chicken *p126*

turkey, chestnut and
barley broth *p128*

marsala chicken with fennel *p125*

Turkey, chestnut and barley broth

When you roast a turkey, don't throw away the carcass. Instead, use it to make this wonderfully rich-tasting soup. Reminiscent of an Italian minestrone, it is packed with vegetables, barley, turkey meat and chestnuts – a really satisfying bowl of soup. Serve with warm, crusty wholemeal bread.

Preparation time **15 minutes**   Cooking time **about 2¼ hours**   *Serves 6*

Stock

1 roast turkey carcass

1 onion, cut into quarters

1 carrot, chopped

2 celery sticks, chopped

few sprigs of parsley

few sprigs of fresh thyme

1 bay leaf

Soup

1 large carrot, chopped

1 large parsnip, chopped

3 celery sticks, chopped

4–6 Brussels sprouts, chopped

1 large leek, chopped

100 g (3½ oz) freshly cooked or vacuum-packed chestnuts, roughly chopped

75 g (2½ oz) pearl barley

3 tbsp chopped parsley

100 g (3½ oz) cooked turkey meat, without skin, chopped or shredded

salt and pepper

1 First, make the stock. Break up the turkey carcass, discarding any skin, and place in a very large saucepan. Add the quartered onion, carrot and celery. Tie the herb sprigs and bay leaf into a bouquet garni and add to the pan. Cover generously with water and bring to the boil, skimming any scum from the surface with a draining spoon. Reduce the heat, cover the pan and simmer gently for 1½ hours. Strain the stock, and discard the bones and vegetables.

2 Measure the stock and, if necessary, make up to 1.7 litres (3 pints) with water. Skim off any fat and pour back into the cleaned saucepan.

3 Bring the stock back to the boil. Add the chopped vegetables, chestnuts and pearl barley, and simmer for 35 minutes or until the pearl barley is tender.

4 Add the parsley and turkey, and heat through thoroughly. Season with salt and pepper and serve.

Another idea

For a **turkey, lentil and sweet potato soup**, add red lentils instead of pearl barley and use 1 large orange-fleshed sweet potato, 1 large parsnip and 225 g (8 oz) celeriac instead of the carrot, parsnip, celery, sprouts and leek. Flavour the soup with 1 tbsp redcurrant jelly, stirred in just before serving.

Plus points

● Barley is believed to be the world's oldest cultivated grain. It is low in fat and rich in starchy carbohydrate. It contains traces of gluten, but is useful for those on wheat-free diets.

● Turkey is even lower in fat than chicken. Use skinless turkey wherever possible.

● Unlike other nuts, chestnuts are high in complex carbohydrates and low in fat – Brazil nuts, hazelnuts and walnuts have 20 times as much fat as chestnuts. Chestnuts also provide useful amounts of vitamins E and B_6.

photo, page 127

Each serving provides   kcal 115, protein 7 g, fat 1.2 g (of which saturated fat 0.2 g), carbohydrate 20 g (of which sugars 3.5 g), fibre 2 g. Useful source of folate, vitamin B_6, vitamin C, vitamin E.

Roast turkey with lemon couscous

A small turkey like this is amazingly economical. It will give enough meat for at least 8 portions, or you can serve 4 people and have plenty of leftovers for sandwiches, salads and other dishes. Don't forget to keep the turkey carcass to make stock for soup.

Preparation time **20 minutes, plus 10 minutes soaking**   Cooking time **about 1¾ hours**   *Serves 8*

4 large lemons

340 g (12 oz) couscous

1 tsp turmeric

1 tsp ground cumin

1 tsp ground cinnamon

900 ml (1½ pints) hot chicken or turkey stock, preferably home-made (see page 212)

115 g (4 oz) ready-to-eat dried apricots, chopped

4 tbsp chopped fresh mint

1 turkey, about 2.25 kg (5 lb), without giblets

150 ml (5 fl oz) dry sherry

salt and pepper

sprigs of fresh mint to garnish

1 Halve the lemons lengthways and squeeze out all the juice into a jug. Pull the membranes and pulp from each lemon half to leave a smooth clean shell. Cut a thin slice off the base of each shell so that it will stand firmly. Set aside.

2 Place the couscous in a medium-sized mixing bowl. Add 4 tbsp of the lemon juice, the spices, 750 ml (1¼ pints) of the stock, the apricots and mint, and stir to mix well. Leave to soak for 10 minutes or until the couscous has absorbed all the stock.

3 Preheat the oven to 200°C (400°F, gas mark 6). Place the turkey on a rack in a medium-sized roasting tin and pour over 150 ml (5 fl oz) hot water.

4 When the couscous is ready, use a spoon to stuff some of it into the neck end of the turkey. Secure the skin flap underneath the bird with the wing tips. Spoon 2 tbsp of the lemon juice over the bird. Cover the turkey loosely with oiled foil and roast for 1¾ hours. Baste with roasting juices occasionally to keep it moist, and remove the foil for the last 30 minutes of cooking to allow the skin to brown. At the end of the cooking time, test the turkey by pushing a metal skewer into the thickest part of the thigh; the juices should run clear.

If they are still pink, continue to roast the bird, testing every 10 minutes.

5 Meanwhile, fill the lemon halves with couscous. Spread the rest of the couscous in a small ovenproof dish and sit the lemon halves on top. Cover loosely with foil and place in the oven for the last 20 minutes of the turkey's roasting time.

6 When the turkey is cooked, remove it from the tin and leave it to rest on a carving board for 10 minutes. Skim all the fat from the surface of the juices in the tin, then add the sherry and remaining stock. Bring to the boil on top of the cooker, scraping up the browned bits from the tin. Boil for 5 minutes. Season to taste.

7 Carve the turkey and serve with the couscous-filled lemons, garnished with mint sprigs, the extra couscous and the sauce from the pan.

Plus points

• Couscous is low in fat and high in starchy carbohydrate. It scores fairly low on the Glycaemic Index scale, which means that it breaks down slowly in the body, releasing energy gradually into the bloodstream.

photo, page 133

Each serving provides   kcal 310, protein 36 g, fat 4 g (of which saturated fat 1 g), carbohydrate 28 g (of which sugars 6.5 g), fibre 1 g. Excellent source of vitamin B$_6$, vitamin B$_{12}$. Good source of iron, niacin. Useful source of copper, potassium, vitamin B$_1$, vitamin B$_{12}$, zinc.

Turkey kebabs with fennel and red pepper relish

Here lean little bites of turkey are marinated with wine and herbs to add juiciness and flavour, and then threaded onto skewers to be grilled or barbecued. A colourful raw-vegetable relish provides a nice splash of vitamin C as well as a delightful taste contrast. Serve with a complex carbohydrate such as steamed Basmati rice or couscous.

Preparation time **20 minutes, plus at least 10 minutes marinating**   Cooking time **15 minutes**   *Serves 4*

450 g (1 lb) skinless turkey breast steak

3 garlic cloves, chopped

1½ tbsp lemon juice

2 tbsp dry white wine

1 tbsp chopped fresh sage or 2 tsp dried sage, crumbled

1 tbsp chopped fresh rosemary

1½ tsp fresh thyme leaves or ½ tsp dried thyme

1 tsp fennel seeds, lightly crushed

2½ tbsp extra virgin olive oil

1 red pepper, seeded and finely diced

1 bulb of fennel, finely diced

1 tbsp black olive paste (tapenade) or 10 black Kalamata olives, finely diced

8 stalks of fresh rosemary (optional)

8 shallots or button onions

salt and pepper

1 Cut the turkey into 24 pieces, each about 5 x 2 cm (2 x ¾ in). Combine the turkey pieces with 2 of the chopped garlic cloves, 1 tbsp lemon juice, the wine, sage, rosemary, thyme, fennel seeds, 2 tbsp of the olive oil and seasoning. Toss so that all the turkey pieces are covered with the herb mixture. Leave to marinate for at least 10 minutes, or up to 1 hour if you have the time.

2 Meanwhile, make the relish. Put the red pepper, diced fennel and olive paste or diced olives in a bowl together with the remaining garlic, ½ tbsp lemon juice and ½ tbsp olive oil. Season to taste. Mix well, then set aside.

3 Preheat the grill to high, or prepare a charcoal fire in the barbecue. Thread the marinated turkey pieces onto the rosemary stalks if using, or onto skewers, and top each one with a shallot or button onion.

4 Grill or barbecue the kebabs for about 15 minutes or until cooked through and the turkey pieces are lightly browned in spots. Turn the kebabs and baste with the remaining marinade frequently. Serve the kebabs hot, with the red pepper relish.

Some more ideas

Add red pepper and fennel to the kebabs. Cut the pepper and fennel into 2.5 cm (1 in) chunks. Alternate the vegetable chunks with pieces of turkey on the skewers, and brush with the marinade. Grill as above, then serve drizzled with the remaining lemon juice.

To make an oil-free **roasted red pepper and tomato relish**, cut a large red pepper in half and grill until charred. Leave to cool, then peel off the skin. Finely dice the flesh and mix with 1 diced tomato, 1 finely chopped shallot, 2 chopped garlic cloves, 2 tbsp chopped fresh basil or parsley and a splash of balsamic vinegar, then season to taste.

Plus points

• The vegetable relish is a low-fat condiment that is high in vitamin C and beta-carotene from the red peppers. These nutrients are powerful antioxidants that can help to protect against many diseases including cancer and heart disease.

• Fennel provides useful amounts of potassium and folate. It is also low in calories – 100 g (3½ oz) contains 12 kcal.

photo, page 133

Each serving provides   kcal 224, protein 28 g, fat 9.5 g (of which saturated fat 1.5 g), carbohydrate 7 g (of which sugars 6 g), fibre 2.5 g. Excellent source of vitamin B$_6$, vitamin B$_{12}$, vitamin C. Good source of niacin, vitamin A. Useful source of copper, folate, iron, potassium, vitamin E, zinc.

Turkey and lentil pâté

This coarse-textured pâté, deliciously flavoured with garlic and fresh coriander, combines minced turkey and turkey livers with lentils for a starter that has considerably less fat than a traditional pâté. Serve with toasted slices of brioche or other bread, plus some crisp vegetable sticks and crunchy radishes.

Preparation time 1¼ hours, plus about 2 hours chilling *Serves 6*

55 g (2 oz) green lentils

1½ tbsp sunflower oil

4 shallots, finely chopped

1 garlic clove, crushed

450 g (1 lb) minced turkey

115 g (4 oz) turkey livers, chopped

3 tbsp dry Marsala wine

30 g (1 oz) fresh coriander leaves

salt and pepper

sprigs of fresh coriander to garnish

1 Put the lentils in a saucepan, cover generously with water and bring to the boil. Simmer for about 45 minutes or until tender. Drain well and set aside to cool.

2 Heat the oil in a large frying pan and fry the shallots and garlic over a moderately high heat for 2 minutes or until they have softened. Reduce the heat to moderate and add the minced turkey and the livers. Cook, stirring, for 8–10 minutes.

3 Pour in the Marsala, bring to the boil and allow the mixture to bubble for 1–2 minutes. Season with salt and pepper.

4 Transfer the mixture to a food processor. Add the coriander leaves and cooked lentils, and then process for a few seconds until the mixture becomes a coarse paste. Alternatively, finely chop the coriander, and mash all the ingredients together thoroughly using a fork.

5 Spoon into 6 ramekins, pressing down well with the back of the spoon. Cover and chill for about 2 hours before serving, garnished with fresh coriander sprigs.

Some more ideas

Use chicken livers instead of turkey livers, or a mixture of the two.

Replace the Marsala with medium sherry.

For a **turkey and apricot pâté**, omit the lentils and instead use 55 g (2 oz) dried apricots, diced, and 115 g (4 oz) mushrooms, finely chopped. Cook with the minced turkey and livers in step 2. Replace the Marsala with 2 tbsp brandy. Dried apricots are a useful source of vitamin A (through beta-carotene) and one of the richest fruit sources of iron.

Plus points

• Turkey livers are a rich source of iron, zinc, vitamin A and many of the B vitamins, especially B_{12}. The iron present in the livers is in a form that is easily absorbed by the human body.

• Lentils can be used as a substitute for meat in recipes such as hamburgers. Just replace about half the meat with cooked lentils and follow the recipe as usual. This cuts the amount of fat and cholesterol, and increases the fibre content.

photo, page 133

Each serving provides kcal 245, protein 33 g, fat 9 g (of which saturated fat 2.5 g), carbohydrate 6 g (of which sugars 1 g), fibre 1 g. Excellent source of folate, iron, niacin, vitamin A, vitamin B_2, vitamin B_6, vitamin B_{12}. Good source of copper, vitamin B_1, vitamin C, zinc. Useful source of potassium, selenium, vitamin E.

Turkey sausage and bean hotpot

Having diabetes doesn't mean giving up favourite family meals. Here, lean turkey sausages replace the more traditional pork in a hearty hotpot, with a spicy bean sauce and a covering of thinly sliced root veggies.

Preparation time **about 1 hour**   Cooking time **30–35 minutes**   *Serves 4*

400 g (14 oz) potatoes, peeled and thinly sliced

1 large carrot, about 200 g (7 oz), thinly sliced on a diagonal

1 medium parsnip, about 200 g (7 oz), thinly sliced on a diagonal

1½ tbsp sunflower oil

8 turkey sausages, about 450 g (1 lb) in total

1 onion, finely chopped

2 tsp paprika

2 tbsp plain flour

450 ml (15 fl oz) chicken stock, preferably home-made (see page 212)

1 tbsp Worcestershire sauce

3 tsp wholegrain mustard

1 tsp light soft brown sugar

1 can red kidney beans, about 400 g, drained and rinsed

20 g (¾ oz) butter, melted

pepper

1 Preheat the oven to 190°C (375°F, gas mark 5). Boil the potato, carrot and parsnip slices for 3–4 minutes or until just tender. Drain and set aside.

2 Heat the oil in a frying pan. Cook the sausages over a moderate heat for 10 minutes, turning occasionally. Remove the sausages from the pan and reserve.

3 Add the onion to the pan and sauté for 5 minutes, stirring, until golden. Stir in the paprika and flour, then gradually mix in the stock. Bring to the boil, stirring, then reduce the heat to moderate and simmer until thickened and smooth. Stir in the Worcestershire sauce, 2 tsp of the mustard and the sugar. Add pepper to taste. Add the beans. Cut the sausages into thick slices and stir into the sauce. Bring to the boil.

4 Spoon the sausage and bean mixture into a 1.5 litre (2¾ pint) shallow baking dish. Arrange the sliced root vegetables over the top, starting in the centre and working out in overlapping rings to cover the surface completely. Mix the remaining 1 tsp of mustard with the melted butter and brush over the vegetables.

5 Bake for 30–35 minutes or until the sauce is bubbling and the vegetable topping is golden brown. Serve hot.

Some more ideas

For a **vegetarian hotpot**, use meat-free sausages and vegetable stock. Replace the Worcestershire sauce with mild chilli sauce.

Make a **mash topping**: cut the potatoes, carrot and parsnip into chunks and cook in boiling water for 15–20 minutes. Drain well, then mash with 200 g (7 oz) virtually fat-free fromage frais and add pepper to taste. Spread over the sausage and bean mixture, then dot with 15 g (½ oz) butter and sprinkle with a little paprika. Bake as above.

Plus points

● Red kidney beans – and all other pulses – are a good source of dietary fibre, particularly soluble fibre which can help to reduce high blood cholesterol levels.

● Both parsnips and potatoes provide useful amounts of potassium. Parsnips also contain useful quantities of some of the B vitamins, particularly folate and B_1.

● Since the sausages and stock are quite salty, there's no need to add extra salt.

Each serving provides   kcal 486, protein 39 g, fat 12 g (of which saturated fat 4 g), carbohydrate 58 g (of which sugars 15 g), fibre 12 g. Excellent source of vitamin A, vitamin B_6, vitamin B_{12}. Good source of copper, folate, iron, niacin, potassium, vitamin B_1, vitamin C, vitamin E. Useful source of calcium, selenium.

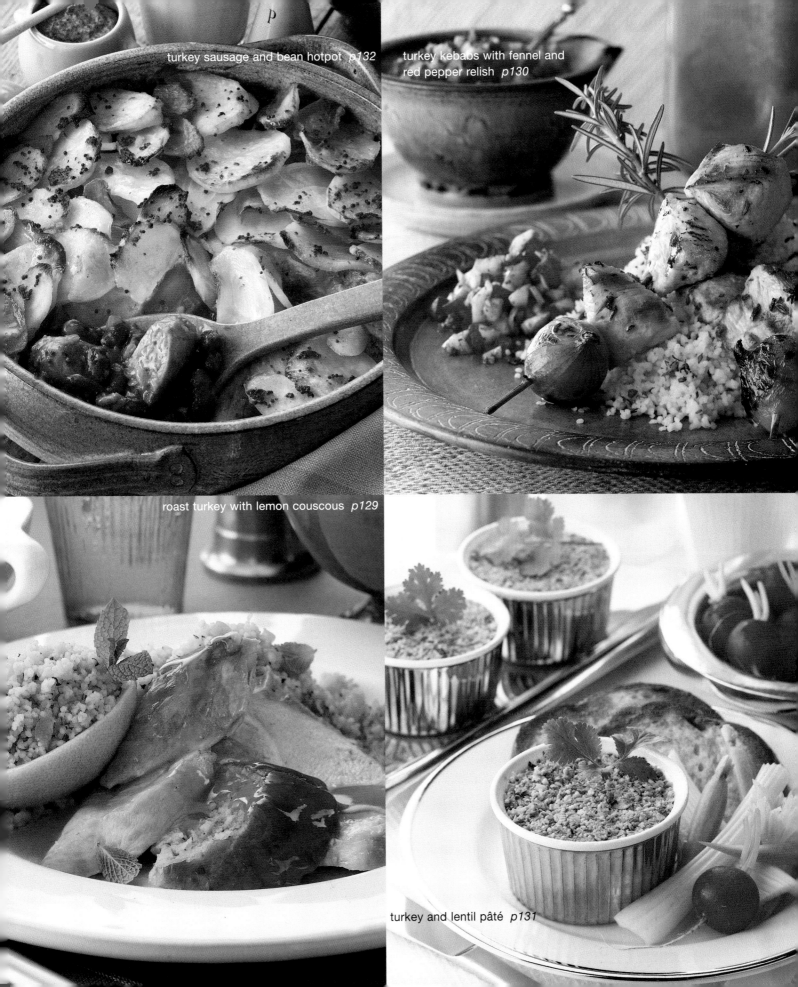

turkey sausage and bean hotpot *p132*

turkey kebabs with fennel and
red pepper relish *p130*

roast turkey with lemon couscous *p129*

turkey and lentil pâté *p131*

Turkey drumsticks braised with baby vegetables

This is a simple dish to prepare and makes an economical, healthy mid-week family meal, low in calories and fat. Roasted in the French style, in stock with a few herbs, the meat from the turkey legs turns out wonderfully moist and tender. Serve with baked or boiled potatoes to add starchy carbohydrate.

Preparation time **10 minutes**   Cooking time **1½ hours**   *Serves 4*

2 tbsp sunflower oil

4 medium leeks, thickly sliced

12 baby carrots

12 baby courgettes

12 baby corn

300 ml (10 fl oz) turkey or chicken stock, preferably home-made (see page 212)

2 sprigs of fresh rosemary

1 bay leaf

2 large turkey drumsticks, about 600 g (1 lb 5 oz) each, skinned

pepper

1 Preheat the oven to 200°C (400°F, gas mark 6). Heat the oil in a large flameproof casserole over a moderately high heat. Add the leeks, carrots, courgettes and baby corn, and fry for 3–4 minutes, stirring all the time, until beginning to brown.

2 Pour in the stock, and then add the rosemary and bay leaf. Season the turkey drumsticks with pepper and put on top of the vegetables.

3 Transfer to the oven and braise for about 1½ hours or until the turkey is golden brown and cooked. Baste the turkey about halfway through the cooking, and stir the vegetables. Test by piercing the thickest part of a drumstick with a sharp knife; the juices that run out should be clear.

4 Carve the meat from the drumsticks into slices. Serve with the vegetables and a little of the stock spooned over.

Some more ideas

Instead of turkey drumsticks, use 8 chicken drumsticks. Braise for about 1 hour.

Replace 150 ml (5 fl oz) of the stock with the same quantity of white wine.

Use 4 large carrots and 4 large courgettes, all cut into 5 cm (2 in) chunks, instead of the baby vegetables.

Roast the turkey on a bed of root vegetables: include the carrots, but replace the leeks, courgettes and baby corn with 12 baby parsnips, 12 baby turnips and ½ small swede, cut into thick fingers. Or use 4 large carrots, parsnips and turnips with the swede, and cut all the vegetables into chunks.

Plus points

● Carrots may be one of the earliest foods eaten by man. Native to Asia, they were being cultivated long before the birth of Christ. The beta-carotene found in carrots is much better absorbed by the body (and converted into vitamin A) after the carrots have been cooked, and even more so if they are eaten along with a little fat or oil.

● The corn in this recipe provides good amounts of fibre and vitamin A.

photo, page 137

Each serving provides   kcal 250, protein 32 g, fat 10 g (of which saturated fat 2 g), carbohydrate 9 g (of which sugars 8 g), fibre 6 g. Excellent source of folate, vitamin A, vitamin B$_6$, vitamin B$_{12}$, vitamin C. Good source of iron, niacin, potassium, vitamin B$_1$, vitamin E, zinc. Good source of calcium, copper, vitamin B$_2$.

Pan-fried turkey escalopes with citrus honey sauce

The tanginess of citrus fruit marries well with poultry. Here, orange and lemon, with honey and shallots, create a tasty sauce for turkey escalopes, served on a stack of green beans. Serve with steamed new potatoes in their skins.

Preparation time **15 minutes**   Cooking time **about 15 minutes**   *Serves 4*

4 small skinless turkey breast steaks, about 115 g (4 oz) each

30 g (1 oz) butter

4 large shallots, thinly sliced

1 garlic clove, crushed

400 g (14 oz) fine French beans, trimmed

2 tbsp clear honey

grated zest and juice of 1 orange

grated zest and juice of 1 lemon

salt and pepper

1 Put the turkey steaks between sheets of cling film and pound them to flatten to about 5 mm (¼ in) thickness. Set these escalopes aside.

2 Melt the butter in a large frying pan, add the shallots and garlic, and cook, stirring, for 2–3 minutes or until softened but not brown. Remove the shallots from the pan with a draining spoon and set aside.

3 Put the turkey escalopes in the pan, in one layer, and fry them for 2–3 minutes on each side.

4 Meanwhile, cook the beans in a saucepan of boiling salted water for 3–4 minutes or until just tender. Drain and rinse briefly in cold water to stop the cooking. Keep the beans warm.

5 Mix the honey with the zest and juice of the orange and lemon. Remove the turkey escalopes from the pan and keep hot. Pour the honey mixture into the pan, return the shallots and garlic, and add seasoning to taste. Bring to the boil and bubble for about 2 minutes, stirring constantly.

6 Make a pile of beans on 4 plates and place a turkey escalope on top of each pile. Spoon over the sliced shallots and pan juices, and serve.

Some more ideas

Use 4 skinless boneless turkey breast fillets, about 125 g (4½ oz) each. Being a bit thicker than escalopes, they will need to be cooked for 5 minutes on each side.

Replace the turkey steaks with 4 small boneless duck breasts, about 550 g (1¼ lb) in total. Remove the skin and all fat from the breasts. Pan-fry for 3 minutes on each side, if you like duck a little pink, or a little longer for well-done duck. For the sauce, use the zest and juice from a pink grapefruit instead of the orange and lemon. Also add a piece of stem ginger, cut into fine slivers, and 1 tbsp of the stem ginger syrup.

Plus points

• In this recipe, only a touch of butter is used in the sauce, making it smooth and glossy. The healthy citrus fruits contribute most of the flavour in this zesty sauce.

• All citrus fruits are an excellent source of vitamin C. Vitamin C is often lost in the cooking water, so remember to mop up the pan juices with potatoes or bread.

photo, page 137

Each serving provides   kcal 245, protein 27 g, fat 9 g (of which saturated fat 5 g), carbohydrate 14 g (of which sugars 13 g), fibre 2.5 g. Excellent source of vitamin B$_{12}$. Good source of folate, iron, niacin, vitamin B$_6$, vitamin C, zinc. Useful source of copper, potassium, vitamin A.

Turkey mole

This is a simplified, quite mild version of the classic spicy-hot Mexican recipe, made with lean turkey, raisins and almonds. Serve with boiled rice and salad.

Preparation time **10 minutes**   Cooking time **25 minutes**   *Serves 4*

2 tbsp sunflower oil

1 large onion, chopped

2 garlic cloves, crushed

1 fresh red chilli, seeded and sliced (optional)

2 tbsp sesame seeds

500 g (1 lb 2 oz) skinless turkey breast steaks, cut into thin strips

1½ tbsp mild chilli powder, or more to taste

½ tsp ground cloves

1 can chopped tomatoes, about 400 g

40 g (1½ oz) raisins

150 ml (5 fl oz) chicken stock, preferably home-made (see page 212)

3 tbsp toasted flaked almonds

2 tbsp chopped fresh coriander

salt and pepper

sprigs of fresh coriander to garnish

1 Heat the oil in a large wide pan over a moderately low heat. Add the onion and garlic with the sliced chilli and sesame seeds and cook, stirring frequently, for 10 minutes or until the onion is soft and golden.

2 Add the strips of turkey and stir them briefly round the pan to mix with the onion. Sprinkle over the chilli powder and cloves, and add the canned tomatoes with their juice and the raisins. Stir well to mix.

3 Pour in the stock. Bring to the boil, then reduce the heat to low, cover the pan and leave to simmer gently for 10 minutes.

4 Add the almonds and chopped coriander, and mix well. Season to taste. Spoon into a serving dish, garnish with sprigs of coriander and serve immediately.

Some more ideas

Diced cooked turkey can be used as an alternative to the raw turkey. Add to the sauce with the raisins.

For **turkey mole tacos**, mix 1 tsp cornflour with 1 tbsp cold water and stir into the sauce before the almonds in step 4. Bubble, stirring, until thickened, then add the almonds and coriander. Make a salad with 1 red onion, thinly sliced, 2 tomatoes, chopped, 1 large avocado, sliced, a wedge of iceberg lettuce, shredded, and a handful of fresh coriander leaves. Heat 12 taco shells in the oven preheated to 180°C (350°F, gas mark 4) for 3 minutes or according to the instructions on the packet. To serve, place a little salad in the warmed taco shells, then spoon over the turkey mole. Eat with your fingers and plenty of napkins!

Plus points

• Research has shown that lycopene – the natural pigment that gives tomatoes their red colour – can reduce the risk of heart disease and prostate cancer. A six-year study of 48,000 men, conducted at Harvard medical school, found that consuming tomato products more than twice a week was associated with a reduced risk of prostate cancer of up to 34 per cent. Processed tomatoes contain much higher concentrations of lycopene than fresh.

• Raisins contain a useful amount of fibre and potassium.

Each serving provides kcal 400, protein 34 g, fat 21 g (of which saturated fat 3.5 g), carbohydrate 22 g (of which sugars 15 g), fibre 3.5 g. Excellent source of copper, vitamin B_6, vitamin B_{12}, vitamin E. Good source of iron, niacin, potassium, vitamin C, zinc. Useful source of folate, vitamin B_1, vitamin B_2.

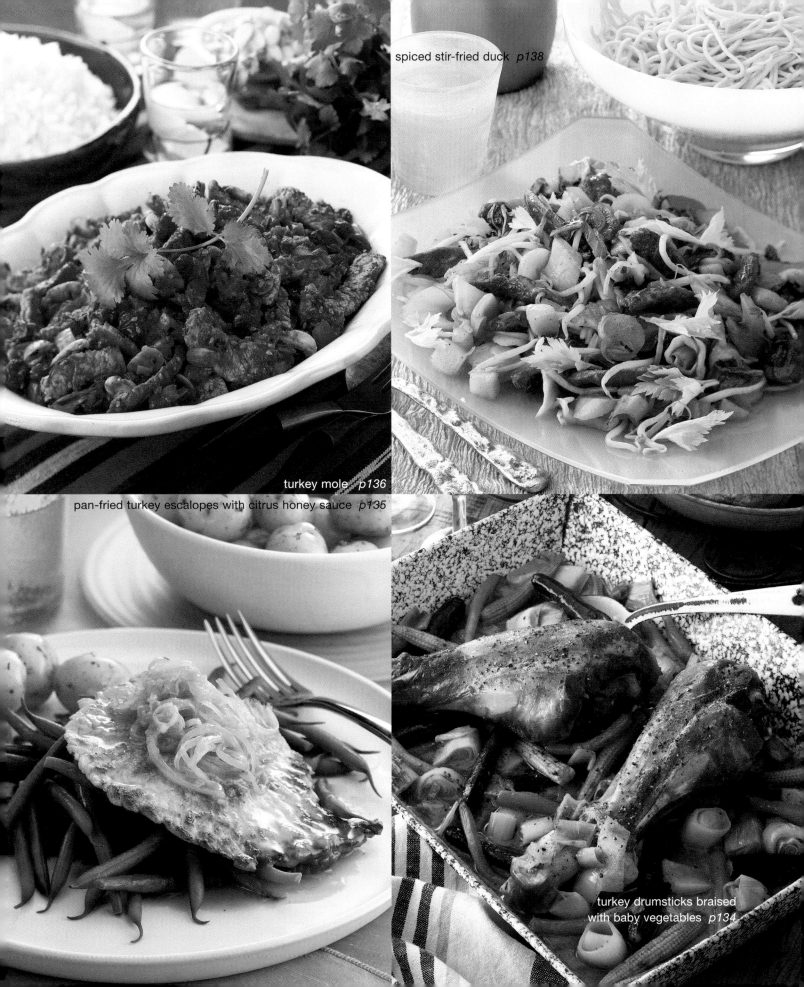

spiced stir-fried duck *p138*

turkey mole *p136*

pan-fried turkey escalopes with citrus honey sauce *p135*

turkey drumsticks braised
with baby vegetables *p134*

Spiced stir-fried duck

Here, strips of duck are stir-fried in the Chinese fashion, with onions, water chestnuts, pak choy, bean sprouts and – a sweet touch – fresh pear. Very little oil is needed for a stir-fry, and adding lots of vegetables keeps the quantity of meat down. Serve with rice noodles or with plain boiled or steamed rice.

Preparation time **about 15 minutes**   Cooking time **about 10 minutes**   *Serves 4*

400 g (14 oz) boneless duck breasts

2 tsp five-spice powder

100 g (3½ oz) button onions, thinly sliced

4 small celery sticks, thinly sliced, plus a few leaves to garnish

1 large firm pear, peeled, cored and diced

1 can water chestnuts, about 225 g, drained and sliced

1 tbsp clear honey

3 tbsp rice vinegar or sherry vinegar

1 tbsp light soy sauce

200 g (7 oz) pak choy, shredded

150 g (5½ oz) bean sprouts

1 Remove the skin and all fat from the duck breasts, then cut them across into thin strips. Sprinkle with the five-spice powder and toss to coat. Set aside for a few minutes while the vegetables are prepared.

2 Heat a wok or heavy-based frying pan until really hot. Add the duck pieces and dry-fry for 2 minutes. Add the onions and celery and continue to fry for 3 minutes or until softened. Add the pear and water chestnuts and stir to mix.

3 Add the honey, rice vinegar and soy sauce. When the liquid is bubbling, reduce the heat to low and simmer for 2 minutes.

4 Turn the heat up to high again. Add the pak choy and bean sprouts, and stir-fry for 1 minute or until the pak choy is just wilted and the bean sprouts are heated through.

5 Transfer the stir-fry to a warmed serving dish and serve immediately, garnished with celery leaves.

Some more ideas

For a less piquant sauce, replace the rice vinegar or sherry vinegar with red wine or apple or orange juice.

If in season, use an Asian pear instead of an ordinary pear. Or substitute 3–4 ripe but firm plums, sliced, for the pear.

For a **duck stir-fry with a citrus flavour**, use ground star anise instead of five-spice powder, and 170 g (6 oz) sliced and seeded kumquats instead of the pear. Replace the pak choy with ½ head Chinese leaves, shredded. Instead of rice vinegar, use orange juice or red wine.

Plus points

* Removing the skin and fat from duck lowers the fat content substantially. Skinless duck breast contains only a fraction more fat than skinless chicken breast.

* Dark green, leafy vegetables such as pak choy provide good amounts of vitamin C, as well as vitamin B_6, folate and niacin.

* Bean sprouts are a good source of vitamin C and also offer B vitamins.

* Water chestnuts provide small amounts of potassium, iron and fibre, but their big advantage is that they contain no fat and very few calories.

photo, page 137

Each serving provides   kcal 150, protein 13 g, fat 5 g (of which saturated fat 1 g), carbohydrate 17 g (of which sugars 13 g), fibre 2.5 g. Excellent source of vitamin B_{12}. Good source of copper, folate, iron, vitamin B_6, vitamin C, vitamin E. Useful source of calcium, niacin, potassium, vitamin B_1, vitamin B_2, zinc.

Piquant pasta and tuna salad

The dressing for this simple, colourful salad has a sweet-sour flavour, which perfectly complements the lightly cooked courgette, tuna, tomatoes and al dente pasta. Serve the salad cool, but not chilled, or try it while it is still warm. Mini pitta bread is good served alongside, to mop up the dressing.

Preparation time **20–25 minutes, plus cooling**   *Serves 4*

250 g (9 oz) pasta twists or spirals, such as cavatappi, fusilli or rotini, or other shapes

2 tbsp extra virgin olive oil

1 onion, chopped

1 garlic clove, chopped

2 courgettes, thinly sliced

2 tsp caster sugar

2 tbsp red pesto sauce

1 tbsp white or red wine vinegar

2 tbsp capers

6 tomatoes, skinned, halved and cut into thin wedges

1 can tuna fish in brine, about 200 g, drained and roughly flaked

6 black olives, stoned and halved

fresh flat-leaf parsley to garnish (optional)

1 Cook the pasta in boiling water for 10–12 minutes, or according to the packet instructions, until al dente. Drain well, rinse with cold water and drain again very thoroughly.

2 While the pasta is cooking, heat half the oil in a saucepan. Add the onion and garlic, and fry for 3 minutes, stirring often. Add the remaining oil and the courgettes and cook, stirring occasionally, for 3 minutes.

3 Add the sugar, red pesto, vinegar and capers to the onion and courgettes. Heat for a few seconds, stirring until the ingredients have combined to form a dressing. Stir in the tomatoes, then transfer the mixture to a large mixing bowl and set aside to cool.

4 Add the drained pasta to the bowl, then gently mix in the tuna fish and black olives. Divide among 4 plates or transfer to a large serving bowl. Serve garnished with some flat-leaf parsley leaves, if liked.

Some more ideas

To increase the fibre content and make a more substantial meal, add 1 can borlotti beans, about 400 g, drained, with the pasta. Omit the tuna for a vegetarian dish.

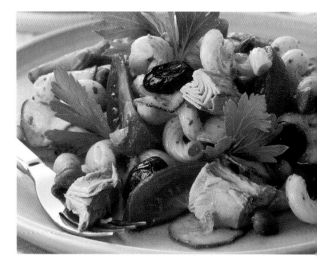

Canned anchovies can be used instead of tuna. Use the oil from 1 can, about 50 g, to cook the ingredients in step 1.

Use 225 g (8 oz) small patty pan squash instead of courgettes. Trim their tops and bases, then slice them in half.

Plus points

* Using tuna canned in water or brine, rather than in oil, keeps the fat content of the dish low.

* Tomatoes and courgettes together ensure that this simple salad provides an excellent supply of vitamin C.

Each serving provides   kcal 420, protein 25 g, fat 12 g (of which saturated fat 2 g), carbohydrate 57 g (of which sugars 10 g), fibre 4 g. Excellent source of selenium, vitamin C. Good source of vitamin A. Useful source of copper, folate, niacin, potassium, vitamin B_1, vitamin E.

Provençal tuna and pepper salad

This colourful salad is full of varied flavours and textures. Chunks of tuna, wedges of potato, crisp beans and tangy tomatoes – one bite is like a visit to Provence. Serve with crusty baguettes or oatmeal crackers.

Preparation time **45 minutes**   *Serves 4*

400 g (14 oz) new potatoes, with skins

55 g (2 oz) fine green beans

6 quail's eggs

225 g (8 oz) mixed salad leaves

1 tbsp chopped parsley

1 tbsp snipped fresh chives

1 small red onion, thinly sliced

1 tbsp tapenade (black olive paste)

2 garlic cloves, chopped

2 tbsp extra virgin olive oil

1 tbsp red wine vinegar

1 tsp balsamic vinegar

10–15 radishes, thinly sliced

1 can tuna in spring water, about 200 g, drained

100 g (3½ oz) cherry tomatoes

1 red pepper, seeded and thinly sliced

1 yellow pepper, seeded and thinly sliced

1 green pepper, seeded and thinly sliced

8 black olives

salt and pepper

fresh basil leaves to garnish

1 Place the potatoes in a saucepan and cover with boiling water. Cook over a moderate heat for 10 minutes. Add the beans and cook for a further 5 minutes or until the potatoes are tender and the beans are just cooked. Drain well and set aside to cool.

2 Put the quail's eggs into a saucepan with cold water to cover and bring to the boil. Reduce the heat and cook at a low simmer for 3 minutes. Rinse well in cold water. Peel the eggs carefully and place in cold water.

3 Toss the salad leaves together with the parsley, chives and red onion in a large shallow bowl.

4 To make the dressing, mix the tapenade with the garlic, olive oil, red wine vinegar and balsamic vinegar, and season with salt and pepper to taste. Then pour two-thirds of the dressing over the salad leaves and toss well to mix.

5 Halve the potatoes and arrange them on top of the leaves with the green beans, radishes, chunks of tuna, tomatoes, peppers and olives. Halve the quail's eggs and add them to the salad. Pour over the remaining dressing, garnish with basil leaves and serve.

Some more ideas

For a classic **Italian cannellini bean and tuna salad**, omit the potatoes and quail's eggs and add 1 can cannellini beans, about 400 g, well drained, to the salad leaves. Use the juice of ½ lemon in the dressing instead of balsamic vinegar.

Try this salad using different varieties of tomatoes, such as yellow cherry tomatoes, baby plum tomatoes or quartered vine-ripened plum tomatoes.

Plus points

• Canned tuna retains a high vitamin content, particularly vitamins B_{12} and D.

• In common with many other salad ingredients, radishes are a useful source of vitamin C and are very low in calories. The radish has a very hot flavour due to an enzyme in the skin that reacts with another substance to form a mustard type of oil.

• Green beans are a good source of dietary fibre and provide valuable amounts of folate.

photo, page 143

Each serving provides kcal 296, protein 20 g, fat 13 g (of which saturated fat 2 g), carbohydrate 26 g (of which sugars 10 g), fibre 5 g. Excellent source of niacin, selenium, vitamin B_1, vitamin B_6, vitamin B_{12}, vitamin C. Good source of folate, iron, potassium, vitamin A. Useful source of calcium, copper, vitamin B_2, vitamin E, zinc.

Grilled salmon salad

Conjure up the colours and flavours of a tropical island with this unusual warm salad. The rich flavour of salmon is perfectly balanced by the gentle acidity of orange and the sweetness of mango and papaya. Serve with an accompanying salad of mixed long-grain and wild rice or bulghur wheat.

Preparation and cooking time **30 minutes, plus 30 minutes marinating**   *Serves 4*

8 cardamom pods, crushed

1 tsp cumin seeds

finely grated zest and juice of 1 lime

juice of 1 large orange

1 tbsp light soy sauce

1 tbsp clear honey

4 pieces of skinless salmon fillet, about 115 g (4 oz) each

150 g (5½ oz) mixed colourful salad leaves, such as Lollo Rosso, Oak Leaf lettuce and baby red chard

1 mango, peeled and cut into 1 cm (½ in) cubes

1 papaya, peeled, seeded and cut into 1 cm (½ in) cubes

1 orange, peeled and segmented

salt and pepper

1 Heat a small frying pan. Scrape the seeds from the cardamom pods, and add them to the hot pan with the cumin seeds. Toast for a few seconds to release the aromas, then tip the cardamom and cumin seeds into a shallow non-metallic dish.

2 Add the lime zest and juice, orange juice, soy sauce and honey to the seeds, and season with salt and pepper to taste. Lay the pieces of salmon fillet in the dish. Turn them over to coat both sides. Cover and leave to marinate for about 30 minutes.

3 Preheat the grill to high. Lift the salmon out of the marinade, place on the grill rack and grill for 4–5 minutes on one side only; the salmon fillets should still be slightly translucent in the centre. Meanwhile, pour the marinade into a small saucepan and bring just to the boil.

4 Arrange the salad leaves in the middle of 4 plates. Scatter the mango and papaya cubes and orange segments over and around the salad. Place the cooked salmon on top of the salad and spoon over the warm marinade. Serve immediately.

Another idea

For an **Oriental-style halibut salad**, use 4 pieces of skinless halibut fillet, about 140 g (5 oz) each, instead of the salmon. Make a marinade with 2 crushed garlic cloves, 1 tsp grated fresh root ginger, 1 tsp ground cumin, 1 tsp ground coriander, 2 tbsp rice wine or dry sherry, 1 tbsp fish sauce, the grated zest of 1 lime, the juice of 2 limes and salt to taste. Marinate the halibut for 30 minutes, then grill for 5–6 minutes. Strain the marinade and bring just to the boil. Serve on a salad of bean sprouts, shredded Chinese cabbage, carrot, red pepper and sliced mushrooms, with the warm marinade spooned over.

Plus points

* Salmon is a useful source of potassium, which is needed for the regulation of fluid balance in the body, to help to prevent high blood pressure. Salmon also contains heart-protective omega-3 fats.

* Papaya is a useful source of vitamin A, which helps to maintain good vision. It has a vital role to play in preventing blindness in parts of the world where few other foods with a vitamin A content are eaten regularly.

photo, page 143

Each serving provides   kcal 330, protein 25 g, fat 13 g (of which saturated fat 2 g), carbohydrate 29 g (of which sugars 29 g), fibre 5 g. Excellent source of niacin, vitamin A, vitamin B$_1$, vitamin B$_6$, vitamin B$_{12}$, vitamin C. Good source of potassium, selenium, vitamin E. Useful source of calcium, copper, folate, iron, zinc.

Crab and avocado salad

Fresh crab is a real summertime treat. It is rich in flavour and combines well in a salad with crunchy apples and bean sprouts, chunks of perfectly ripe avocados and nutty-flavoured bulghur wheat.

Preparation time **40 minutes, plus cooling** *Serves 4*

Bulghur wheat salad

200 g (7 oz) bulghur wheat

1 tbsp extra virgin olive oil

3 tbsp lemon juice

3 tbsp chopped fresh flat-leaf parsley

1 tbsp snipped fresh chives

2 medium-sized tomatoes, diced

salt and pepper

Crab salad

340 g (12 oz) fresh white crab meat

2 avocados

2 crisp green dessert apples

125 g (4½ oz) bean sprouts

3 tbsp reduced-fat mayonnaise

3 tbsp plain low-fat yogurt

1 tbsp lemon juice

small pinch of cayenne pepper

2 Little Gem lettuces, separated into leaves

30 g (1 oz) walnut halves, toasted and roughly chopped

1 Put the bulghur wheat in a large saucepan with 1.3 litres (2¼ pints) cold water. Bring to the boil over a high heat, then reduce the heat and simmer for 10–15 minutes or until the grains are just tender. Drain in a large sieve, pressing down well to squeeze out all the excess water. Leave to cool.

2 Combine the oil, lemon juice, parsley, chives and diced tomatoes in a large mixing bowl. Add the bulghur wheat and mix thoroughly, then season with salt and pepper to taste. Leave to stand at room temperature while preparing the crab salad.

3 Pick over and flake the crab meat, discarding any fragments of shell. Halve, stone and peel the avocados, then chop the flesh. Add to the crab. Quarter and core the apples, then thinly slice them. Add to the crab meat with the bean sprouts.

4 Mix the mayonnaise with the yogurt until smooth. Add the lemon juice and cayenne pepper. Spoon onto the crab mixture and toss gently until just combined.

5 Pile the bulghur salad onto a serving platter and arrange the Little Gem leaves on top. Spoon the crab salad onto the leaves and scatter over the walnuts. Serve immediately.

Some more ideas

Canned crab meat makes an excellent salad base. Use 2 cans, about 170 g each, well drained, instead of the fresh crab.

Use 200 g (7 oz) basmati rice instead of the bulghur wheat. Cook the rice in boiling water for 10–12 minutes, or according to the packet instructions. Drain, rinse with cold water and drain again, then leave to dry before mixing with the dressing and tomatoes.

Plus points

● Although yogurt has been used for its nutritional and medicinal properties for hundreds of years in the Middle and Far East and Eastern Europe, it has only become popular in the UK in the past few decades. It is a good source of calcium and helps to maintain healthy bones, as well as being vital for the proper functioning of muscles and nerves and for blood clotting.

● Walnuts are a good source of the antioxidant nutrients selenium, zinc, copper and vitamin E. Nuts should be used in moderation in diabetic cooking for their beneficial monounsaturated fat.

Each serving provides kcal 553, protein 28 g, fat 26 g (of which saturated fat 4 g), carbohydrate 52 g (of which sugars 12.5 g), fibre 5 g. Excellent source of copper, niacin, vitamin B$_1$, vitamin B$_6$. Good source of iron, potassium, vitamin B$_2$, vitamin C, vitamin E, zinc. Useful source of calcium, folate, selenium, vitamin A.

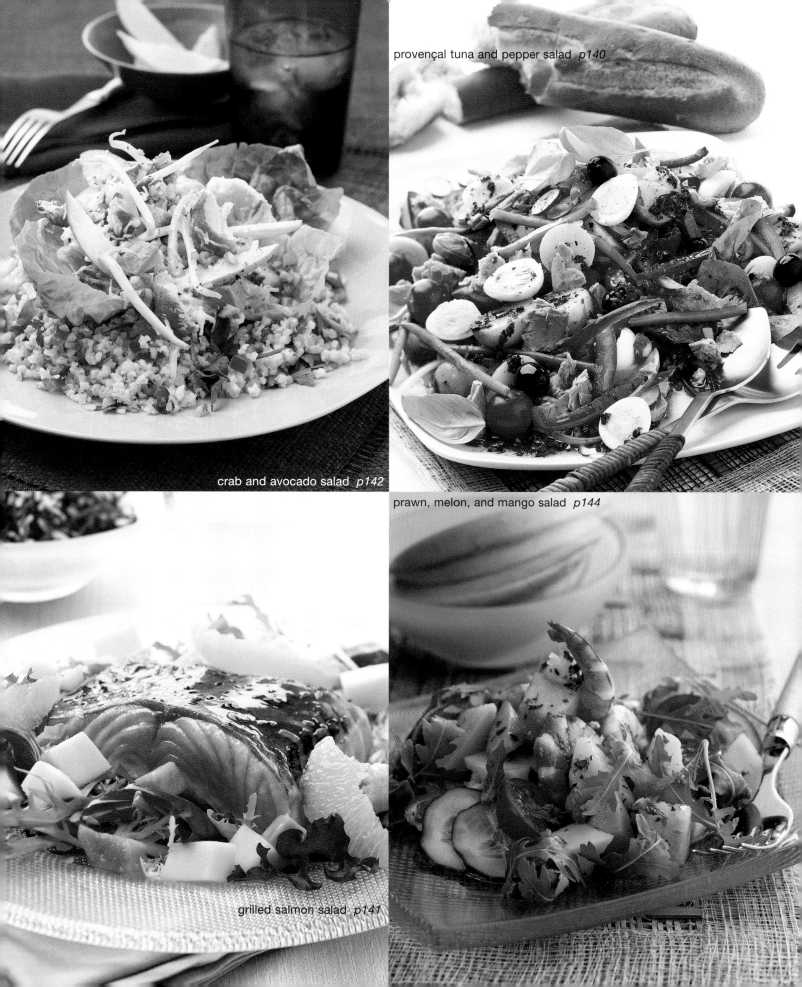

provençal tuna and pepper salad *p140*

crab and avocado salad *p142*

prawn, melon, and mango salad *p144*

grilled salmon salad *p141*

Prawn, melon and mango salad

A very pretty salad, this combines tiger prawns with colourful, juicy fruits tossed in a light dressing flavoured with honey and fresh mint. It makes a lovely light summer meal, served with bread or rolls.

Preparation time **20 minutes, plus at least 30 minutes marinating**   *Serves 4*

400 g (14 oz) cooked peeled tiger prawns

1 mango, about 600 g (1 lb 5 oz)

¼ honeydew or ½ Charentais melon, about 340 g (12 oz), cubed

8 cherry tomatoes, halved

100 g (3½ oz) rocket leaves

¼ cucumber, sliced

salt and pepper

fresh mint leaves to garnish

Mint and honey dressing

2 tbsp extra virgin olive oil

juice of 1 lemon

1 tbsp clear honey

2 tbsp chopped fresh mint

1 Whisk together all the ingredients for the dressing in a large bowl and season with salt and pepper to taste. Add the prawns to the dressing, cover and leave to marinate in the fridge for 30 minutes to 1 hour.

2 Halve the mango lengthways, cutting down round each side of the stone. Cut the flesh on each half in a criss-cross fashion to make cubes, then cut the cubes away from the skin.

3 Remove the prawns from the fridge. Add the mango, melon and tomatoes and gently stir together. Arrange the rocket leaves and cucumber slices around the edge of a shallow serving dish, and spoon the prawn salad into the centre. Garnish with sprigs of mint and serve.

Some more ideas

Use mixed seafood instead of the prawns. Another idea is crabsticks, cut in half.

To add a slightly spicy note to the salad, mix 15 g (½ oz) fresh root ginger, cut into very fine strips, into the dressing.

Other fruits can be used in place of the melon and mango. Good combinations include chopped nectarine and halved, seedless white grapes or sliced kiwi fruit with cubes of fresh pineapple.

For an attractive presentation, serve the salad in halved Charentais melon shells.

Plus points

● Fresh mangoes are an excellent source of the important antioxidant beta-carotene, which the body can convert to vitamin A. The amount of beta-carotene on offer varies according to the ripeness of the fruit – levels can range from 300 to 3000 mcg per 100 g (3½ oz) raw mango flesh.

● Melons have an exceptionally high water content, averaging at least 90 per cent, which makes them very refreshing. The varieties with orange flesh, like Charentais, contain beta-carotene.

● Although prawns contain cholesterol, this generally has very little effect on your blood cholesterol levels.

photo, page 143

Each serving provides   kcal 253, protein 24 g, fat 7 g (of which saturated fat 1 g), carbohydrate 25 g (of which sugars 24 g), fibre 4 g. Excellent source of niacin, vitamin B$_1$, vitamin B$_{12}$, vitamin C. Good source of copper, iron, selenium, vitamin A, zinc. Useful source of potassium, vitamin E.

Lobster salad with lime dressing

A ready-cooked lobster makes a luxurious salad for 2 people to share. The firm, sweet flavoured lobster meat is here served on a bed of peppery salad leaves, shredded mange-tout, grapes and tiny new potatoes cooked in their skins, all tossed with a dressing spiked with lime zest. Serve with country-style bread.

Preparation time **1 hour**   *Serves 2*

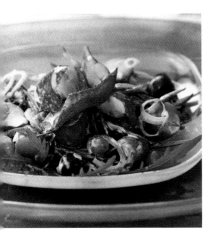

250 g (8½ oz) baby red-skinned new potatoes, scrubbed

2 tbsp reduced-fat mayonnaise

2 tbsp 0% Greek-style yogurt

finely grated zest of ½ lime

1 cooked lobster, about 500 g (1 lb 2 oz)

2 small shallots, thinly sliced

85 g (3 oz) mange-tout, shredded

85 g (3 oz) seedless red grapes

85 g (3 oz) seedless green grapes

30 g (1 oz) watercress

55 g (2 oz) rocket leaves

salt and pepper

1 Put the potatoes in a saucepan and cover with boiling water. Cook for about 15 minutes or until just tender. Drain and leave to cool, then cut the potatoes in half.

2 While the potatoes are cooling, mix together the mayonnaise, yogurt and lime zest, and season with salt and pepper to taste. Set aside.

3 Pull and twist off the lobster claws and set aside. With a sharp knife, cut the body in half lengthways, from tail end through the head. Remove the meat from the body/tail shell and the claws. Chop all the meat into chunks. (The meat from the spindly legs can also be removed with tweezers, but this takes a lot of effort for the small amount of meat inside them.)

4 Toss the potatoes with the shallots, mange-tout, grapes, watercress and lime dressing. Arrange the rocket on large plates and add the watercress and potato salad. Scatter the lobster meat on top and serve.

Some more ideas

For a **lightly curried lime and honey dressing**, mix 2 tbsp groundnut oil with 1 tbsp lemon juice, ½ tsp curry paste and ½ tsp clear honey.

To make a **lobster and papaya salad**, instead of the mange-tout and grapes, toss 1 large ripe papaya, seeded and sliced, and 1 chopped avocado with the potatoes, watercress and shallots. Pile the papaya salad onto 85 g (3 oz) herb salad leaves (containing sprigs of fresh coriander) rather than rocket. Drizzle with the curried lime and honey dressing and scatter over the lobster meat and 30 g (1 oz) toasted cashew nuts.

Chicory or shredded romaine or cos lettuce can be used instead of the rocket.

Plus points

● Lobster is an excellent source of the antioxidant selenium, which helps to protect cells from damage by free radicals.

● Some varieties of grape are cultivated for wine, others for drying to become raisins, currants and sultanas, and others for eating. The nutrient content of different coloured grapes is very similar. Grapes are a good source of potassium and the skin provides fibre but they have a high sugar content. However, it is easier to limit the amount you eat when you use them in cooking.

Each serving provides kcal 338, protein 27 g, fat 10 g (of which saturated fat 3 g), carbohydrate 39 g (of which sugars 20 g), fibre 4 g. Excellent source of copper, niacin, selenium, vitamin B_1, vitamin B_6, vitamin B_{12}, vitamin C. Good source of calcium, iron, potassium, vitamin A, vitamin E, zinc. Useful source of folate, vitamin B_2.

Italian seafood stew

Any fish or shellfish is delicious in this Italian fisherman's stew – make the bubbling tomato mixture and add whatever is tasty and fresh from the sea. Serve with triangles of polenta grilled at the last minute.

Preparation time **20 minutes** Cooking time **1 hour** *Serves 4*

2 tbsp extra virgin olive oil

1 medium-sized leek, chopped

1 onion, chopped

4 garlic cloves, chopped

½ green pepper, seeded and chopped

½ medium bulb of fennel, diced

360 ml (12 fl oz) dry white wine

300 ml (10 fl oz) fish stock

1 can chopped tomatoes, 400 g

2 tbsp tomato purée

¼ tsp dried herbes de Provence

1 medium-sized courgette, sliced

3 tbsp coarsely chopped parsley

55 g (2 oz) peas

85 g (3 oz) spinach leaves

200 g (7 oz) skinless cod fillet, cut into chunks

400 g (14 oz) peeled or shelled mixed shellfish, such as raw king prawns, scallops and mussels

salt and pepper

Polenta

225 g (8 oz) instant polenta

2 tsp extra virgin olive oil

1 Heat the oil in a large saucepan, add the leek and onion, and cook for 2 minutes or until starting to soften. Add the garlic, pepper and fennel and cook for a further 5–10 minutes or until softened.

2 Add the wine, stock and tomatoes with their juice, and season with salt and pepper to taste. Simmer for 30 minutes or until the mixture has thickened slightly. Stir in the tomato purée, herbes de Provence and courgette, and continue simmering for 10 minutes, adding a little water if the mixture becomes too thick.

3 Meanwhile, cook the polenta according to the packet instructions until it is thick. Season with salt and pepper to taste. Pour the polenta into a lightly oiled 18 x 28 cm (7 x 11 in) shallow tin. Leave until cool and firm, then cut the polenta into triangles. Preheat the grill to high.

4 Stir the parsley, peas, chard or spinach, fish and shellfish into the tomato mixture. Cover and simmer gently over a moderate heat for about 5 minutes or until all the seafood is just cooked.

5 Lightly brush the polenta triangles with the oil and grill until lightly browned. Serve the fish stew in bowls with the polenta triangles.

Some more ideas

For an **Italian clam stew with asparagus**, use 3 medium onions, chopped, and omit the leek and green pepper. In step 2, omit the stock. Replace the seafood with 1 kg (2¼ lb) clams in their shells. Add them to the mixture, cover and bring to the boil, then simmer over a low heat for about 2 minutes. Add 125 g (4½ oz) asparagus spears, cut into bite-sized pieces, cover and cook for 5 minutes or until all the clams have opened (discard any that remain shut) and the asparagus is just tender. Serve the stew with the polenta triangles.

Plus points

• Cod provides excellent quantities of iodine. Fish is one of the most reliable sources of this essential mineral because of the consistent iodine content of sea water. Other foods depend on the iodine in soil, which can vary.

• Polenta, which is finely milled corn or maize meal, is a good gluten-free source of starchy carbohydrate.

• You can use either fresh or frozen peas in this recipe. The nutritional content of frozen peas is very similar to that of fresh as long as they are not overcooked.

photo, page 149

Each serving provides kcal 356, protein 33 g, fat 9 g (of which saturated fat 1 g), carbohydrate 22 g (of which sugars 9 g), fibre 5 g. Excellent source of copper, niacin, selenium, vitamin B$_1$, vitamin B$_6$, vitamin B$_{12}$, vitamin C. Good source of folate, iron, potassium, vitamin A, vitamin E, zinc. Useful source of calcium.

Chunky fish soup

Even though this soup contains bacon and root vegetables, it has a delicate flavour that makes it an appealing first course at any time of the year. Rich in B-complex vitamins, it is also low in fat and contains a good amount of fibre. Serve with crusty wholegrain rolls.

Preparation time **15 minutes**   Cooking time **about 20 minutes**   *Serves 4*

pinch of saffron threads

2 tsp extra virgin olive oil

55 g (2 oz) lean smoked back bacon rashers, rinded and chopped

85 g (3 oz) waxy potatoes, such as Charlotte, scrubbed and finely diced

85 g (3 oz) parsnips, finely diced

2 celery sticks, finely chopped

85 g (3 oz) onion, finely chopped

1 bay leaf

1 strip of finely pared lemon zest

750 ml (1¼ pints) fish stock, preferably home-made

250 g (8½ oz) skinless haddock fillet, cut into bite-sized pieces

salt and pepper

4 spring onions, finely chopped, to garnish

1 Put the saffron threads in a small frying pan over a moderate heat and stir until they just begin to give off their aroma. Immediately tip the saffron threads onto a small plate and set aside.

2 Heat the oil in a large non-stick saucepan, add the bacon and cook over a moderate heat, stirring, for about 2 minutes. Add the potatoes, parsnips, celery and onion, and cook gently for about 1 minute, stirring frequently.

3 Add the saffron threads, bay leaf and lemon zest, and season with salt and pepper to taste. Pour in the stock and slowly bring to the boil. Reduce the heat to moderately low, half cover the pan and simmer, stirring occasionally, for about 8 minutes or until the vegetables are almost tender when pierced with the tip of a knife.

4 Lay the pieces of haddock on top of the vegetables. Reduce the heat to low and cover the pan tightly. Simmer for 7–8 minutes or until the fish will flake easily and all the vegetables are tender. Remove and discard the bay leaf and lemon zest.

5 Ladle the soup into bowls, sprinkle with the chopped spring onions and serve immediately.

Some more ideas

For a thicker soup, use floury potatoes such as King Edward or Maris Piper. They will fall apart as they cook and thicken the soup.

Vary the vegetables to use what is in season. Green beans are an excellent alternative to the celery, and turnips can replace the parsnips. Other suitable vegetables include carrots, courgettes, fennel and peppers.

Plus points

• White fish such as haddock is an important source of good-quality protein. On a weight for weight basis, white fish provides similar amounts of protein to that found in lean meat.

• Potatoes do not have as much vitamin C as some other vegetables, but they are an important source because of the large quantity normally eaten.

• Celery was originally grown as a medicinal herb, only being used as a cooked vegetable and salad ingredient in the late 17th century. Green celery contains beta-carotene, which the body converts into vitamin A.

photo, page 149

Each serving provides   kcal 148, protein 16 g, fat 5 g (of which saturated fat 1 g), carbohydrate 11 g (of which sugars 4 g), fibre 3 g. Excellent source of niacin, vitamin B_1, vitamin B_6. Good source of selenium. Useful source of folate, potassium, calcium, vitamin B_{12}, vitamin C.

Mixed seafood and noodle broth

In China soups are not served at the beginning of the meal but in between courses or dishes. This is why they are made with a light stock, so they are more appropriate as a starter in a Western meal. You can part-prepare this soup ahead, then add the scallops, vegetables and noodles just before serving.

Preparation and cooking time **25 minutes**   *Serves 6*

55 g (2 oz) fine stir-fry rice noodles, broken into 10 cm (4 in) lengths

2 tsp groundnut oil

2.5 cm (1 in) piece fresh root ginger, finely chopped

75 g (2½ oz) shiitake mushrooms, stalks discarded and caps thinly sliced

1.2 litres (2 pints) chicken stock

1 tbsp dry sherry

2 tbsp light soy sauce

125 g (4½ oz) cooked mixed seafood, such as prawns, squid and queen scallops

75 g (2½ oz) Chinese leaves, shredded

4 spring onions, thinly sliced

75 g (2½ oz) beansprouts

fresh coriander leaves to garnish

chilli sauce to serve

1 Put the noodles in a bowl and pour over plenty of boiling water. Set aside to soak for 4 minutes.

2 Meanwhile, heat the groundnut oil in a large saucepan, add the ginger and mushrooms, and cook for about 2 minutes to soften slightly. Add the stock, sherry and soy sauce, and bring to the boil.

3 Halve the scallops if they are large. Add the mixed seafood to the boiling stock together with the Chinese leaves, spring onions and beansprouts. Bring back to the boil and cook for 1 minute or until the seafood is heated through.

4 Drain the noodles and add to the soup. Bring back to the boil, then ladle into large soup bowls. Scatter over a few fresh coriander leaves and serve with chilli sauce, to be added to taste.

Another idea

For a **crab and noodle broth**, use 1 can white crab meat, about 170 g, drained, instead of the mixed seafood. Replace the mushrooms with 100 g (3½ oz) thinly sliced baby corn and 100 g (3½ oz) diced courgettes, cooking them with the ginger for 1 minute. In step 3, omit the Chinese leaves. After adding the rice noodles in step 4, bring to the boil and season with 1 tbsp fish sauce.

Plus points

* Scallops are a good source of selenium and B_{12}, and a useful source of phosphorus and potassium. Prawns provide calcium, while squid is an excellent source of B_{12}.

* Shiitake mushrooms contain the B vitamins B_2, niacin and pantothenic acid. They also provide potassium and good quantities of copper.

* Rice noodles are both gluten-free and wheat-free, making them useful for people with gluten intolerances or wheat allergies. They also have a fairly low Glycaemic Index.

Each serving provides   kcal 80, protein 5 g, fat 1.5 g (of which saturated fat 0.3 g), carbohydrate 9 g (of which sugars 1 g), fibre 0.5 g. Good source of vitamin B_{12}. Useful source of copper, selenium.

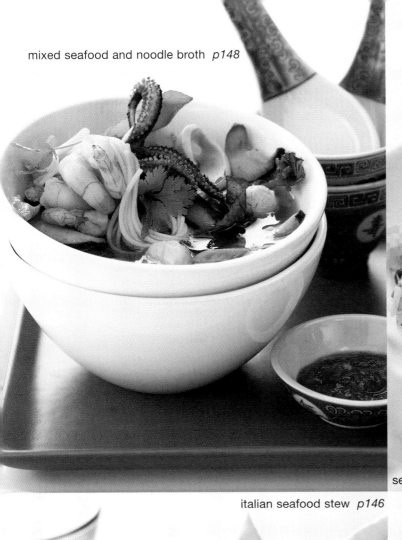

mixed seafood and noodle broth *p148*

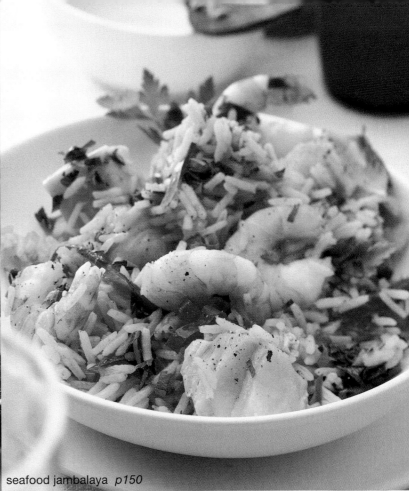

seafood jambalaya *p150*

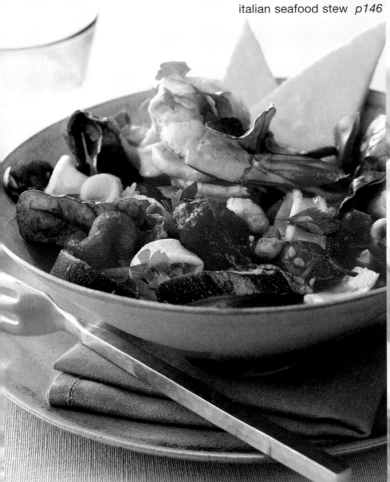

italian seafood stew *p146*

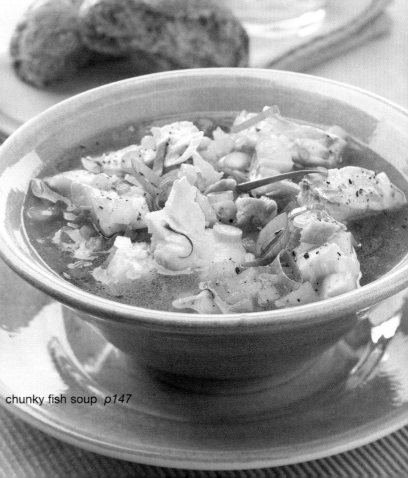

chunky fish soup *p147*

Seafood jambalaya

Mixed with rice and plenty of vegetables, a small amount of succulent salmon and prawns goes a long way, making a good balance of protein and carbohydrate in this temptingly spicy, Louisiana-style dish. As an added bonus for the busy cook, it is cooked in just one pan and makes a complete meal on its own.

Preparation and cooking time **30 minutes**   *Serves 4*

1½ tbsp extra virgin olive oil

1 onion, chopped

2 celery sticks, sliced

1 green or red pepper, seeded and cut into strips

2 garlic cloves, crushed

½ tsp ground ginger

½ tsp cayenne pepper

1 tsp mild chilli powder

340 g (12 oz) basmati white rice

900 ml (1½ pints) hot vegetable stock

1 can chopped tomatoes, about 225 g

3 tbsp coarsely chopped parsley

100 g (3½ oz) peeled large raw prawns

200 g (7 oz) skinned salmon fillet, cut into 2.5 cm (1 in) cubes

dash of Tabasco sauce (optional)

salt and pepper

1 Heat the oil in a large, wide pan over a moderately high heat. Add the onion and cook, stirring, for about 3 minutes. Add the celery, green or red pepper, garlic, ginger, cayenne, chilli powder and rice, and cook, stirring, for 2 minutes.

2 Pour in the hot stock and stir well, then reduce the heat so that the stock is simmering gently. Cover the pan with a tight-fitting lid and simmer for 15 minutes.

3 Stir in the chopped tomatoes with their juice and 2 tbsp of the parsley, then add the prawns and salmon. Cover again and simmer for 3–4 minutes or until the seafood is just cooked and the rice has absorbed most of the liquid and is tender.

4 Add the Tabasco sauce, if using, and salt and pepper to taste. Sprinkle with the remaining 1 tbsp parsley and serve hot.

Some more ideas

Use brown rice instead of white. It will take 30–40 minutes to cook and will need about 150 ml (5 fl oz) more stock.

For a **pork and smoked sausage jambalaya**, cut 200 g (7 oz) pork fillet (tenderloin) into thin strips and brown in 1 tbsp olive oil, then remove from the pan

and set aside. Add 1 chopped red onion to the pan and cook for 5 more minutes, or until almost soft. Stir in the rice and cook for 2–3 minutes, then pour in 750 ml (1¼ pints) vegetable stock. Cover and simmer for 10 minutes. Stir in 1 can tomatoes with added peppers and basil, about 400 g, with the juice, and 200 g (7 oz) sliced courgettes. Cover and cook for a further 5 minutes. Return the pork to the pan together with 115 g (4 oz) sliced smoked sausage and cook, covered, for 5 more minutes or until all the liquid has been absorbed and the rice is tender. Serve sprinkled with 2 tbsp chopped parsley.

Plus points

• Prawns are low in fat and high in protein. They are also an excellent source of the antioxidant mineral selenium, which helps to protect the cardiovascular system.

• Salmon provides vitamins B_6 and B_{12} and the minerals selenium and potassium.

• Of all types of rice, basmati has the lowest Glycaemic Index.

photo, page 149

Each serving provides   kcal 483, protein 22 g, fat 11 g (of which saturated fat 2 g), carbohydrate 80 g (of which sugars 5 g), fibre 2 g. Excellent source of vitamin B_{12}, vitamin C. Good source of copper, niacin, selenium, vitamin B_6, vitamin E, zinc. Useful source of folate, iron, potassium, vitamin B_1.

Cod with a gremolata crust

Here's a delicious recipe for jazzing up plain cod fillets. Gremolata is an Italian mixture of parsley, lemon zest and garlic (and sometimes chopped anchovy). This recipe uses the gremolata with breadcrumbs to make a tasty topping for the fish, which is baked with juicy tomatoes and courgettes and served with saffron mash.

Preparation time **20 minutes** Cooking time **25 minutes** *Serves 4*

2 lemons

55 g (2 oz) fresh white bread-crumbs

3 tbsp chopped parsley

2 garlic cloves, crushed

4 chunky pieces of skinless cod fillet, about 550 g (1¼ lb) in total

2 tsp wholegrain mustard

3 plum tomatoes, quartered

1 large courgette, thinly sliced diagonally

1 tbsp extra virgin olive oil

900 g (2 lb) potatoes, peeled and cut into chunks

1 tsp saffron threads

3 tbsp semi-skimmed milk

salt and pepper

1 Preheat the oven to 200°C (400°F, gas mark 6). Finely grate the zest and squeeze the juice from one of the lemons. Mix the zest with the breadcrumbs, parsley and garlic, and season to taste.

2 Place the cod fillets in a lightly oiled, large ovenproof dish. Then spread the mustard evenly over the top of the fish and sprinkle over the lemon juice. Arrange the tomatoes and courgette around the fish. Cut the remaining lemon into 4 wedges and put them into the dish too.

3 Spoon the breadcrumb mixture over the fish and press down lightly. Drizzle with the olive oil. Bake the fish for 25 minutes or until the topping is crisp.

4 Meanwhile, place the potatoes in a saucepan, cover with boiling water and add the saffron. Cook for 15–20 minutes or until tender. Drain the potatoes and mash with the milk. Season to taste. Serve with the saffron mash, tomatoes and courgettes.

Some more ideas

For a special occasion, bake the cod in individual ovenproof dishes. Slice the tomatoes, and replace the courgette with

1 red or yellow pepper, seeded and chopped. Put a piece of fish in each dish and arrange the sliced tomatoes on top. Scatter over the pepper and then the breadcrumb mixture, and bake for 20 minutes. Garnish with wedges of lemon.

For an oaty topping, replace 20 g (¾ oz) of the breadcrumbs with jumbo porridge oats.

Pieces of skinless salmon fillet can be used instead of cod. Replace the lemon zest with orange zest and add some snipped fresh chives to the breadcrumb topping.

Plus points

• Although wholemeal bread is in many ways healthier than white bread, the latter contains twice as much calcium – 110 mg per 100 g (3½ oz) compared with 54 mg for the same weight. White breadcrumbs are particularly appealing for this recipe, but people with diabetes should choose wholegrain breads wherever possible.

• Citrus fruits are nutritionally important for their vitamin C content.

photo, page 153

Each serving provides kcal 362, protein 33 g, fat 5 g (of which saturated fat 1 g), carbohydrate 48 g (of which sugars 5 g), fibre 5 g. Excellent source of niacin, selenium, vitamin B$_1$, vitamin B$_6$, vitamin C. Good source of folate, iron, potassium, vitamin B$_{12}$. Useful source of copper, vitamin A, vitamin E, zinc.

Cod with spicy Puy lentils

Dark green Puy lentils, grown in the south of France, have a unique, peppery flavour that is enhanced by chilli. They do not disintegrate during cooking and their texture is a perfect complement for the flakiness of fresh cod. Serve this satisfying dish with warm crusty bread and a mixed salad.

Preparation and cooking time **about 35 minutes**   *Serves 4*

2 tbsp extra virgin olive oil

1 onion, chopped

2 celery sticks, chopped

2 medium-sized leeks, chopped

1–2 fresh red chillies, seeded and finely chopped

170 g (6 oz) Puy lentils, rinsed and drained

750 ml (1¼ pints) vegetable stock

1 sprig of fresh thyme

1 bay leaf

juice of 1 lemon

pinch of cayenne pepper

4 pieces of skinless cod fillet or cod steaks, about 140 g (5 oz) each

salt and pepper

lemon wedges to serve

1 Preheat the grill to moderately high. Heat 1 tbsp of the olive oil in a saucepan, add the onion, celery, leeks and chillies, and cook gently for 2 minutes. Stir in the lentils. Add the vegetable stock, thyme and bay leaf and bring to the boil. Lower the heat and simmer for about 20 minutes or until the lentils are tender. If at the end of this time the lentils have not absorbed all the stock, drain them (you can use the excess stock to make a soup).

2 While the lentils are cooking, mix together the remaining 1 tbsp oil, the lemon juice and cayenne pepper. Lay the cod in the grill pan, skinned side up, season with salt and pepper, and brush with the oil mixture. Grill for 6–7 minutes or until the fish will flake easily. There is no need to turn the fish over.

3 Spread the lentils in a warmed serving dish and arrange the pieces of cod on top. Serve immediately, with lemon wedges.

Another idea

For **cod with mustard lentils**, cook the lentils as in the main recipe, omitting the chillies. Mix 125 g (4½ oz) fromage frais or half-fat crème fraîche with 1–2 tbsp Dijon mustard and stir into the cooked lentils. Spread a thin layer of Dijon mustard over the seasoned cod, drizzle with olive oil and grill. Serve on top of the lentils, garnished with grilled cherry tomatoes.

Plus points

• White fish such as cod is low in calories. Frying it in batter more than doubles the calorie content, whereas brushing it with a little oil and grilling it keeps the fat and therefore calories at healthy levels.

• Lentils are classified as pulses, but unlike other pulses they do not need to be soaked before cooking. Lentils are a good source of protein, starch, dietary fibre and B vitamins. Iron absorption from lentils is poor, but vitamin C-rich foods, such as the lemon juice in this recipe, can improve this considerably. Lentils have a low Glycaemic Index.

• Thyme has been used as an antiseptic since Greek and Roman times.

Each serving provides kcal 324, protein 38 g, fat 7.5 g (of which saturated fat 1 g), carbohydrate 26 g (of which sugars 6 g), fibre 7.5 g. Excellent source of niacin, selenium, vitamin B_1, vitamin B_6. Good source of vitamin B_{12}, vitamin C. Useful source of folate, iron, potassium, vitamin A, vitamin E.

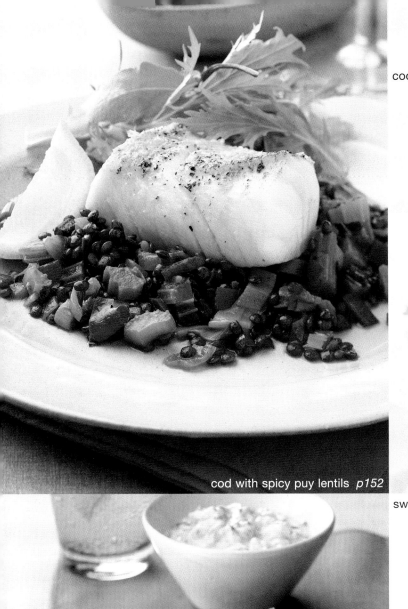

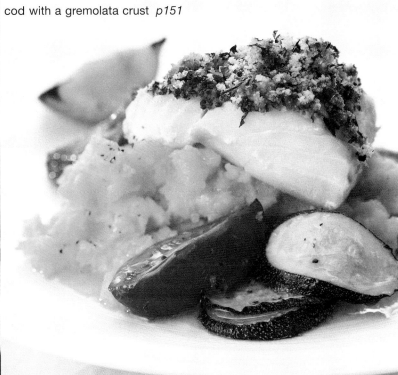

cod with a gremolata crust *p151*

cod with spicy puy lentils *p152*

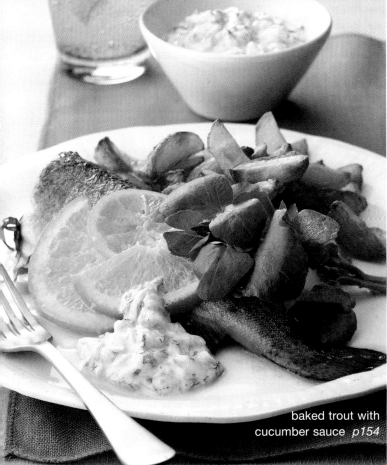

baked trout with
cucumber sauce *p154*

swordfish with salsa dressing *p155*

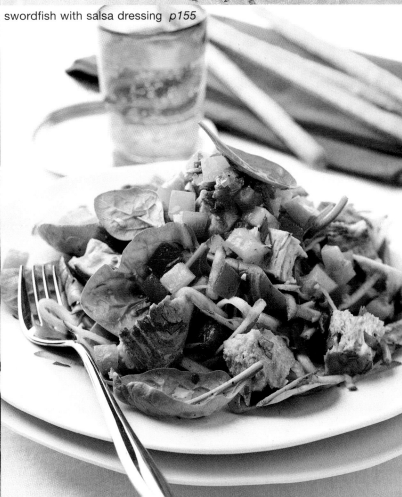

Baked trout with cucumber sauce

Orange and lemon slices add a great flavour to this simple recipe for baked fish, and a cucumber and yogurt sauce provides a refreshing contrast. New potatoes are roasted in the oven with the fish.

Preparation and cooking time **40 minutes**   *Serves 4*

750 g (1 lb 10 oz) new potatoes, quartered lengthways, unpeeled

1 tbsp extra virgin olive oil

4 small trout, about 280 g (10 oz) each, cleaned

4 sprigs of fresh tarragon

1 orange, cut into 8 slices

1 lemon, cut into 8 slices

4 tbsp orange juice

100 g (3½ oz) watercress to garnish

Cucumber sauce

200 g (7 oz) cucumber

150 g (5½ oz) plain low-fat yogurt

2 tbsp chopped fresh mint

salt and pepper

1 Preheat the oven to 200°C (400°F, gas mark 6) and put 2 baking sheets in the oven to heat up. Put the potatoes in a large saucepan and pour over enough boiling water to cover them. Bring back to the boil, then simmer for 5 minutes. Drain and return to the pan.

2 Drizzle the oil over the potatoes and toss them quickly to coat. Spread them out on one of the hot baking sheets and roast for 10 minutes. Turn the potatoes over and roast for another 10 minutes, then turn them again and roast for a further 5 minutes or until crisp and tender.

3 Meanwhile, season inside the fish and tuck in the sprigs of tarragon. Cut out 4 squares of foil, each large enough to wrap up a fish. Cut the orange and lemon slices in half. Divide half the fruit slices among the foil squares, lay the fish on top and cover with the remaining slices. Sprinkle 1 tbsp orange juice over each fish.

4 Wrap up the foil to enclose the fish completely, twisting the ends to seal. Lay the parcels on the second hot baking sheet and bake for 20 minutes.

5 While the fish and potatoes are cooking, make the sauce. Grate the cucumber, put it into a sieve and press to squeeze out the water. Mix together the cucumber, yogurt and mint, and season with salt and pepper to taste.

6 Arrange the fish, orange and lemon slices and roasted potatoes on warm plates. Add a garnish of watercress and serve with the cucumber sauce.

Some more ideas

For a speedy trout dish, buy 2 fillets of trout per person. Sprinkle with a little olive oil and grill, skin side down, for 2–4 minutes. Serve with new potatoes.

Vary the flavour of the sauce by adding 1 tsp horseradish relish. Or, instead of mint, use 1 tbsp chopped fresh chives or green olives.

Plus points

• Like other oily fish, trout contains beneficial fats from the omega-3 family of essential fatty acids. These help to protect the body against strokes and heart disease.

• Plain yogurt is often used as an alternative to cream. This has the advantage of helping to lower the fat content of a recipe. In addition, yogurt provides more calcium than cream on a weight for weight basis.

photo, page 153

Each serving provides kcal 440, protein 43 g, fat 13 g (of which saturated fat 3 g), carbohydrate 40 g (of which sugars 12 g), fibre 3.5 g. Excellent source of niacin, potassium, vitamin B_1, vitamin B_6, vitamin B_{12}, vitamin C. Good source of calcium, iron, selenium, vitamin E. Useful source of copper, folate, vitamin A, vitamin B_2, zinc.

Swordfish with salsa dressing

Orange juice adds a refreshing note to the salsa-style tomato and pepper dressing for this vibrant-looking salad. As the dressing can be made well in advance and the swordfish steaks take only minutes to cook, this is a very quick dish to prepare, ideal when you are entertaining. Serve with lots of sesame breadsticks or crusty wholegrain bread.

Preparation and cooking time **30 minutes, plus at least 20 minutes marinating**   *Serves 4*

4 swordfish steaks, about 1 cm (½ in) thick, 140 g (5 oz) each

1½ tsp extra virgin olive oil

250 g (8½ oz) baby spinach leaves

2 courgettes, coarsely grated

1 tbsp chopped parsley

Tomato salsa dressing

1 large orange

600 g (1 lb 5 oz) ripe tomatoes, seeded and cut into 5 mm (¼ in) dice

4 large spring onions, green parts only, finely chopped

1 orange pepper, seeded and cut into 5 mm (¼ in) dice

1 yellow pepper, seeded and cut into 5 mm (¼ in) dice

1 tsp ground cumin, or to taste

1 tbsp extra virgin olive oil

1 fresh green chilli, seeded and finely chopped

salt and pepper

2 tbsp finely chopped fresh coriander

1 Prepare the salsa dressing at least 20 minutes (or up to 8 hours) before serving. Finely grate the zest from the orange and squeeze out 4 tbsp juice. Put the zest and juice in a large mixing bowl and add the tomatoes, spring onions, peppers, cumin, olive oil and chilli. Season to taste. Stir, then cover and chill.

2 Preheat the grill to high. Lightly brush the swordfish steaks with some of the olive oil and place on the grill rack. Grill, about 7.5 cm (3 in) from the heat, for 2½ minutes. Turn the swordfish steaks over, brush with the rest of the olive oil and grill for a further 2½–3 minutes or until the edges are lightly charred and the flesh is just firm. Don't overcook or the swordfish will be tough and dry. Remove from the heat and set aside to cool slightly.

3 Meanwhile, put the spinach leaves, courgettes and parsley in a bowl and toss to mix. Divide among 4 plates.

4 Stir the coriander into the dressing. Break the swordfish into bite-sized pieces, add to the dressing and gently mix in, taking care not to break up the fish. Spoon the dressed fish on top of the spinach salad and serve.

Another idea
Make a **warm Mediterranean tuna salad**, using 4 tuna steaks, 2 cm (¾ in) thick, about 140 g (5 oz) each. Grill the steaks, basting with a mixture of 1½ tsp olive oil and 1 tbsp orange juice, for 2–3½ minutes on each side. Instead of using the tomatoes in the salsa dressing, slice them. Make the salsa dressing omitting the cumin, chilli and coriander, and toss with 200 g (7 oz) shredded radicchio and 100 g (3½ oz) rocket. Arrange the tomato and salad on 4 plates, top with the tuna, broken into pieces, and scatter over fresh basil.

Plus points
• Swordfish is a good low-fat source of protein and provides excellent amounts of vitamin B_{12}, niacin, selenium and potassium.

• Peppers are native to tropical America and have been cultivated in Europe since the 16th century. They are a good source of beta-carotene and contain over twice as much vitamin C as oranges.

• Courgettes provide the B vitamins B_6, folate and niacin. The greatest concentration of these nutrients is found in the skin, which is also rich in the antioxidant beta-carotene.

photo, page 153

Each serving provides kcal 280, protein 31 g, fat 11 g (of which saturated fat 2 g), carbohydrate 16 g (of which sugars 15 g), fibre 6 g. Excellent source of folate, niacin, selenium, vitamin A, vitamin B_1, vitamin B_6, vitamin B_{12}, vitamin C, vitamin E. Good source of calcium, iron, potassium, vitamin B_2.

Salmon with tarragon mayonnaise

Salmon is readily available all year round and is keenly priced, making it an affordable treat. This dish can be served warm or cold, with a green leaf salad tossed with mange-tout or green beans, and some crusty bread.

Preparation and cooking time **35 minutes**   *Serves 4*

4 salmon steaks or pieces of fillet, about 125 g (4½ oz) each

150 ml (5 fl oz) dry white wine

1–2 bay leaves

strip of pared lemon zest

Tarragon mayonnaise

4 tbsp reduced-fat mayonnaise

150 g (5½ oz) plain low-fat yogurt

finely grated zest of 1 lemon

2 tbsp chopped fresh tarragon

Couscous

250 g (8½ oz) couscous

4 tomatoes, roughly chopped

3 spring onions, chopped

55 g (2 oz) watercress, roughly chopped

1 tbsp extra virgin olive oil

juice of 1 lemon

salt and pepper

1 Place the salmon in a deep-sided, non-stick frying pan. Pour over the wine and add the bay leaves, lemon zest and seasoning to taste. Bring to the boil, then reduce the heat, cover and poach the salmon for 5–6 minutes or until just cooked – it should still be very slightly translucent in the centre.

2 Meanwhile, stir together the yogurt, mayonnaise, grated lemon zest and tarragon. Season to taste and spoon the mixture into a serving bowl.

3 When the fish is cooked, drain off most of the cooking liquid into a measuring jug and add enough boiling water to make 360 ml (12 fl oz). Cover the pan with a lid to keep the salmon warm, off the heat.

4 Pour the diluted fish stock over the couscous in a bowl and leave for 3–4 minutes for the liquid to be absorbed. Fluff up the couscous with a fork and stir in the chopped tomatoes, spring onions and watercress. Drizzle over the olive oil and lemon juice, and stir to blend everything together. Season to taste.

5 Serve warm with the couscous salad and the tarragon mayonnaise.

Some more ideas

The aniseed flavour of Pernod works well with the tarragon mayonnaise. Poach the salmon in 100 ml (3½ fl oz) water or stock mixed with 4 tbsp Pernod or pastis.

Half-fat crème fraîche and 0% Greek-style yogurt can be used to make a sauce with an even lower fat content.

For a special occasion, cook a whole salmon and serve it garnished with twists of lemon and sprigs of fresh tarragon. To cook salmon, season and wrap loosely in a large sheet of lightly oiled foil, then bake in a preheated 180°C (350°F, gas mark 4) oven, allowing 10 minutes per 450 g (1 lb).

Plus points

- Combining reduced fat mayonnaise with plain low-fat yogurt makes a lighter sauce that is lower in calories and fat than standard mayonnaise alone.

- Couscous is the staple food in many North African countries. It is low in fat and high in starchy carbohydrate. For a lower Glycaemic Index, use pasta or rice noodles instead.

photo, page 159

Each serving provides   kcal 500, protein 32 g, fat 22 g (of which saturated fat 5 g), carbohydrate 39 g (of which sugars 6 g), fibre 1 g. Excellent source of iron, niacin, vitamin B$_1$, vitamin B$_6$, vitamin B$_{12}$, vitamin E. Good source of selenium, vitamin A, vitamin C. Useful source of calcium, folate, potassium, vitamin B$_2$, zinc.

Griddled halibut steaks with tomato and red pepper salsa

Fish steaks make ideal fast food and a vibrant salsa transforms the plain cooked fish into an exciting dish. Cooking the halibut on a ridged grill pan produces attractive markings. Serve with rice, a mixed leaf salad and wholegrain bread.

Preparation time **15 minutes**   Cooking time **4–6 minutes**   *Serves 4*

4 halibut steaks, about 140 g (5 oz) each

2 tbsp extra virgin olive oil

juice of 1 small orange

1 garlic clove, crushed

1 orange, cut into wedges, to garnish

Tomato and red pepper salsa

200 g (7 oz) ripe plum tomatoes, diced

½ red pepper, seeded and diced

½ red onion, finely chopped

juice of 1 small orange

15 g (½ oz) fresh basil, chopped

1 tbsp balsamic vinegar

1 tsp caster sugar

salt and pepper

1 Place the halibut steaks in a shallow non-metallic dish. Mix together the oil, orange juice, garlic and salt and pepper to taste, and spoon over the fish steaks.

2 Combine all the salsa ingredients and season with salt and pepper to taste. Spoon into a serving bowl.

3 Heat a lightly oiled ridged cast-iron grill pan or heavy-based frying pan over a high heat. Place the fish steaks on the grill pan or in the frying pan and cook for 2–3 minutes on each side, basting from time to time with the oil mixture, until the fish will just flake easily.

4 Place the fish steaks on warm serving plates and grind over some black pepper. Garnish with wedges of orange and serve with the salsa.

Some more ideas

Other white fish steaks such as cod, haddock, hoki or swordfish, or monkfish fillets, can be cooked in the same way.

For a **tomato and olive salsa**, combine the diced tomatoes with ½ diced cucumber, 4 chopped spring onions, 45 g (1½ oz) chopped stoned green or black olives and 15 g (½ oz) chopped fresh basil. Or use 1 tbsp drained and rinsed capers instead of olives.

In summer, the fish can be cooked on a barbecue. Lay the steaks on foil to prevent the delicate flesh slipping through the grid.

Plus points

● Halibut is a good source of niacin, which has an important role to play in the release of energy inside cells. Niacin is one of the most stable vitamins, and there are little or no losses during preparation or cooking.

● In restaurants, fish is often pan-fried in a good amount of oil. This contributes added fat to the dish. When grilling fish at home, limit the amount of cooking fat you use for a much healthier meal.

photo, page 159

Each serving provides   kcal 225, protein 31 g, fat 8 g (of which saturated fat 2 g), carbohydrate 7.5 g (of which sugars 6.5 g), fibre 1 g. Excellent source of niacin, vitamin B$_1$, vitamin B$_6$, vitamin C. Good source of vitamin A, vitamin B$_{12}$, vitamin E. Useful source of iron, potassium.

Haddock with parsley sauce

When made with the freshest fish and parsley, this simple supper dish is a real winner. Served with mashed potatoes mixed with leeks and courgettes and a salad, it is a satisfying meal that all the family will enjoy.

Preparation and cooking time **45–50 minutes**   *Serves 4*

4 pieces of haddock fillet, about 140 g (5 oz) each

20 g (¾ oz) parsley

1 small onion, thinly sliced

1 carrot, thinly sliced

6 black peppercorns

300 ml (10 fl oz) semi-skimmed milk

750 g (1 lb 10 oz) potatoes, peeled and cut into chunks

1 large leek, thinly sliced

2 courgettes, cut into thin sticks

25 g (scant 1 oz) butter

25 g (scant 1 oz) plain flour

finely grated zest and juice of ½ lemon

salt and pepper

chopped parsley to garnish

lemon wedges to serve

1 Put the fish in a large frying pan. Tear the leaves from the parsley stalks and add the stalks to the pan with the onion, carrot, peppercorns and milk. Bring just to the boil, then cover and simmer very gently for 5 minutes. Remove the pan from the heat and leave for 5 minutes to complete the cooking.

2 Meanwhile, put the potatoes in a saucepan, cover with boiling water and simmer for 15 minutes or until tender. About 5 minutes before the end of the cooking time, add the white part of the leek to the potatoes. Also, set a colander on top of the pan and steam the courgettes with the green part of the leek over the potatoes.

3 Transfer the fish to a plate and remove the skin. Keep warm. Strain the cooking liquid and reserve.

4 Melt the butter in a medium saucepan, stir in the flour and cook for 1 minute. Gradually stir in the cooking liquid and bring to the boil, stirring until the sauce is thick and smooth. Finely chop the parsley leaves and stir into the sauce with the lemon zest. Season to taste and keep hot.

5 Drain the potatoes and white leeks and mash with the lemon juice and seasoning. Stir in the green leek tops and courgettes. Transfer the fish fillets to serving plates and spoon over the sauce. Garnish with parsley and serve with the mash and lemon wedges.

Another idea

Make a **haddock and spinach gratin**. Cook the fish and potatoes as above. Slice 3 tomatoes and arrange in a shallow flameproof dish. Steam 280 g (10 oz) spinach leaves until wilted, then squeeze dry and sprinkle with 1 tbsp lemon juice. Spread over the tomatoes and top with the fish. Pour over the parsley sauce and spread over the mashed potatoes. Sprinkle with 2 tbsp grated mature Cheddar cheese and grill until golden.

Plus points

• Courgettes provide niacin and vitamin B_6. It is the tender skins that contain the greatest concentration of these nutrients.

• Parsley was used in Greek times for its medicinal purposes, but the Romans used it as a herb and introduced it into this country. Parsley is rich in nutrients, particularly vitamin C. Just a teaspoon of chopped parsley can make a significant contribution to the daily requirement for vitamin C.

Each serving provides kcal 389, protein 36 g, fat 8 g (of which saturated fat 4 g), carbohydrate 46 g (of which sugars 9 g), fibre 5 g. Excellent source of niacin, selenium, vitamin A, vitamin B_1, vitamin B_6, vitamin B_{12}, vitamin C. Good source of folate, iron, potassium. Useful source of calcium, copper, vitamin B_2, vitamin E, zinc.

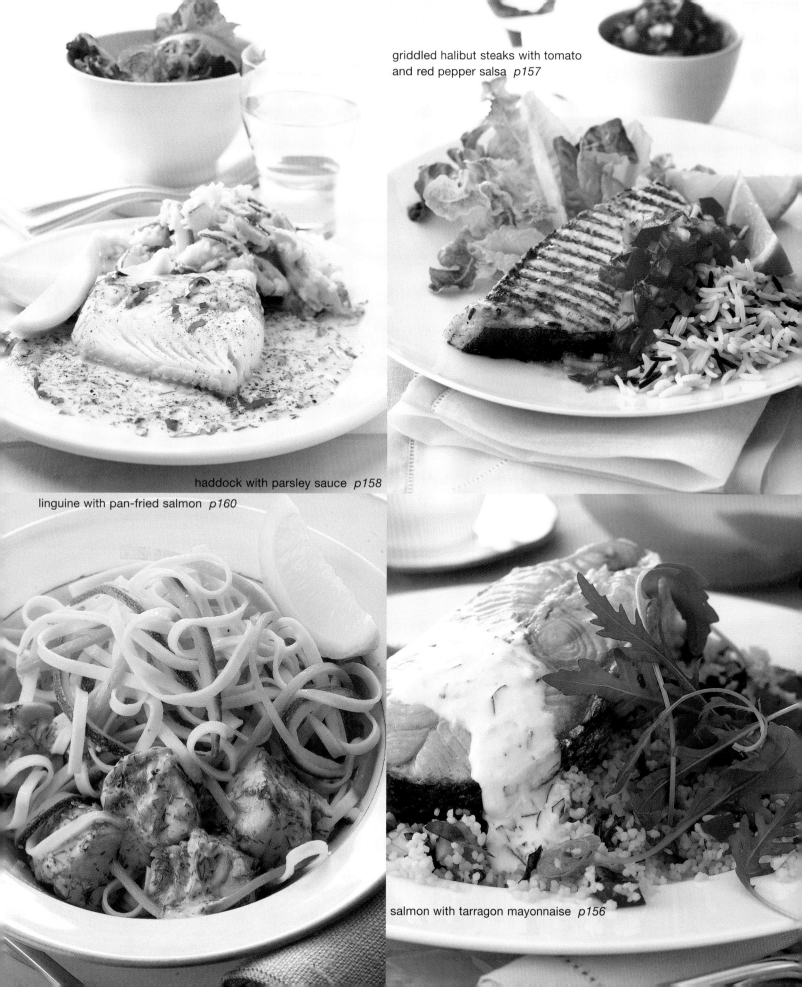

griddled halibut steaks with tomato
and red pepper salsa *p157*

haddock with parsley sauce *p158*

linguine with pan-fried salmon *p160*

salmon with tarragon mayonnaise *p156*

Linguine with pan-fried salmon

All the ingredients for this dish are quickly assembled and cooked, and the result is truly delicious as well as visually impressive. This is definitely a dish to convince anyone who has doubts about the taste benefits of well-balanced eating. With bread and salad, it makes a hearty meal.

Preparation time **10 minutes, plus optional marinating**   Cooking time **15 minutes**   *Serves 4*

400 g (14 oz) salmon fillet, skinned

grated zest and juice of 1 lemon

2 tbsp chopped fresh dill

340 g (12 oz) linguine

225 g (8 oz) carrots, cut into matchstick strips

225 g (8 oz) courgettes, cut into matchstick strips

1 tsp sunflower oil

100 g (3½ oz) reduced-fat crème fraîche

salt and pepper

To garnish

sprigs of fresh dill (optional)

1 lemon, cut into wedges

1 Cut the salmon into chunks and place in a dish. Add the lemon zest and juice, and the dill. Turn the chunks of salmon to coat them evenly. Cover and marinate in the fridge for at least 10 minutes.

2 Cook the linguine in boiling water for 10 minutes, or according to the packet instructions, until al dente. Add the carrots to the pasta after 8 minutes cooking, then add the courgettes 1 minute later.

3 Meanwhile, brush a non-stick or heavy-based frying pan with the oil and heat thoroughly. Drain the salmon, reserving the lemon juice marinade. Add the salmon to the hot pan and cook, turning the pieces occasionally, for 3–4 minutes, or until the fish is firm and just cooked.

4 Add the reserved marinade and the crème fraîche to the salmon, and cook for a few seconds. Remove from the heat and stir in seasoning to taste.

5 Drain the pasta and vegetables, and transfer them to a serving dish or to individual plates. Add the salmon mixture, garnish with fresh dill, if liked, and serve with lemon wedges.

Some more ideas

Trout fillets, asparagus tips and broad beans are an excellent alternative combination to the salmon, carrot and courgette. Cook the asparagus tips and beans with the pasta for the last 4–5 minutes.

Use the recipe as a basis for a quick, healthy storecupboard supper dish, adding frozen green beans and sweetcorn to the pasta, and using well-drained canned salmon instead of the fresh fish. There is no need to marinate or cook the canned salmon: the heat of the pasta will bring out its flavour beautifully.

Plus points

• Using reduced-fat crème fraîche makes a deceptively creamy lemon sauce for a fish that tastes deliciously decadent.

• Cutting the courgettes and carrots into thin, pasta-like strips and mixing them with pasta is a good way of presenting them to children who are reluctant to eat vegetables.

photo, page 159

Each serving provides kcal 560, protein 33 g, fat 18 g (of which saturated fat 5 g), carbohydrate 70 g (of which sugars 6 g), fibre 4.5 g. Excellent source of niacin, vitamin A, vitamin B$_{12}$. Good source of copper, selenium, vitamin B$_1$, vitamin B$_6$, vitamin C. Useful source of folate, potassium, vitamin E.

Spaghetti with clams

This popular trattoria dish is easily made at home. A classic tomato sauce, flavoured with chilli and fresh herbs in true Italian style, is delicious with clams, especially if tossed with perfectly cooked spaghetti. Serve with chunks of ciabatta bread and a green salad – and a glass of red wine.

Preparation time **15 minutes**   Cooking time **20 minutes**   *Serves 4*

1 tbsp extra virgin olive oil

1 onion, chopped

2 garlic cloves, chopped

1 small fresh red chilli, seeded and chopped

150 g (5½ oz) chestnut mushrooms, chopped

1 can plum tomatoes, about 400 g

1 tbsp chopped fresh basil

1 tbsp chopped parsley

½ tsp sugar

340 g (12 oz) spaghetti

48 clams in their shells, about 900 g (2 lb) in total, rinsed

4 tbsp red or white wine

1 Heat the oil in a medium-sized saucepan, add the onion, garlic and chilli, and cook over a moderate heat for 5 minutes. Stir in the mushrooms and cook for 2 minutes, then add the tomatoes and their juice, crushing them down with a wooden spoon. Sprinkle in the basil, parsley and sugar and stir. Cover and simmer for 10 minutes.

2 Meanwhile, cook the spaghetti in boiling water for 10–12 minutes, or according to the packet instructions, until al dente. Drain the pasta in a colander.

3 Put the empty pasta pan back on the heat, add the clams and splash in the wine. Tip the pasta back in. Cover and cook for 3 minutes, shaking the pan occasionally. All the shells should have opened; discard any clams that remain shut.

4 Pour the tomato sauce into the spaghetti and clam mixture, and stir and toss over the heat for 1–2 minutes or until it is all bubbling. Season with salt and pepper to taste, then serve.

Another idea

Make a **tomato, olive and caper sauce with canned clams**. Heat 2 tsp extra virgin olive oil in a saucepan and fry 2 rashers of unsmoked lean back bacon, rinded and chopped. Add 1 chopped onion, 1 small red pepper, seeded and chopped, and 1 chopped garlic clove. Cook for 5 minutes, then add a can of tomatoes, about 400 g, with the juice, crushing them down. Cover and cook for 10 minutes. Stir a can of baby clams in brine, about 280 g, into the tomato sauce (with the brine), and add 8 black olives, roughly chopped, 1 tbsp capers and a handful of freshly torn basil leaves. Season with black pepper. Simmer for 2 minutes, then serve the sauce over the spaghetti.

Plus points

• Clams are a good source of phosphorus, needed for healthy bones and teeth.

• Contrary to popular belief, pasta is not a 'fattening' food. It is only when excessive amounts of oil, cream or butter are added to the accompanying sauces that the calorific value is considerably increased. Spaghetti has a low Glycaemic Index.

• All mushrooms are a good source of copper, which has many important functions, including maintaining healthy bones and helping to prevent anaemia by improving the absorption of iron from food.

photo, page 165

Each serving provides   kcal 448, protein 25 g, fat 7 g (of which saturated fat 1 g), carbohydrate 73 g (of which sugars 10 g), fibre 6 g. Excellent source of copper, iron, niacin, vitamin B$_1$, vitamin B$_6$. Good source of folate, potassium, vitamin C, zinc. Useful source of calcium, vitamin A, vitamin E.

Parmesan-topped mussels

Make this stylish starter when you can buy large mussels, such as the green-lipped mussels from New Zealand, as smaller ones can toughen when grilled. Although you only need 24 mussels for this recipe, buy at least 30 because some might have to be discarded. Serve the mussels with chunks of wholemeal bread.

Preparation and cooking time **30 minutes**   *Serves 4*

100 ml (3½ fl oz) white wine or fish stock, preferably home-made

1 large onion, very finely chopped

3 large garlic cloves, crushed

about 30 large mussels, scrubbed and beards removed

50 g (1¾ oz) fresh wholemeal bread

30 g (1 oz) parsley, chopped

30 g (1 oz) Parmesan cheese, freshly grated

½ tbsp finely grated lemon zest

pinch of cayenne pepper

1 tbsp extra virgin olive oil

lemon wedges to serve

1 Pour the wine or stock into a large saucepan, add the onion and garlic, and bring to the boil over a high heat. Boil rapidly for 1 minute. Add the mussels, cover the pan tightly and cook for 2–3 minutes, shaking the pan occasionally. Uncover the pan and give the mussels a good stir. Using tongs, remove the mussels from the pan as soon as they open and set them aside. Discard any mussels that remain shut.

2 When the mussels are cool enough to handle, remove and discard the top shell. Place 24 mussels on the half shell in a single layer in a shallow flameproof dish, loosening the mussels from the shells but leaving them in place. Set the dish aside.

3 Preheat the grill to high. Put the bread in a food processor or blender and process to fine crumbs. Add the parsley, Parmesan, lemon zest, cayenne pepper and olive oil, and process until well blended.

4 Using your fingers, put a mound of the cheese and crumb mixture on each mussel and pack it down firmly so the mussel is completely covered. Put the dish under the grill and cook for 2–3 minutes or until the crumb topping is lightly browned. Divide the mussels among individual plates and serve with lemon wedges.

Another idea

For **French-style mussels in cider**, put 1 litre (1¾ pints) dry cider in the pan with the onion and garlic and boil until reduced to 600 ml (1 pint). Stir in the parsley, lemon zest and cayenne pepper. Add the mussels and steam them open. Transfer the mussels to serving bowls. Season the cooking liquid to taste and ladle it over the mussels.

Plus points

● Mussels are a good source of iron, an essential component of haemoglobin in red blood cells responsible for transporting oxygen around the body.

● Parmesan cheese is a very hard cheese made from unpasteurised skimmed cow's milk. Although Parmesan has a high fat content, it also has a strong flavour and a little goes a long way in a recipe.

● Cayenne pepper, made from one of the smallest and hottest chillies, is often used in herbal medicine to stimulate the circulation.

photo, page 165

Each serving provides kcal 167, protein 12 g, fat 7 g (of which saturated fat 2 g), carbohydrate 12 g (of which sugars 4 g), fibre 2 g. Excellent source of iron, niacin, vitamin B_1, vitamin B_6, vitamin B_{12}. Good source of selenium. Useful source of calcium, copper, folate, potassium, vitamin A, vitamin C, zinc.

Tiger prawns with pepper salsa

A salsa is a Mexican-style vegetable or fruit sauce with a fresh zingy flavour. A tomato, pepper and chilli salsa makes a wonderful accompaniment for grilled prawn kebabs, here served with sweet melon and grainy bread.

Preparation and cooking time **30 minutes**   *Serves 4*

32 large raw tiger prawns, peeled but tails left on

1 Charentais melon, seeded and cut into cubes

Marinade

2 tbsp lime juice

1 tsp bottled chopped garlic in oil, drained

1 tsp bottled chopped root ginger in oil, drained

Salsa

6 vine-ripened tomatoes, chopped

1 small red onion, finely chopped

1 red pepper, seeded and chopped

1 tsp bottled chopped garlic in oil, drained

1 fresh green chilli, seeded and finely chopped

2 tbsp lime juice

2 tbsp chopped fresh coriander

salt and pepper

shredded spring onions to garnish

1 Preheat the grill. Soak 8 bamboo skewers in cold water (to prevent them from burning under the grill). Combine all of the ingredients for the marinade in a shallow dish. Add the prawns and stir to coat them with the marinade. Cover and chill while preparing the salsa.

2 Mix together all the salsa ingredients and season with salt and pepper to taste. Pile into a serving bowl. Thread the cubes of melon onto 8 unsoaked wooden skewers and place on a serving dish. Set aside.

3 Thread 4 prawns onto each of the soaked skewers, piercing them through both ends (this will help to keep them flat). Place under the grill and cook for 3–4 minutes or until they are pink, turning them once. Do not overcook or they will become tough.

4 Garnish the salsa with the shredded spring onions. Place the prawn kebabs on the serving dish with the melon and serve immediately, with the salsa alongside.

Some more ideas

Make **grilled chicken kebabs with a fresh citrus salsa**. Cut 550 g (1¼ lb) skinless boneless chicken breasts (fillets) into cubes and marinate as described in the main recipe. Grill the chicken on skewers for 10 minutes or until tender and cooked through. For the salsa, chop the flesh from 1 pink grapefruit and 1 orange and 1 crisp juicy apple, and mix with 2 chopped spring onions, 1 finely chopped fresh green chilli and 1 tbsp chopped fresh mint.

Cubes of fresh pineapple can be speared onto skewers to accompany the prawn or chicken kebabs in place of melon.

Plus points

* The raw fruit and vegetables in the salsa are packed with vitamins. The tomatoes and red peppers are excellent sources of the antioxidants beta-carotene and vitamin C. Red peppers, in particular, are an excellent source of vitamin C. Weight for weight, they provide over twice as much vitamin C as oranges.

* Prawns are a high-protein, low-fat food.

photo, page 165

Each serving provides kcal 150, protein 24 g, fat 1.5 g (of which saturated fat 0.5 g), carbohydrate 11 g (of which sugars 10 g), fibre 3 g. Excellent source of vitamin A, vitamin B$_{12}$, vitamin C. Good source of iron, vitamin B$_6$. Useful source of folate, niacin, potassium, selenium, zinc.

Prawn gumbo

A bowl of steaming gumbo – a thick and spicy cross between a soup and a stew, full of peppers, tomatoes, okra, herbs and prawns – brings you all the good tastes of the Louisiana bayou. Serve with steamed rice or crusty bread so you can enjoy all the sauce.

Preparation time **25 minutes**   Cooking time **40 minutes**   *Serves 4*

1 tbsp extra virgin olive oil

2 onions, chopped

1 red pepper, seeded and chopped

2 celery sticks, chopped

3 garlic cloves, chopped

75 g (2½ oz) lean smoked back bacon rashers, rinded and diced

1 tbsp plain flour

1 tbsp paprika

1 litre (1¾ pints) fish stock, preferably home-made

1 tsp chopped fresh thyme

1 can chopped tomatoes, about 225 g

2 tbsp chopped parsley

2 bay leaves

2 tsp Worcestershire sauce

Tabasco sauce to taste

100 g (3½ oz) okra, sliced crossways

340 g (12 oz) peeled raw prawns

55 g (2 oz) fine green beans, cut into bite-sized lengths

salt and pepper

3 spring onions, thinly sliced, to garnish

1 Heat the oil in a large saucepan, add the onions, pepper and celery, and cook for 5–6 minutes or until lightly browned. Stir in the garlic and bacon and cook for a further 3–4 minutes. Stir in the flour, increase the heat slightly and cook for 2 minutes, stirring. Stir in the paprika and cook for 2 more minutes. Gradually add the stock, stirring well to dissolve the flour mixture.

2 Add the thyme, tomatoes with their juice, parsley, bay leaves and the Worcestershire sauce. Bring to the boil, then reduce the heat to a simmer and add Tabasco sauce to taste. Add the okra and simmer for 15 minutes or until the okra is tender and the mixture has thickened.

3 Add the prawns and green beans and cook for 3 minutes or until the prawns turn pink and the beans are tender. Remove the bay leaves and season the gumbo with salt and pepper to taste. Serve in bowls, sprinkled with spring onions.

Some more ideas

Try a **Jamaican-style gumbo**. Instead of lean bacon, use 75 g (2½ oz) lean smoked sausage such as kabanos. In step 2, add 1 tsp chopped fresh root ginger, ½ tsp Angostura bitters, 1 small can red kidney beans, about 200 g, drained, and 1 tbsp dark rum with the tomatoes and other ingredients. Replace half the parsley with fresh coriander.

Use a mixture of 170 g (6 oz) prawns and 170 g (6 oz) canned crab meat, adding the crab at the very end, with the final seasoning.

Plus points

● Okra contains a mucilaginous substance that is used to thicken the liquid in dishes such as this (the name gumbo comes from the African word for okra). The nutrient content of okra is very similar to other green vegetables in that it provides useful amounts of dietary fibre, potassium, calcium, folate and vitamin C.

● Bacon is a good source of vitamin B_1, which is essential for maintaining a healthy nervous system. Always choose lean varieties and be aware of the salt content.

Each serving provides   kcal 206, protein 23 g, fat 6 g (of which saturated fat 1 g), carbohydrate 17 g (of which sugars 10 g), fibre 4 g. Excellent source of niacin, vitamin B_1, vitamin B_6, vitamin B_{12}, vitamin C. Good source of iron, potassium, vitamin A, vitamin E. Useful source of calcium, copper, folate, selenium, zinc.

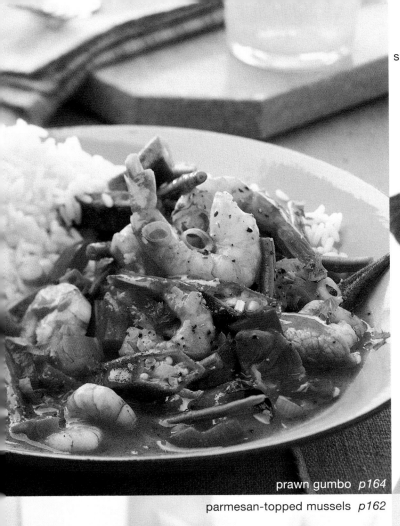

prawn gumbo *p164*

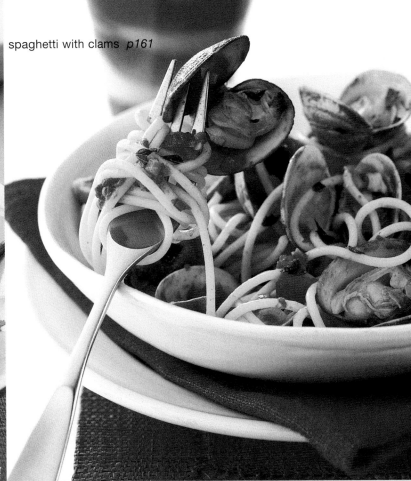

spaghetti with clams *p161*

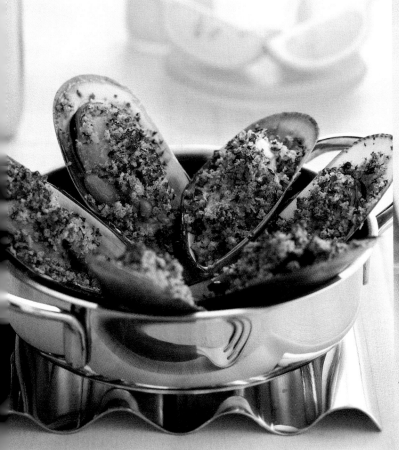

parmesan-topped mussels *p162*

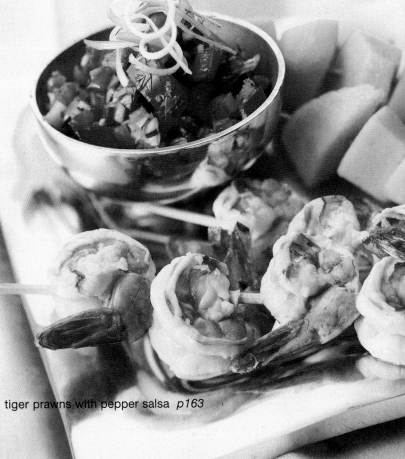

tiger prawns with pepper salsa *p163*

Scampi provençal

The ideal accompaniment to this stylish dish is a simple salad of sliced tomatoes drizzled with a little vinaigrette and served on a bed of fresh baby spinach leaves – perfect for a quick supper.

Preparation and cooking time **30 minutes**   *Serves 4*

1 tbsp extra virgin olive oil

1 large onion, chopped

1 bulb of fennel, chopped

1 large garlic clove, crushed

1 can chopped tomatoes, about 400 g

120 ml (4 fl oz) fish stock, preferably home-made

½ tbsp fennel seeds

finely grated zest and juice of ½ orange

pinch of saffron threads

250 g (8½ oz) long-grain rice

400 g (14 oz) peeled raw scampi (langoustines)

salt and pepper

fresh basil leaves to garnish

1 Heat the oil in a large non-stick frying pan with a tight-fitting lid. Add the onion, fennel and garlic and cook over a moderate heat, stirring occasionally, for 5 minutes or until softened but not browned. Add the tomatoes with their juice, the stock, fennel seeds, and orange zest and juice, and season with salt and pepper to taste. Bring to the boil, stirring, then reduce the heat to low and half cover the pan. Simmer for 12 minutes.

2 Meanwhile, crumble the saffron threads into a saucepan of boiling water. Add the rice and boil for 10–12 minutes, or according to the packet instructions.

3 Bring the tomato sauce back to the boil. Place the scampi on top of the sauce, cover the pan tightly and cook over a low heat for 3–4 minutes or until the scampi are cooked through and opaque. Do not boil the mixture or the scampi may toughen.

4 Drain the rice and divide among serving bowls. Spoon in the scampi and tomato sauce. Sprinkle with basil and serve at once.

Some more ideas
This combination of seafood and tomatoes also makes a delicious sauce for 400 g (14 oz) wholemeal spaghetti.

For **tuna provençal**, make the tomato sauce and, just before serving, stir in 2 cans tuna in spring water, about 200 g each, drained and flaked. This makes a great sauce for cooked pasta shells. Serve garnished with fresh dill.

If you can't find scampi, you can use peeled raw tiger or king prawns, scallops or 400 g (14 oz) shellfish cocktail mix.

For extra flavour, add a pinch of crushed dried chillies with the tomatoes. Or, stir in 3–4 diced canned anchovy fillets.

Plus points
• Called scampi in Italy, but known in Britain by their French name, langoustine, or as Dublin Bay prawns, this crustacean is a rich source of vitamin E. Vitamin E is actually a group of several related compounds which have powerful antioxidant properties.

• The vitamin C in tomatoes is concentrated in the jellylike substance surrounding the seeds. Vitamin C is an important nutrient for maintaining immunity and healthy skin.

• Fennel seeds are thought to aid digestion, and fennel tea is often recommended to ease flatulence.

photo, page 169

Each serving provides kcal 377, protein 25 g, fat 4 g (of which saturated fat 0.5 g), carbohydrate 64 g (of which sugars 8 g), fibre 3 g. Excellent source of niacin, vitamin B$_1$, vitamin B$_6$, vitamin B$_{12}$. Good source of copper, iron, selenium, vitamin C, vitamin E, zinc. Useful source of calcium, folate, potassium.

Seafood with watercress dressing

Scallops and strips of salmon fillet are briefly poached in a little wine and stock, then lifted onto a colourful crunchy salad. The poaching liquid provides the base for a creamy dressing. Serve with crusty bread.

Preparation and cooking time **about 40 minutes**   *Serves 4*

300 g (10½ oz) piece of skinless salmon fillet, cut into 4 strips

200 g (7 oz) small scallops without coral

3 tbsp dry white wine

200 ml (7 fl oz) fish stock

thin slice of fresh root ginger (there is no need to peel it)

225 g (8 oz) sugarsnap peas

140 g (5 oz) radishes

150 g (5½ oz) mixed salad leaves, including baby spinach, watercress, and cos and Oak Leaf lettuces

Watercress dressing

85 g (3 oz) watercress

1 shallot, chopped

thin strip of lemon zest

2 tbsp snipped fresh chives

1 tsp lemon juice

2 tbsp half-fat crème fraîche

salt and pepper

1 Put the strips of salmon into a non-aluminium saucepan or sauté pan with a well-fitting lid. Arrange the scallops on top of the salmon. Pour over the wine and fish stock, and add the slice of ginger. Bring to the boil over a moderate heat, then lower the heat until the liquid is simmering gently. Cover and poach for 5–8 minutes or until the salmon and scallops are cooked and feel just firm to the touch.

2 While the seafood is cooking, drop the sugarsnap peas into a pan of boiling water and cook for 3–4 minutes or until just tender but still crunchy. Drain, then refresh under cold running water. Set aside.

3 To make radish flowers, cut 5 slits round each radish, cutting down from the top almost to the base. Put the flowers into a bowl of iced water and leave until the 'petals' open slightly. Alternatively, simply slice the radishes.

4 Put the mixed leaves into a salad bowl. Add the sugarsnap peas and the drained radishes and mix well.

5 With a draining spoon, lift the seafood out of the pan onto a plate. Reserve the poaching liquid. Cut each strip of salmon in half, or flake into large chunks. Arrange the salmon and scallops on top of the salad.

6 To make the dressing, remove the tough stalks from the watercress and reserve. Drop the leaves into a pan of boiling water and bring back to the boil. Immediately drain and refresh under cold running water. Squeeze out excess water, then chop finely.

7 Put the reserved watercress stalks in a pan with the shallot, lemon zest and 120 ml (4 fl oz) of the poaching liquid. Half cover the pan and simmer for 5 minutes. Strain, discarding the zest and vegetables. Stir in the watercress, chives, lemon juice and crème fraîche, and season to taste. Spoon over the warm dressing and serve.

Plus points

• Scallops are an excellent source of selenium, a powerful antioxidant that protects the body against disease, and of vitamin B$_{12}$. They also provide useful amounts of phosphorus and potassium.

• Watercress is a positive powerhouse of disease-fighting nutrients. It contains phytochemicals that help to protect against cancer and help to neutralise the damaging effects of smoking. It is also an excellent source of vitamin C and beta-carotene.

photo, page 169

Each serving provides   kcal 217, protein 30 g, fat 12 g (of which saturated fat 2 g), carbohydrate 6 g (of which sugars 4 g), fibre 2 g. Excellent source of niacin, selenium, vitamin A, vitamin B$_1$, vitamin B$_6$, vitamin B$_{12}$, vitamin C, vitamin E. Good source of folate, potassium, vitamin B$_2$, zinc. Useful source of calcium, iron.

Steamed sea bass fillets with spring vegetables

Oriental steamer baskets are most handy for this dish – you can stack them so that everything can be steamed together. The moist heat from steaming ensures that the fish doesn't dry out. If using a liquid fish stock base or a cube, make up the stock half strength as it will get a lot of flavour from the marinade.

Preparation and cooking time **30 minutes**   *Serves 4*

1 tsp grated fresh root ginger

1 tbsp light soy sauce

½ tsp toasted sesame oil

1 garlic clove, finely chopped

1 tbsp dry sherry, dry white wine or vermouth

4 sea bass fillets, 3.5 cm (1¼ in) thick, about 140 g (5 oz) each

700 ml (24 fl oz) fish stock

200 g (7 oz) couscous

1 strip of lemon zest

225 g (8 oz) baby carrots

12 spring onions, trimmed to about 10 cm (4 in) long

200 g (7 oz) asparagus tips

2 tbsp chopped parsley

salt and pepper

1 First make the marinade. Combine the ginger, soy sauce, sesame oil, garlic and sherry, wine or vermouth in a bowl. Add the fish and coat in the marinade. Set aside.

2 Bring 250 ml (8½ fl oz) of the stock to the boil in a saucepan that will accommodate the steamer basket(s). Put the couscous in a bowl and pour over the boiling stock. Cover and leave to stand for about 15 minutes or until the couscous has swelled and absorbed the liquid.

3 Pour the remaining stock into the saucepan. Add the lemon zest and bring to the boil. Add the carrots. Reduce the heat so the stock simmers.

4 Place the fish, skin side down, in a steamer basket. Add the spring onions and asparagus, or put them in a second stacking steamer basket. Place the steamer basket(s) over the gently boiling stock and cover. Steam for 10–12 minutes or until the fish is opaque throughout and begins to flake, and the vegetables are tender.

5 When the couscous is ready, add the parsley and fluff the grains with a fork to mix the couscous and parsley. Season with salt and pepper to taste.

6 Lift the steamer basket(s) off the pan. Drain the carrots, reserving the cooking liquid. Arrange the fish, carrots and steamed vegetables on warm plates together with the couscous. Discard the lemon zest from the cooking liquid. Serve the liquid as a sauce.

Some more ideas

If you don't have a steamer, place the fish and vegetables in a colander, then place inside a large pan and cover with a lid.

Use salmon or cod fillets instead of sea bass. The cooking time may need to be reduced by a minute or two for thinner fish fillets; check for doneness after 8–9 minutes.

Plus points

• White fish such as sea bass are low in fat and calories and they offer many B-complex vitamins. Sea bass is also a good source of calcium, an essential mineral with many important functions in the body, including keeping bones and teeth strong.

• The active ingredient in asparagus, called asparagine, has a strong diuretic effect. Herbalists recommend eating asparagus as a treatment for rheumatism, arthritis and the bloating associated with PMT.

Each serving provides kcal 320, protein 34 g, fat 5 g (of which saturated fat 1 g), carbohydrate 35 g (of which sugars 8 g), fibre 3 g. Excellent source of vitamin A, vitamin B$_{12}$. Good source of calcium, folate, iron, vitamin C. Useful source of vitamin B$_1$, vitamin B$_6$.

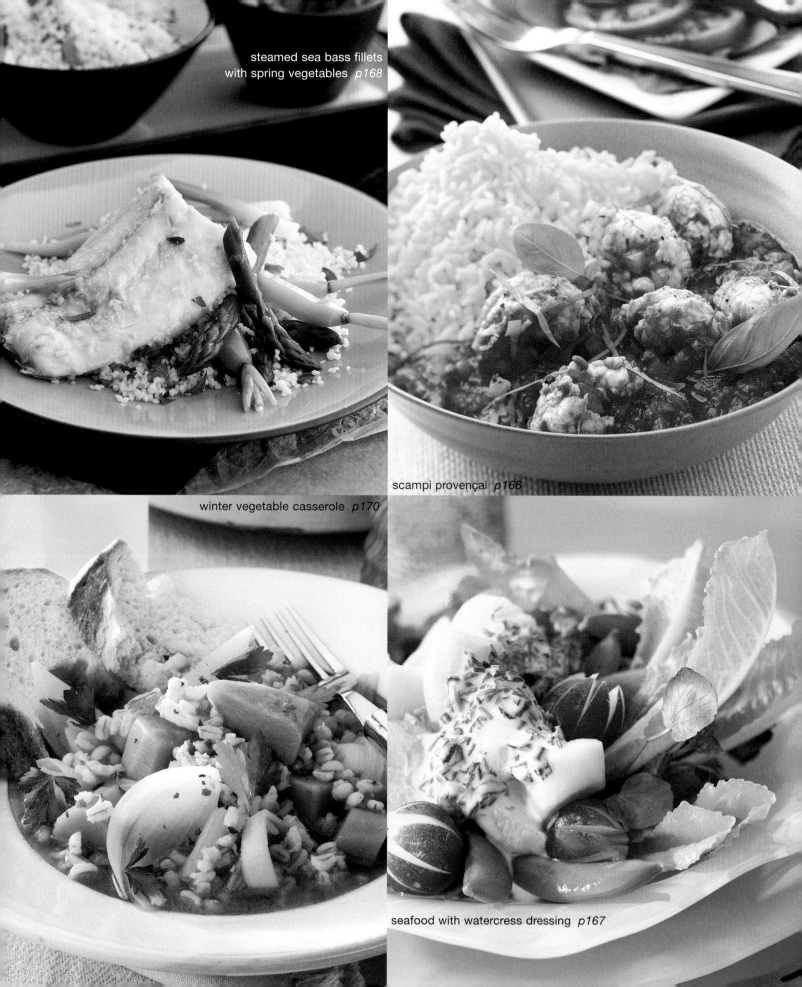

steamed sea bass fillets
with spring vegetables *p168*

scampi provençal *p166*

winter vegetable casserole *p170*

seafood with watercress dressing *p167*

Winter vegetable casserole

Good food does not have to be complicated or time-consuming. This simple, homely casserole is made without a lengthy shopping list of exotic fresh ingredients or hours of precise slicing and chopping. Raid the storecupboard and use everyday vegetables from the refrigerator for a warming and heart-healthy meal.

Preparation time **15 minutes**   Cooking time **1 hour**   *Serves 4*

2 onions, each cut into
6 wedges

3 carrots, cut into chunks

3 celery sticks, cut into chunks

400 g (14 oz) sweet potato or
swede, cut into chunks

1 litre (1¾ pints) hot vegetable
stock, preferably home-made
(see pages 224–225)

2 garlic cloves, finely chopped

3 leeks, about 300 g (10½ oz) in
total, thickly sliced

150 g (5½ oz) pearl barley

2 tsp dried sage

salt and pepper

3 tbsp coarsely chopped fresh
flat-leaf parsley to garnish

1 Preheat the oven to 180°C (350°F, gas mark 4). Put the onions, carrots, celery and sweet potato or swede in a large flameproof casserole. Pour in the stock and bring to the boil.

2 Add the garlic, leeks, pearl barley, sage and seasoning. Stir to mix the vegetables together. Cover and transfer to the oven to cook for about 1 hour or until the vegetables are just soft, and the barley is tender.

3 Sprinkle with the parsley and serve. Thick slices of farmhouse bread are an excellent accompaniment.

Some more ideas

A combination of Puy lentils and barley works well in this casserole. Use 100 g (3½ oz) pearl barley with 55 g (2 oz) Puy lentils. Cook for 30 minutes, then add 1 Golden Delicious apple, cored and sliced, to the casserole. Sprinkle the finished casserole with 50 g (1¾ oz) hazelnuts, toasted and coarsely chopped, with the chopped parsley garnish.

Other vegetables to add include parsnips, turnips and peeled chunks of butternut or kabocha squash.

Use dry cider instead of the stock, and add 50 g (1¾ oz) ready-to-eat dried pears, chopped, for a hint of sweetness.

The casserole can be simmered gently on the hob for 45–50 minutes, instead of cooking in the oven. Stir occasionally.

Plus points

● Barley is renowned for having a soothing effect on the intestines and urinary tract. It has long been considered a nourishing food for people convalescing after illness, and it is also beneficial for anyone suffering from stress or fatigue. For people with diabetes, barley is particularly good because it is absorbed very slowly.

● Some gummy fibres present in the barley grain (beta-glucans) appear to have dramatic cholesterol-lowering ability.

● Instead of frying the vegetables in oil, they are simmered in broth. This makes the dish extremely low in fat. With some bread to accompany it, the meal also offers a healthy balance of starchy carbohydrates.

photo, page 169

Each serving provides   kcal 205, protein 6 g, fat 2 g (of which saturated fat 0.1 g), carbohydrate 45 g (of which sugars 12 g), fibre 5 g. Excellent source of vitamin A. Good source of folate, vitamin B$_1$, vitamin B$_6$, vitamin C, vitamin E. Useful source of niacin, potassium.

Caribbean butternut squash and sweetcorn stew

Butternut squash has a lovely firm texture, ideal for cooking in stews. Combined with black-eyed beans, sweetcorn and red pepper it makes a nutritious family supper dish that is perfect for cold winter days. Serve with boiled rice or warm crusty bread.

Preparation and cooking time **30 minutes**   *Serves 4*

1 tbsp extra virgin olive oil

1 onion, sliced

2 garlic cloves, crushed

1 butternut squash, about 675 g (1½ lb), peeled and cut into 1 cm (½ in) cubes

1 red pepper, seeded and sliced

1 bay leaf

1 can chopped tomatoes, about 400 g

1 can black-eyed beans, about 410 g, drained and rinsed

1 can sweetcorn kernels, about 200 g, drained

300 ml (10 fl oz) vegetable stock, preferably home-made (see pages 224–225)

1 tbsp Worcestershire sauce, or to taste

1 tsp Tabasco sauce, or to taste

1 tbsp dark muscovado sugar

1–2 tsp balsamic vinegar

chopped parsley to garnish

1 Heat the oil in a large saucepan and add the onion, garlic, butternut squash, red pepper and bay leaf. Stir well, then cover the pan and allow the vegetables to sweat for 5 minutes, stirring occasionally.

2 Add the tomatoes with their juice, the black-eyed beans and sweetcorn, and stir to mix. Add the stock, Worcestershire sauce, Tabasco sauce, sugar and vinegar and stir again. Cover and simmer for 15 minutes or until the squash is tender.

3 Sprinkle the parsley over the stew and serve at once.

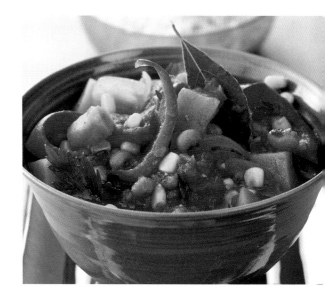

Some more ideas

For an **Indian stew**, soften the sliced onion and garlic in the olive oil for 2–3 minutes, then stir in 2 tbsp medium balti paste. Add the butternut squash with 150 g (5½ oz) thickly sliced baby corn. Cover and cook for 5–6 minutes. Replace the black-eyed beans with borlotti beans, adding them with the canned tomatoes and stock (omit the sweetcorn). Garnish with 2 tbsp chopped fresh coriander instead of parsley, and serve with boiled jasmine rice or warm naan bread.

For a vegetarian alternative, use mushroom ketchup instead of Worcestershire sauce.

Plus points

● There are more than 25 species of squash and pumpkin, some of which have been cultivated for 9000 years. All the varieties are rich in beta-carotene and contain useful amounts of vitamin C.

● If you have the time, leave the freshly crushed garlic cloves to stand for 10 minutes or so before starting to cook. Researchers at Penn State University in the USA have found that this maximises the formation and retention of cancer-fighting compounds.

Each serving provides   kcal 335, protein 15 g, fat 4 g (of which saturated fat 1 g), carbohydrate 62 g (of which sugars 21 g), fibre 9 g. Excellent source of folate, vitamin A, vitamin B$_6$, vitamin C. Good source of copper, iron, potassium, vitamin B$_1$, vitamin E. Useful source of calcium, zinc.

Roast vegetable and bean stew

This easy, one-pot dish of root vegetables and pinto beans makes a nourishing winter main course, and needs no accompaniments. It's particularly enjoyable with a glass of dry cider or apple juice.

Preparation time **20 minutes**   Cooking time **50–55 minutes**   *Serves 4*

1 acorn squash, about 600 g (1 lb 5 oz)

500 g (1 lb 2 oz) new potatoes, scrubbed and cut into 4 cm (1½ in) chunks

200 g (7 oz) carrots, cut into 4 cm (1½ in) chunks

200 g (7 oz) parsnips, cut into 4 cm (1½ in) chunks

2 large courgettes, about 400 g (14 oz) in total, cut into 4 cm (1½ in) chunks

2 tbsp extra virgin olive oil

1 garlic clove, finely chopped

4 large sprigs of fresh rosemary, plus extra sprigs to garnish

2 cans pinto beans, about 410 g each, drained and rinsed

240 ml (8 fl oz) dry cider

240 ml (8 fl oz) hot vegetable stock, preferably home-made (see pages 224–225)

salt and pepper

1 Preheat the oven to 200°C (400°C, gas mark 6). Halve the squash and remove the seeds and fibres, then cut off the hard skin and cut the flesh into 4 cm (1½ in) chunks.

2 Put the squash in a bowl and add the potatoes, carrots, parsnips and courgettes. Drizzle over the olive oil and toss to coat the vegetables evenly. Stir in the garlic and season to taste.

3 Lay the rosemary sprigs on the bottom of a large roasting tin and spread the vegetables on top in a single layer. Roast for about 30 minutes, turning once, until lightly browned.

4 Remove from the oven and stir in the pinto beans, cider and stock. Cover the tin tightly with foil, then return to the oven and cook for a further 20–25 minutes or until the vegetables are tender. Before serving, remove the rosemary stalks and garnish with fresh rosemary sprigs.

Some more ideas

You can also cook the stew on top of the stove. Heat the oil in a large saucepan, add the vegetables and fry for 4–5 minutes, stirring, then add the garlic, rosemary and seasoning. Stir in the beans, cider and stock, and bring to the boil. Cover and simmer for 30–35 minutes or until tender.

Replace the acorn squash with butternut squash and use canned ful medames beans instead of the pinto beans. Omit the potatoes from the stew and reduce the stock to 150 ml (5 fl oz). Bake 4 medium-sized potatoes in their jackets alongside the stew for 40–50 minutes or until tender. Serve the stew spooned into the split jacket potatoes.

Plus points

• Parsnips are a very nutritious starchy vegetable, providing useful amounts of potassium, the B vitamins B_1 and folate, and vitamin C.

• Use freshly dug potatoes whenever possible, as they can contain as much as ten times more vitamin C than potatoes that have been stored.

Each serving provides kcal 452, protein 17 g, fat 8 g (of which saturated fat 1 g), carbohydrate 76 g (of which sugars 13 g), fibre 9 g. Excellent source of copper, folate, potassium, vitamin A, vitamin B_1, vitamin B_6, vitamin C. Good source of calcium, iron, zinc. Useful source of niacin, selenium, vitamin E.

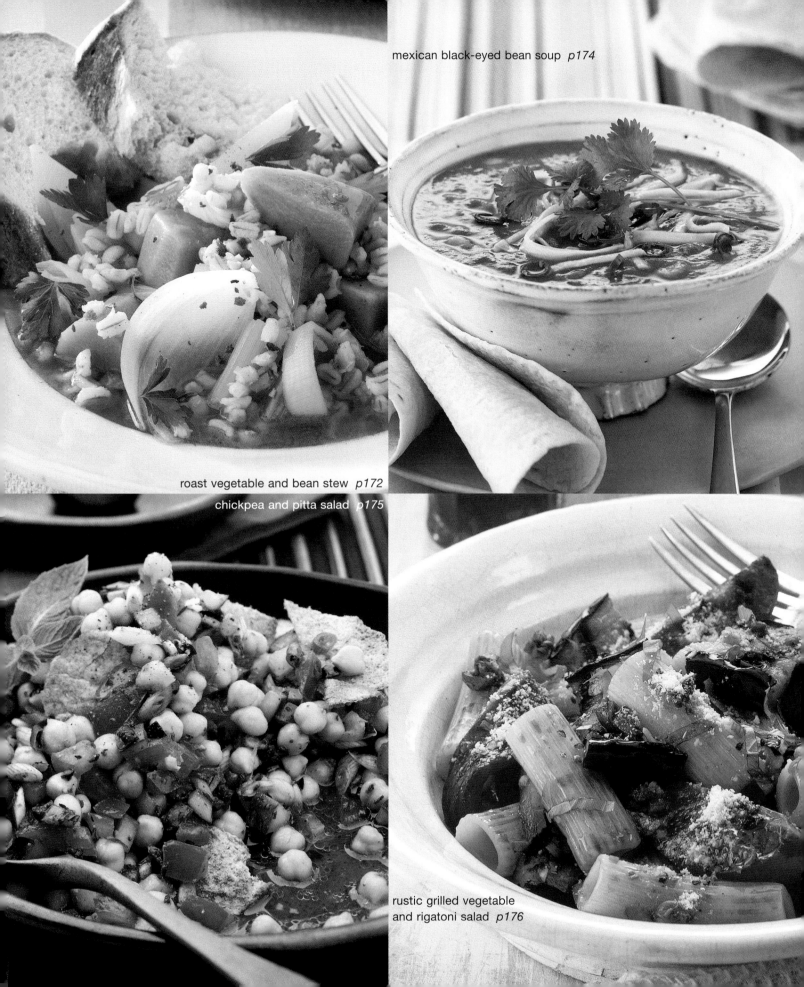

mexican black-eyed bean soup *p174*

roast vegetable and bean stew *p172*

chickpea and pitta salad *p175*

rustic grilled vegetable
and rigatoni salad *p176*

Mexican black-eyed bean soup

The creamy texture of black-eyed beans works particularly well in warming, spicy soups. This one is filling enough to make a hearty main course. A scattering of grated cheese melting into the soup is the finishing touch.

Preparation time **20 minutes**   Cooking time **20 minutes**   *Serves 6*

1 tbsp sunflower oil

1 large fresh green chilli, seeded and finely chopped

2 green peppers, seeded and chopped

1 tsp ground cumin

1 can chopped tomatoes, about 400 g

1 tsp sun-dried tomato paste

600–750 ml (1–1¼ pints) vegetable stock, preferably home-made (see pages 224–225)

1 bay leaf

2 cans black-eyed beans, about 410 g each, drained and rinsed

170 g (6 oz) frozen sweetcorn

3 tbsp chopped fresh coriander

salt and pepper

To serve

12 large flour tortillas

50 g (1¾ oz) mature Cheddar cheese, coarsely grated

sprigs of fresh coriander (optional)

thinly sliced fresh green chilli (optional)

1 Heat the oil in a large saucepan, add the chilli and green peppers, and cook gently for 5 minutes or until almost soft, stirring frequently. Stir in the ground cumin and cook for a few seconds longer.

2 Add the canned tomatoes with their juice, the tomato paste, 600 ml (1 pint) of the stock, the bay leaf and 1½ cans of the beans. Bring slowly to the boil, then turn down the heat, cover and simmer gently for 15 minutes. Discard the bay leaf.

3 Purée the soup, either in batches in a blender or food processor, or using a hand-held blender directly in the pan. Stir in the remaining beans, plus the sweetcorn and chopped coriander. Add enough of the remaining 150 ml (5 fl oz) stock to thin the soup to the desired consistency. Season with salt and pepper to taste, then heat through gently until piping hot.

4 Meanwhile, heat the tortillas in the oven or microwave, according to the packet instructions.

5 Ladle the soup into bowls and sprinkle over the cheese. Garnish with coriander sprigs and green chilli, if liked. Serve with the tortillas.

Some more ideas

For a **roasted vegetable and kidney bean soup**, peel, seed and cube ½ butternut squash, about 350 g (12½ oz). Put on a baking tray with 1 halved onion, 1 halved parsnip and 1 thickly sliced leek. Drizzle over 1 tbsp olive oil, then add 2 sprigs of fresh thyme. Roast in a preheated 200ºC (400ºF, gas mark 6) oven for 45 minutes, turning occasionally. Discard the thyme, then tip the vegetables into a saucepan. Mix in 1 can red kidney beans, about 410 g, drained and rinsed, and 900 ml (1½ pints) vegetable stock. Purée, then stir in a second can of kidney beans and season. Heat thoroughly, then ladle into bowls and swirl 1 tsp pesto in each.

Plus points

● Using canned beans rather than dried beans has little effect on the nutritional value of a dish, and it certainly saves time. Beans are an excellent source of dietary fibre. Rinse canned beans well to help to remove the sugars that can cause wind and bloating.

● The mature Cheddar cheese adds a rich flavour, so you don't need to use much of it.

photo, page 173

Each serving provides   kcal 428, protein 19 g, fat 8 g (of which saturated fat 3.5 g), carbohydrate 75 g (of which sugars 6 g), fibre 7 g. Excellent source of folate, vitamin C. Good source of copper, iron, vitamin B$_1$, vitamin E, zinc. Useful source of calcium, niacin, potassium, selenium, vitamin A, vitamin B$_6$.

Chickpea and pitta salad

This is based on fattoush, the popular salad enjoyed in the Lebanon and Syria, and it makes a satisfying main dish. It's important to grill the pitta bread until it is really crisp and golden or it will quickly become soggy when mixed with the other ingredients. The dressing adds the distinctive flavours of olives, anchovy and garlic.

Preparation and cooking time **20 minutes**   *Serves 4*

4 sesame pitta breads

2 cans chickpeas, about 410 g each, rinsed and drained

½ cucumber, diced

4 large beefsteak tomatoes, about 900 g (2 lb) in total, chopped

6 spring onions, chopped

55 g (2 oz) stoned black olives, preferably Kalamata olives

sprigs of fresh mint to garnish

Tapenade dressing

2 tbsp extra virgin olive oil

1 tbsp balsamic vinegar

2 tsp tapenade

1 tbsp chopped fresh mint

pepper

1 Preheat the grill to high. Split the pitta breads in half and open with a sharp knife. Toast under the grill until golden brown and crisp, turning once, then leave to cool. Tear into bite-sized pieces.

2 Put the chickpeas, cucumber, tomatoes, spring onions and olives in a serving bowl. For the dressing, whisk together the olive oil, vinegar, tapenade, mint and pepper to taste. Drizzle over the vegetables and toss.

3 Just before serving, add the pieces of pitta bread and mix well. Serve garnished with sprigs of fresh mint.

Some more ideas

Instead of toasted pitta bread, try **polenta croutons**. Bring 750 ml (1¼ pints) vegetable stock to the boil and add 170 g (6 oz) instant polenta, stirring. Cook for 4–5 minutes, or according to packet instructions, until the mixture is thick and pulling away from the sides of the pan. Stir in 15 g (½ oz) freshly grated Parmesan cheese, 3 tbsp chopped fresh coriander, and season to taste. Quickly spread the polenta in a greased 18 x 28 cm (7 x 11 in) shallow tin and leave to cool for about 30 minutes or until set. Then turn out and cut into 1 cm (½ in) cubes. Spread out the croutons on foil in a grill pan and toast under a preheated moderate grill for 5–8 minutes, turning several times. Add most of the croutons to the salad and toss. Scatter over the remaining few croutons and serve.

Make a **chickpea and aubergine salad**. Cut a 340 g (12 oz) aubergine into 1 cm (½ in) cubes and fry in 2 tbsp olive oil for 5 minutes. Stir in 1 tsp cumin seeds and continue to cook until the aubergine is lightly browned and tender. Tip into a bowl and mix with 2 cans chickpeas, about 410 g each, drained and rinsed, 1 thinly sliced red onion, 170 g (6 oz) baby spinach leaves and 1 seeded and thinly sliced yellow pepper. For the dressing, whisk together 1 tbsp olive oil, 2 tsp lemon juice, 2 tbsp chopped fresh coriander and pepper to taste.

Plus points

• Although olives have a relatively high fat content, it is mainly unsaturated fat, which is considered to be the healthiest kind of fat to include in the diet.

• Chickpeas are an excellent choice for people with diabetes because of their very low Glycaemic Index.

photo, page 173

Each serving provides kcal 454, protein 18 g, fat 12 g (of which saturated fat 2 g), carbohydrate 72 g (of which sugars 11 g), fibre 10 g. Excellent source of vitamin C, vitamin E. Good source of copper, iron, niacin, potassium, vitamin A, vitamin B_1, zinc. Useful source of calcium, folate, vitamin B_6.

Rustic grilled vegetable and rigatoni salad

Grilled vegetables are delicious with chunky pasta in a tangy dressing. Serve this salad as a light lunch or offer it as an accompaniment for grilled poultry or meat, when it will serve 6 or 8.

Preparation time **35 minutes, plus cooling and 30 minutes marinating**   *Serves 4*

200 g (7 oz) rigatoni

1 large red pepper, seeded and halved

125 g (4½ oz) tomatoes, cut into wedges

1 aubergine, trimmed and sliced lengthways

2 tbsp balsamic vinegar or lemon juice

2 tbsp extra virgin olive oil

2 tbsp shredded fresh basil

1 tbsp chopped capers

1 large garlic clove, crushed (optional)

30 g (1 oz) Parmesan cheese, freshly grated

salt and pepper

1 Cook the rigatoni in boiling water for 10–12 minutes, or according to the packet instructions, until al dente. Drain and rinse under cold running water, then drain thoroughly and set aside to cool.

2 Preheat the grill to high. Grill the pepper halves, skin side up, for 5–10 minutes or until blistered and blackened. Place in a polythene bag, then leave until cool enough to handle.

3 Grill the tomatoes and aubergine for about 5 minutes or until slightly charred. Turn the vegetables so that they cook evenly, and remove the pieces as they are ready. Place the tomato wedges in a large salad bowl. Set the aubergine slices aside on a plate to cool slightly.

4 Cut the aubergine slices into 2.5 cm (1 in) strips and add to the tomatoes. Peel the peppers and cut them into 2.5 cm (1 in) strips, then add to the salad bowl. Mix in the pasta.

5 In a small bowl, mix the balsamic vinegar or lemon juice with the olive oil, basil, capers, garlic, if using, and Parmesan cheese. Lightly toss this dressing into the salad. Season to taste. Set the salad aside to marinate for about 30 minutes so that the flavours can mingle before serving.

Some more ideas

For a hearty vegetarian main course salad, stir in 1 can cannellini or red kidney beans, about 400 g, well drained.

Grilled courgettes and asparagus can be added to the salad. Slice the courgettes lengthways. Grill alongside the aubergine and tomatoes.

Replace the aubergine with well-drained, bottled char-grilled artichokes.

Plus points

● Aubergines are a useful vegetable for making satisfying meals without a high calorie content. They contain just 15 kcal per 100 g (3½ oz).

● Grilling or baking is a healthy cooking method for vegetables like aubergines, which can absorb large amounts of fat when they are fried.

● Pastas of any shape or size have a fairly low Glycaemic Index.

photo, page 173

Each serving provides   kcal 285, protein 10 g, fat 9 g (of which saturated fat 3 g), carbohydrate 42 g (of which sugars 5.5 g), fibre 3 g. Good source of vitamin A, vitamin C. Useful source of calcium, copper, niacin, potassium.

Tagliatelle with green sauce

This simple vegetable and yogurt sauce is ready in as little time as it takes to cook and drain the fresh pasta. It is bursting with fresh flavours and irresistibly creamy, but without the heaviness of a classic cream sauce for pasta. A salad of crisp radicchio and Lollo Rosso lettuce is a good accompaniment.

Preparation time **5 minutes**   Cooking time **7–8 minutes**   *Serves 4*

225 g (8 oz) baby spinach, thick stalks discarded

100 g (3½ oz) watercress, thick stalks discarded

125 g (4½ oz) frozen peas

500 g (1 lb 2 oz) fresh tagliatelle

2 tsp cornflour

200 ml (7 fl oz) Greek-style yogurt

4 tbsp chopped parsley

6 sprigs of fresh basil, torn into pieces

salt and pepper

1 Rinse the spinach and watercress and place in a large saucepan with just the water clinging to the leaves. Cover and cook over a moderate heat for 2 minutes, stirring and turning the vegetables occasionally, until they have wilted.

2 Add the peas and cook uncovered for 2 minutes – there should be enough liquid to cook them. Tip the greens and their liquid into a bowl. Set aside.

3 Cook the pasta in a large saucepan of boiling water for 3 minutes, or according to the packet instructions, until al dente.

4 Meanwhile, blend the cornflour to a smooth paste with the yogurt, and put into the pan used for cooking the vegetables. Stir over a moderate heat until it is just bubbling. Add the vegetables, parsley, basil and seasoning to taste and stir well. Heat the sauce through, then remove the pan from the heat.

5 Drain the pasta and add to the sauce. Toss to mix with the sauce, then serve.

Another idea

For a **creamy broccoli and pea sauce**, replace the spinach and watercress with 200 g (7 oz) broccoli. Cook the broccoli in a little boiling water for 5–8 minutes, then drain, refresh in cold running water, drain well again and return to the pan. Mash the broccoli with a potato masher, then add the yogurt mixed with the cornflour and 5 tbsp semi-skimmed milk. Stir in 125 g (4½ oz) frozen peas and 2 spring onions, finely chopped. Bring to the boil, stirring, and cook for 1–2 minutes to thicken. Season to taste and add a dash of lemon juice if you like. Toss with the freshly cooked pasta, then sprinkle with plenty of chopped parsley.

Plus points

• Cream-based sauces are always popular for pasta dishes. Traditionally, the sauces are made with heavy cream and cheese. This recipe uses low-fat yogurt to create a creamy sauce that is much lower in fat.

• Heat can destroy vitamin C. The best way to cook leafy green vegetables, such as spinach and watercress, and still retain the maximum vitamin C, is to wilt them briefly.

• Peas provide protein. They are also rich in fibre, some of it soluble, and this helps to keep blood sugar levels and cholesterol under control.

photo, page 179

Each serving provides kcal 215, protein 11 g, fat 6 g (of which saturated fat 3 g), carbohydrate 30 g (of which sugars 3 g), fibre 4 g. Excellent source of vitamin A. Good source of calcium, folate, vitamin C, vitamin E. Useful source of copper, iron, niacin, vitamin B$_2$, zinc.

Penne rigati with sesame and orange dressing

This fresh-flavoured pasta salad is ideal as a side dish with grilled chicken or firm fish, such as fresh tuna or swordfish. It makes a healthy change from noodles dressed with oil or butter and Parmesan cheese.

Preparation time **25–30 minutes, plus cooling**   *Serves 4*

200 g (7 oz) penne rigati (ridged penne)

2 large oranges

6 spring onions, cut into short fine strips

55 g (2 oz) bean sprouts

2 tbsp sesame seeds, toasted

Dressing

grated zest and juice of 1 orange

1 tbsp toasted sesame oil

2 tbsp light soy sauce

1 garlic clove, crushed

1 tbsp finely grated fresh root ginger

salt and pepper

1 Cook the pasta in boiling water for 10–12 minutes, or according to the packet instructions, until al dente.

2 While the pasta is cooking, peel the oranges, removing all the pith. Holding the oranges over a bowl to catch any juice, cut out the segments from their surrounding membrane. Set the segments aside, and reserve the juice in the bowl.

3 Place the spring onion strips in a bowl of cold water and set them aside until they curl.

4 To make the dressing, add the orange zest and juice to the juices reserved from segmenting the oranges. Add the sesame oil, soy sauce, garlic, grated fresh ginger and seasoning to taste. Whisk lightly to mix.

5 Drain the pasta and add to the dressing. Mix well, then cover and set aside to cool.

6 When ready to serve, thoroughly drain the spring onions; reserve a few for garnish and add the remainder to the salad together with the orange segments, bean sprouts and toasted sesame seeds. Gently toss the ingredients together, then serve the salad immediately, sprinkled with the reserved spring onions.

Some more ideas

Use Japanese soba noodles, made from buckwheat flour, instead of penne and cook them for 5–7 minutes. Use sunflower oil in the dressing instead of the sesame oil and omit the sesame seeds. Stir in 1 tbsp Thai red curry paste instead of the fresh root ginger. Add 2 tbsp finely chopped fresh coriander with the orange segments, if liked.

To increase the vegetable content of the salad, finely shred ½ bulb fennel and add it to the salad; scatter with the fronds or feathery leaves from the fennel to garnish.

Plus points

• Oranges are an excellent source of vitamin C, with 1 orange providing more than twice the recommended daily intake of the vitamin. Studies have highlighted a connection between a regular intake of vitamin C and the maintenance of intellectual function in elderly people. Those eating a diet rich in vitamin C were also less likely to suffer a stroke.

• Oranges, and other citrus fruit, also contain coumarins, compounds that are believed to help thin the blood and thus prevent stroke and heart attacks.

Each serving provides kcal 280, protein 9 g, fat 8 g (of which saturated fat 1 g), carbohydrate 45 g (of which sugars 8 g), fibre 4 g. Excellent source of vitamin C. Good source of copper. Useful source of folate, niacin, potassium, selenium, vitamin B$_1$.

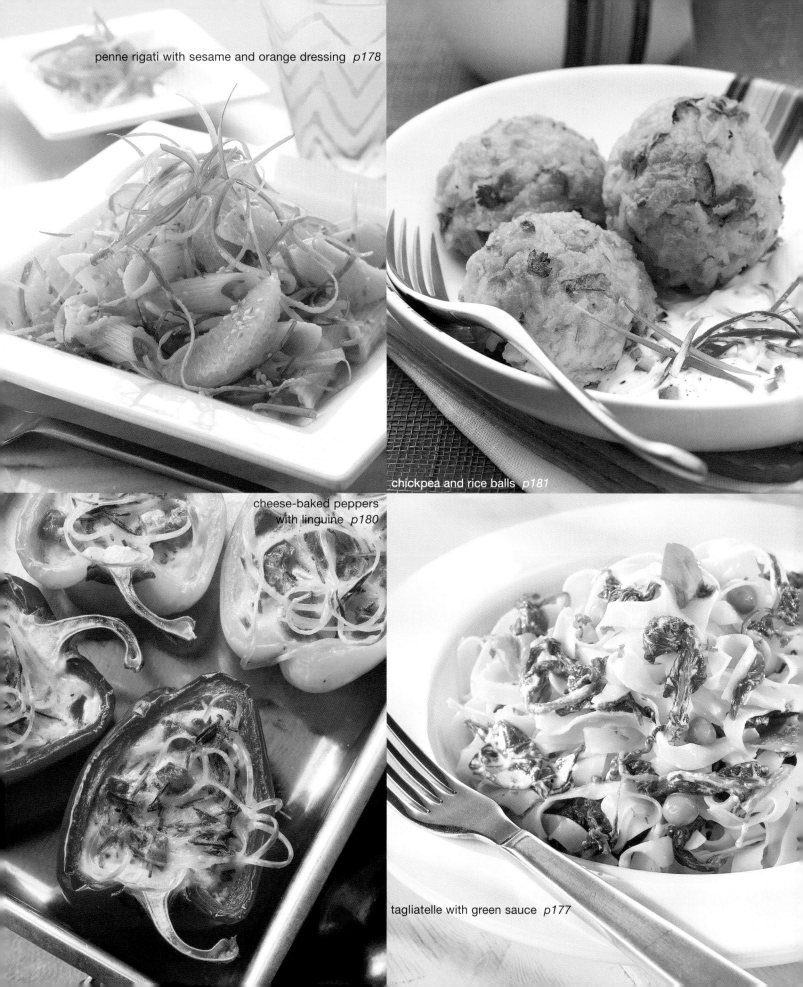

penne rigati with sesame and orange dressing *p178*

chickpea and rice balls *p181*

cheese-baked peppers
with linguine *p180*

tagliatelle with green sauce *p177*

Cheese-baked peppers with linguine

These stuffed peppers, filled with thin noodles in a savoury custard, make an ideal first course to serve 4, or a light vegetarian lunch for 2 served with an assortment of salads and plenty of warm bread. Any colour of pepper suggested can be used, but avoid green peppers which are not as sweet.

Preparation time **about 40 minutes**   Cooking time **20–25 minutes**   *Serves 4*

2 large red, orange or yellow peppers

45 g (1½ oz) linguine

2 eggs, beaten

55 g (2 oz) mature Cheddar cheese, grated

1¼ tsp English mustard powder

3 tbsp semi-skimmed milk

3 tbsp snipped fresh chives

¼ tsp dried marjoram or oregano

2 tomatoes, skinned, seeded and diced

salt and pepper

fresh whole chives to garnish

To serve (optional)

salad leaves

1 Preheat the oven to 180°C (350°F, gas mark 4). Halve the peppers lengthways, carefully cutting through the stalk. Remove the pith and seeds. Cook the pepper shells in boiling water for 6–8 minutes or until tender. Drain thoroughly and place on kitchen paper.

2 Cook the linguine in boiling water for 10 minutes, or according to the packet instructions, until al dente. Drain well and set aside.

3 Beat the eggs with the cheese, mustard, milk, chives and marjoram or oregano. Stir in the tomatoes and seasoning to taste.

4 Place the peppers in an ovenproof dish or roasting tin, supporting them with pieces of crumpled foil, if necessary, to ensure that they are level (otherwise the filling will spill out). Half fill each pepper with linguine, then spoon the egg and cheese mixture over the pasta.

5 Bake for 20–25 minutes or until the filling is set and beginning to turn golden. Serve garnished with whole chives, with an accompaniment of mixed salad leaves, if liked.

Some more ideas

Use 55 g (2 oz) fresh linguine instead of dried. Fresh linguine will only need to be cooked for 2–3 minutes.

For a more substantial dish, cook an extra 140 g (5 oz) linguine while the peppers are baking and toss with 1 tbsp snipped fresh chives. Serve as a base for the peppers.

To make a tasty supper for 2, thoroughly drain and flake 1 can tuna fish in brine, about 100 g, and add it to the egg mixture. Serve 2 pepper halves per person.

Stir 4 stoned green olives, finely chopped, into the egg mixture.

Plus points

- These peppers make an elegant and delicious vegetarian dish. They are a complete meal, since they contain a starch component, protein from the milk and cheese, and several servings of vegetables.

photo, page 179

Each serving provides kcal 180, protein 10 g, fat 9 g (of which saturated fat 4 g), carbohydrate 15 g (of which sugars 7 g), fibre 2 g. Excellent source of niacin, vitamin A, vitamin B$_1$, vitamin B$_6$, vitamin C, vitamin E. Good source of vitamin B$_{12}$.

Chickpea and rice balls

These tasty chickpea-based balls, flavoured with garlic, chilli and lots of fresh coriander, make a delicious alternative to rice or potatoes. Cooked traditionally as an Indian dish the balls would be deep-fried, but here they are baked.

Preparation time **50 minutes**   Cooking time **30 minutes**   *Serves 4 (makes 12)*

100 g (3½ oz) long-grain white rice

1 tbsp sunflower oil

1 small onion, finely chopped

1 garlic clove, crushed

1 fresh red chilli, seeded and finely chopped

2 tomatoes, skinned, seeded and very finely chopped

1 can chickpeas, about 410 g, drained and rinsed

1 egg yolk

3 tbsp chopped fresh coriander

½ tsp paprika

salt and pepper

1 Put the rice in a saucepan, add 240 ml (8 fl oz) water and bring to the boil. Cover and simmer very gently for 10–15 minutes or until the rice is tender and has absorbed all the water. Remove from the heat and leave to cool for a few minutes.

2 Meanwhile, preheat the oven to 180°C (350°F, gas mark 4). Heat the oil in a saucepan, add the onion and fry gently for about 5 minutes, stirring frequently, until soft. Stir in the garlic and chilli, and cook for 2 more minutes. Remove from the heat and stir in the chopped tomatoes.

3 Put the chickpeas in a bowl and mash with a potato masher until fairly smooth, or purée in a food processor. Add the onion mixture, rice, egg yolk, coriander, paprika, and season to taste. Mix together well. Divide the mixture into 12 equal portions and shape each into a ball.

4 Place the chickpea and rice balls on a greased baking sheet and bake for 30 minutes or until beginning to brown, turning them over carefully halfway through the cooking. Serve hot.

Another idea
To make **onion and chickpea bhajia**, gently cook 1 large sliced onion in 1 tbsp sunflower oil for 10 minutes or until very soft. Sift 85 g (3 oz) chickpea (gram) flour into a bowl with 1 tsp ground coriander, 1 tsp turmeric, ½ tsp mild chilli powder and ½ tsp salt. Stir in ½ tsp cumin seeds and make a well in the centre. Add 4 tbsp plain low-fat yogurt, 3 tbsp cold water and 1 tsp lemon juice, and mix to a thick, smooth batter. Stir in the onion and 1 can chickpeas, about 410 g, drained, rinsed and lightly mashed. Heat 1 tbsp sunflower oil in a frying pan, drop in spoonfuls of the batter and flatten them slightly with the back of the spoon. Cook over a moderate heat for 2–3 minutes on each side.

Plus points
• Chickpeas have a very low Glycaemic Index although mashing them increases the index. This dish is nonetheless a good low-calorie, low-fat choice for those with diabetes.

• Eating onions regularly can have several beneficial effects, particularly in helping to reduce blood cholesterol levels and to lessen the risk of blood clots forming.

photo, page 179

Each serving provides kcal 213, protein 7 g, fat 6 g (of which saturated fat 1 g), carbohydrate 34 g (of which sugars 2.5 g), fibre 3 g. Good source of vitamin E. Useful source of iron, vitamin B$_{12}$, vitamin C, zinc.

Dolmades

Here's a new, healthy twist on these delicious and popular little Greek parcels. To boost the fibre and nutrient content, brown rice is used instead of the traditional white. The filling for the vine leaves is flavoured with garlic and fresh herbs, with a hint of sweetness from raisins and crunch from walnuts.

Preparation time **1 hour**   Cooking time **10–15 minutes**   *Serves 8 (makes 24)*

200 g (7 oz) long-grain brown rice

24 large vine leaves preserved in brine, about 115 g (4 oz) in total when drained

3 tbsp extra virgin olive oil

1 onion, finely chopped

1 large garlic clove, finely chopped

1 tbsp chopped parsley

1 tbsp chopped fresh mint

1 tbsp chopped fresh dill

grated zest and juice of 1 lemon

50 g (1¾ oz) raisins

50 g (1¾ oz) walnuts, chopped

salt and pepper

To garnish

lemon wedges

sprigs of fresh dill, parsley or mint

1 Put the rice in a saucepan and add 600 ml (1 pint) water. Bring to the boil. Stir, then cover with a tight-fitting lid and simmer very gently for 30–40 minutes or until the rice is tender and has absorbed all the water. Remove from the heat.

2 While the rice is cooking, drain the vine leaves, rinse with cold water and pat dry with kitchen paper.

3 Heat 2 tbsp of the oil in a saucepan over a moderate heat. Add the onion and garlic, and cook, stirring occasionally, for 5–8 minutes or until soft. Remove from the heat and stir in the parsley, mint, dill, lemon zest and raisins.

4 Put the walnuts in a small frying pan and toast them over a moderate heat, stirring constantly, until lightly browned and aromatic.

5 Add the toasted walnuts to the onion mixture. Stir in the cooked rice and add the lemon juice (you may not need all of it), and salt and pepper to taste. Mix well.

6 Spread one of the vine leaves flat and place about 2 spoonfuls of the rice mixture in the centre. Fold over the stalk end, then fold in the sides. Roll up the leaf into a cylinder shape. Repeat with the remaining vine leaves and filling.

7 Place the rolls seam side down in a steamer and brush the tops with the remaining 1 tbsp olive oil. Cover and steam for 10–15 minutes or until piping hot. Serve hot or at room temperature, garnished with lemon wedges and sprigs of fresh herbs.

Plus points

• Brown rice has only the outer husk removed and therefore contains all the nutrients in the germ and outer layers of the grain. Raw brown rice contains 1.9 g fibre per 100 g (3½ oz) compared with 0.4 g fibre for the same weight of raw white rice. It also contains more B vitamins.

• Raisins, currants and sultanas are all types of dried grapes. Although they are rich in sugars – mostly as glucose and fructos – in this recipe they are mixed with other ingredients, and so are unlikely to cause a rapid rise in blood glucose levels.

photo, page 185

Each serving provides   kcal 199, protein 4 g, fat 9 g (of which saturated fat 1 g), carbohydrate 27 g (of which sugars 6 g), fibre 1 g. Excellent source of copper. Useful source of calcium, folate, iron, vitamin A, vitamin B₁, vitamin C, zinc.

Minted barley and beans

The mild, sweet flavour and chewy texture of pearl barley is combined here with black-eyed beans and lots of colourful vegetables. A fresh-tasting tomato and mint dressing adds a summery feel to this wholesome salad. Serve on its own for lunch or supper, with some fresh fruit to follow.

Preparation and cooking time **1½ hours**   *Serves 4*

1.4 litres (2½ pints) vegetable stock

strip of lemon zest

1 bay leaf

225 g (8 oz) baby leeks

1 tsp sunflower oil

225 g (8 oz) pearl barley

1 can black-eyed beans, about 410 g, drained and rinsed

6 firm, ripe plum tomatoes, about 500 g (1 lb 2 oz) in total, cut into thin wedges

140 g (5 oz) baby spinach leaves, shredded

1 bunch spring onions, 85 g (3 oz), halved and shredded

sprig of fresh mint to garnish

Tomato and mint dressing

2 sun-dried tomatoes packed in oil, drained and finely chopped

1 tbsp oil from the sun-dried tomatoes

1 tbsp red wine vinegar

1 garlic clove, crushed

2 tbsp chopped fresh mint

1 tbsp chopped fresh chervil

salt and pepper

1 Put the stock in a saucepan with the lemon zest and bay leaf. Bring to a rapid boil, then add the leeks and cook for 2–3 minutes or until just tender. Remove with a draining spoon and refresh briefly in cold water. Cut on the diagonal into 2.5 cm (1 in) lengths. Set aside.

2 Add the sunflower oil to the stock in the pan and bring back to the boil. Add the pearl barley, then cover and simmer for 30–40 minutes or until tender.

3 Spoon out 2 tbsp of the stock and reserve, then drain the barley. Discard the lemon zest and bay leaf. Tip the barley into a bowl and leave to cool.

4 Add the leeks, black-eyed beans, plum tomatoes, spinach and spring onions to the barley and stir gently to mix together.

5 To make the dressing, put the sun-dried tomatoes, oil, vinegar, garlic, mint, chervil, reserved stock, and salt and pepper to taste into a screwtop jar. Shake well until combined.

6 Drizzle the dressing over the barley and vegetables and toss to coat thoroughly. Serve at room temperature, garnished with a sprig of fresh mint.

Another idea

For a **spicy barley salad**, add a pinch of saffron strands when cooking the pearl barley and use 1 can red kidney beans, about 410 g, drained and rinsed, rather than black-eyed beans. For the dressing, whisk 1 seeded and finely chopped fresh red chilli and 1 tbsp extra virgin olive oil with the vinegar and garlic, and add chopped fresh coriander and parsley instead of the mint and chervil.

Plus points

● Barley is low in fat and rich in starchy carbohydrate, and is a good source of B vitamins. It is an excellent food for those with diabetes because it is absorbed slowly.

● Although highly refined, weight for weight pearl barley provides more dietary fibre than brown rice.

● Spinach contains oxalic acid, which binds with iron, making most of it unavailable to the body. Eating spinach with something that is a good source of vitamin C, such as tomatoes, can increase iron uptake.

photo, page 185

Each serving provides kcal 442, protein 14 g, fat 16 g (of which saturated fat 2.5 g), carbohydrate 67 g (of which sugars 7 g), fibre 6 g. Excellent source of copper, folate, vitamin A, vitamin C, vitamin E. Good source of iron, potassium, vitamin B_1, vitamin B_6, zinc. Useful source of calcium, niacin.

Quinoa with griddled aubergines

Quinoa, a nutritious grain from South America, has a texture rather like split lentils when cooked. It makes a great alternative to rice. Here it is combined with griddled aubergines, peppers, cherry tomatoes and onions, and then baked with tangy goat's cheese on the top. Serve with a mixed leaf salad.

Preparation time **35 minutes**   Cooking time **35 minutes**   *Serves 4*

300 g (10½ oz) quinoa

3–4 sprigs of fresh thyme

1.2 litres (2 pints) vegetable stock, preferably home-made (see pages 224–225)

250 g (8½ oz) baby aubergines, cut lengthways into quarters

1 red pepper, seeded and cut into chunks

1 red onion, cut into chunks

2 tbsp extra virgin olive oil

200 g (7 oz) cherry tomatoes

2 garlic cloves, crushed

300 ml (10 fl oz) tomato juice

150 g (5½ oz) goat's cheese log with herbs, cut into 8 slices

salt and pepper

1 Preheat the oven to 190°C (375°F, gas mark 5). Put the quinoa in a sieve and rinse thoroughly under cold running water. Place in a saucepan with the thyme sprigs and stock, and bring to the boil. Cover and simmer gently for 20 minutes or until all the stock has been absorbed and the quinoa is tender.

2 Meanwhile, heat a ridged cast-iron grill pan. Brush the aubergines, red pepper and onion with the olive oil, then cook them on the grill pan (in batches if necessary) for 4–5 minutes or until softened and lightly charred on both sides. Transfer to a plate.

3 Put the whole tomatoes on the grill pan and cook for about 2 minutes or until they are just beginning to burst their skins. Remove from the heat.

4 When the quinoa is cooked, tip it into an ovenproof dish. Add the griddled vegetables, garlic and tomato juice, and season with salt and pepper to taste. Fold together gently.

5 Arrange the slices of goat's cheese on top of the quinoa mixture. Cover with foil and bake for 35 minutes or until the vegetables are tender. Serve hot.

Some more ideas

Try **quinoa with fresh tuna**. Marinate 2 fresh tuna steaks, about 300 g (10½ oz) in total, in 1 tbsp olive oil, the grated zest of 1 lemon and ¼ tsp crushed dried chillies. Meanwhile, brush 125 g (4½ oz) asparagus tips and 2 courgettes, sliced on the diagonal, with 1 tbsp olive oil and griddle for 30 seconds on each side. Cook the cherry tomatoes as in the main recipe. Griddle the tuna for 2 minutes on each side. Combine the quinoa, vegetables, garlic and tomato juice in an ovenproof dish. Break the tuna into pieces and scatter over the top. Cover with foil and bake for 25 minutes.

Plus points

● Quinoa is low in fat, high in starchy carbohydrate and has a higher protein content than other grains.

● Aubergines are filling and satisfying without adding many calories – just 15 kcals per 100 g (3½ oz).

● Goat's cheese is a good source of protein and calcium, but has a lower fat content than Cheddar cheese.

Each serving provides   kcal 413, protein 20 g, fat 16 g (of which saturated fat 5 g), carbohydrate 53 g (of which sugars 14 g), fibre 3 g. Excellent source of copper, vitamin A, vitamin C. Good source of calcium, iron, niacin, potassium, vitamin B_2, vitamin B_{12}, zinc. Useful source of folate, vitamin B_1, vitamin B_6, vitamin E.

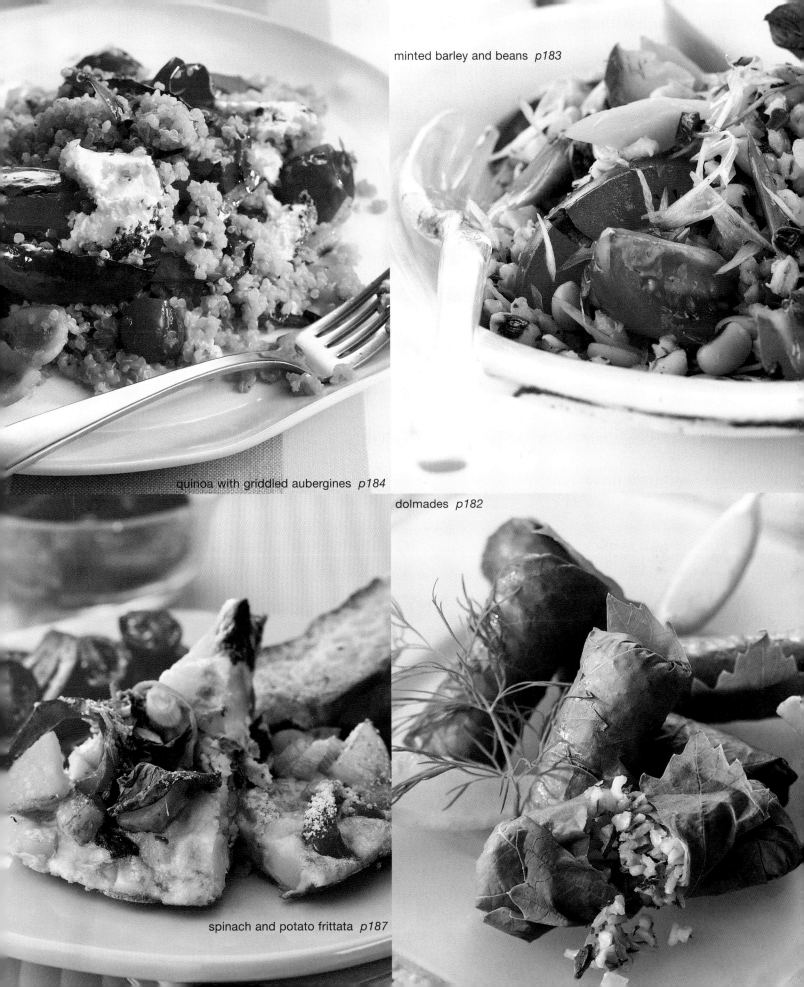

minted barley and beans *p183*

quinoa with griddled aubergines *p184*

dolmades *p182*

spinach and potato frittata *p187*

Rice-stuffed squash

Here's an attractive and fun way to serve small winter squashes – filled with a mixture of wild and white rice, chestnuts, dried cranberries and mozzarella cheese. Individual squashes such as acorn, onion or gem, or small pumpkins, are all suitable. It makes an impressive vegetarian main course for a winter dinner.

Preparation time **25 minutes**   Cooking time **45 minutes**   *Serves 4*

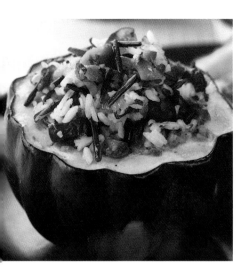

200 g (7 oz) mixed basmati and wild rice

4 small acorn squashes, about 750 g (1 lb 10 oz) each

185 g (6½ oz) cooked chestnuts (canned or vacuum packed), roughly chopped

75 g (2½ oz) dried cranberries

1 small red onion, finely chopped

2 tbsp chopped fresh thyme

2 tbsp chopped parsley

150 g (5½ oz) mozzarella cheese, grated

salt and pepper

1 Put the rice in a saucepan, add 400 ml (14 fl oz) water and bring to the boil. Cover and simmer very gently for about 20 minutes or until the rice is just tender. Drain off any excess water.

2 Meanwhile, preheat the oven to 180°C (350°F, gas mark 4). Using a large, sharp knife, slice off the top quarter (stalk end) of each squash. Set aside these little hats, then scoop out the seeds and fibres from the centre of the squashes using a small spoon. Trim the bases to make them level. Season the cavity of each squash with salt and pepper, then place them in a large ovenproof dish or roasting tin.

3 Mix together the rice, chestnuts, cranberries, onion, thyme, parsley and mozzarella in a large bowl. Season with salt and pepper to taste.

4 Spoon the rice stuffing into the cavity of each squash, pressing it down and mounding it up neatly on top. Replace the reserved 'hats' on top. Bake for about 45 minutes or until the flesh of the squash is tender when pierced with a small, sharp knife. Serve hot.

Another idea

For **feta and sultana rice-stuffed peppers**, cut 2 large red and 2 large yellow peppers in half lengthways and remove the cores and seeds. Make the rice filling as in the main recipe, but omit the salt and replace the cranberries with sultanas and the mozzarella with grated feta cheese. Scoop the stuffing into the pepper halves. Arrange the peppers, side by side, in an ovenproof dish and drizzle over the juice of 1 large orange, 1 tbsp olive oil and pepper to taste. Cover with greased foil and bake in a preheated 190°C (375°F, gas mark 5) oven for about 1 hour.

Plus points

● Acorn squash is a winter variety of squash. Winter squashes are allowed to mature into hard, starchy vegetable fruits, while varieties such as courgettes are eaten while immature and the skins are still edible. Acorn squash is a good source of beta-carotene, which the body can convert to vitamin A.

● Both dried and fresh cranberries are a good source of vitamin C. Cranberries also have the reputation of helping to control urinary tract infections such as cystitis.

Each serving provides kcal 474, protein 19 g, fat 11 g (of which saturated fat 6 g), carbohydrate 79 g (of which sugars 17.5 g), fibre 10 g. Excellent source of calcium, vitamin A, vitamin B_1, vitamin C, vitamin E. Good source of copper, iron, potassium, vitamin B_{12}, zinc. Useful source of folate, niacin, vitamin B_6.

Spinach and potato frittata

This flat omelette makes a delicious vegetarian main course, and can be eaten hot or at room temperature. It is a very versatile recipe, as almost anything can be added to it – a handy way of using up leftovers. Serve with toasted wholemeal bread and sliced tomatoes and/or a mixed green salad for a quick supper.

Preparation and cooking time **30 minutes**   *Serves 4*

500 g (1 lb 2 oz) potatoes, scrubbed and cut into 1 cm (½ in) cubes

225 g (8 oz) baby spinach leaves, trimmed of any large stalks

1 tbsp extra virgin olive oil

1 red pepper, quartered lengthways, seeded and thinly sliced

5–6 spring onions, thinly sliced

5 eggs

2 tbsp freshly grated Parmesan cheese

salt and pepper

1 Cook the potatoes in a saucepan of boiling water for 5–6 minutes or until almost tender. Put the spinach in a steamer or colander over the potatoes and cook for another 5 minutes or until the potatoes are tender and the spinach has wilted. Drain the potatoes. Press the spinach with the back of a spoon to extract excess moisture, then chop.

2 Heat the oil in a non-stick frying pan that is about 25 cm (10 in) in diameter. Add the pepper slices and sauté over a moderate heat for 2 minutes. Stir in the potatoes and spring onions and continue cooking for 2 minutes.

3 Beat the eggs in a large bowl, season with salt and pepper and mix in the spinach. With a draining spoon, remove about half of the vegetables from the pan and add to the egg mixture, leaving the oil in the pan. Stir the egg and vegetables briefly to mix, then pour into the frying pan. Cover and cook, without stirring, for about 6 minutes or until the omelette is almost set but still a little soft on top. Meanwhile, preheat the grill.

4 Dust the top of the frittata with the Parmesan cheese and place under the grill. Cook for 3–4 minutes or until browned and puffed around the edges. Then cut into quarters or wedges and serve.

Some more ideas

For a **courgette and potato frittata**, replace the spinach with 1 large courgette, quartered and sliced, and use 1 sliced small leek in place of the spring onions. Sauté the leek, courgette and pepper for 3–4 minutes. Add the potatoes and stir. Mix a handful of torn fresh basil leaves with the beaten eggs, and cook the omelette as in the main recipe.

Make a **smoked salmon frittata**. Omit the potatoes and red pepper, and sauté a courgette, quartered and sliced, with the spring onions. Add 75 g (2½ oz) slivered smoked salmon to the eggs with the spinach. Finish the frittata under the grill.

Plus points

• Spinach is a good source of several antioxidants, including vitamin C and vitamin E, and it provides useful amounts of folate, niacin and B_6. Contrary to popular belief, it is not a particularly good source of iron.

• Eggs are high in cholesterol, but your blood cholesterol is more affected by the amount of saturated fat you eat. Nevertheless, diabetics should limit intake to 4 eggs a week.

photo, page 185

Each serving provides   kcal 300, protein 19 g, fat 14 g (of which saturated fat 4.5 g), carbohydrate 26 g (of which sugars 6 g), fibre 4 g. Excellent source of vitamin A, vitamin B_6, vitamin B_{12}, vitamin C. Good source of calcium, folate, iron. Useful source of potassium, vitamin B_1, vitamin B_2, vitamin E, zinc.

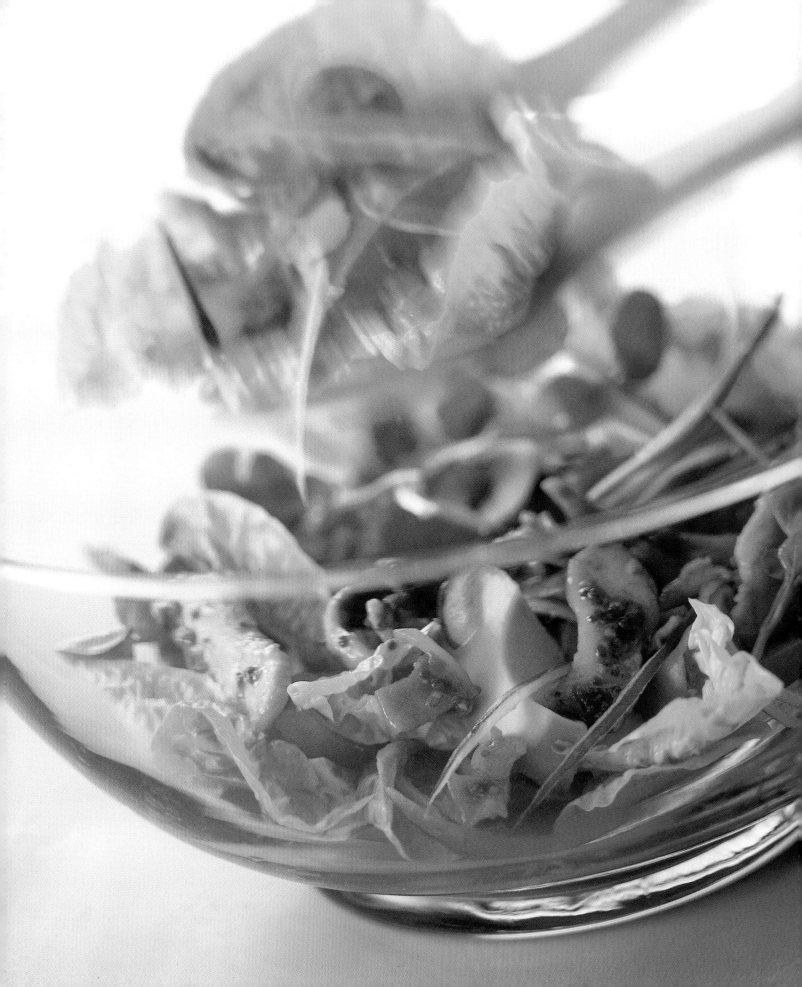

Salads and sides

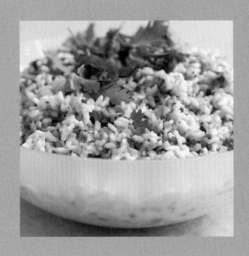

Garlicky tomato salad

When tomatoes are at their peak of sweetness, this salad is particularly delicious. It's eye-catching too if you make it with a mixture of different-coloured tomatoes. New varieties are coming on the market all the time – look for yellow cherry tomatoes as well as small red or yellow pear-shaped plum tomatoes.

Preparation time **15 minutes**   *Serves 4*

1 large soft lettuce, large leaves torn into smaller pieces

4 large or 6 small ripe plum tomatoes, about 500 g
(1 lb 2 oz) in total, sliced

20 cherry tomatoes, about 225 g (8 oz) in total, halved

16 fresh basil leaves

1½ tbsp toasted pumpkin seeds

1½ tbsp toasted sunflower seeds

Garlic vinaigrette

1 small garlic clove, very finely chopped

1½ tsp red wine vinegar

2 tbsp extra virgin olive oil

salt and pepper

1 To make the garlic vinaigrette, whisk together the garlic, vinegar, oil, and salt and pepper to taste in a small mixing bowl.

2 Place a layer of lettuce leaves on a serving platter or on 4 plates and arrange the sliced tomatoes and then the cherry tomatoes on top. Drizzle over the vinaigrette.

3 Scatter the basil leaves and the pumpkin and sunflower seeds over the tomatoes, and serve at once.

Some more ideas

For a **tomato and black olive salad**, slice about 550 g (1¼ lb) ripe tomatoes, preferably beefsteak, and arrange on a serving platter. Top with 100 g (3½ oz) thinly sliced spring onions and drizzle over 1 tbsp extra virgin olive oil and the juice of ¼ lemon. Arrange 8 black olives, halved and stoned, on top and sprinkle with 2 tbsp chopped parsley.

Make a **salad of fresh and sun-dried tomatoes**. Cut 6 ripe plum tomatoes into thin wedges and put them in a mixing bowl. Thinly slice 3 sun-dried tomatoes and add to the bowl. Make a vinaigrette by whisking 1½ tbsp of the oil from the jar of sun-dried tomatoes with 1½ tsp wine vinegar and seasoning to taste. Drizzle over the tomatoes and marinate briefly. Arrange

100 g (3½ oz) rocket on 4 plates and divide the tomatoes among them. Sprinkle with 2 tbsp toasted pine nuts and serve.

Try a **cherry tomato and sugarsnap peas salad**. Trim 250 g (8½ oz) sugarsnap peas and steam for about 3 minutes or until tender but still crisp. Refresh under cold running water, then cool. Mix with 375 g (13 oz) cherry tomatoes, halved if large, and 6 thinly sliced spring onions. Make the garlic vinaigrette as in the main recipe and drizzle it over the tomatoes and peas. Add 3 tbsp chopped fresh mint, or 1 tbsp each chopped fresh tarragon and parsley, and toss to mix.

Plus points

● Pumpkin seeds are one of the richest vegetarian sources of zinc, a mineral that is essential for the functioning of the immune system and for growth and wound healing. They are a good source of protein and unsaturated fat and a useful source of iron, magnesium and fibre.

● Tomatoes are a rich source of vitamin C, important for maintaining immunity and healthy skin. The vitamin C is concentrated in the jellylike substance surrounding the seeds.

photo, page 193

Each serving provides   kcal 160, proteins 5 g, fat 12 g (of which saturated fat 2 g), carbohydrate 9 g (of which sugars 7 g), fibre 3 g. Excellent source of niacin, vitamin A, vitamin B$_1$, vitamin B$_6$, vitamin C, vitamin E. Good source of copper, folate. Useful source of iron, zinc.

Roasted pepper salad

This colourful salad makes a tasty accompaniment to seafood, chicken or lamb, or it can be served as part of a Mediterranean starter selection, with ciabatta bread or baguette. Peppers are an excellent source of vitamin C, and when roasted they still retain substantial amounts of this important vitamin.

Preparation time **45 minutes, plus cooling**   *Serves 6*

2 large red peppers

2 large yellow or orange peppers

2 large green peppers

2½ tbsp extra virgin olive oil

2 tsp balsamic vinegar

1 small garlic clove, very finely chopped or crushed

salt and pepper

To garnish

12 black olives, stoned

a handful of small fresh basil leaves

1 Preheat the oven to 200°C (400°F, gas mark 6). Brush the peppers with 1 tbsp of the olive oil and arrange them in a shallow roasting tin. Roast for about 35 minutes or until the pepper skins are evenly darkened, turning them 3 or 4 times. Place the peppers in a polythene bag and leave until they are cool enough to handle.

2 Working over a bowl to catch the juice, peel the peppers. Cut them in half and discard the cores and seeds (strain out any seeds that fall into the juice), then cut into thick slices.

3 Measure 1½ tbsp of the pepper juice into a small bowl (discard the rest). Add the vinegar, garlic and salt and pepper to taste, and whisk in the remaining 1½ tbsp olive oil.

4 Arrange the peppers on a serving platter or on individual salad plates. Drizzle over the dressing and garnish with the olives and basil leaves.

Another idea

For a **roasted red pepper and onion salad** to serve 4, quarter and seed 4 red peppers and put them in a baking dish with 4 small red onions, quartered. Drizzle over 1½ tbsp extra virgin olive oil and season to taste.

Roast in a preheated 200°C (400°F, gas mark 6) oven for about 35 minutes, turning once, until the vegetables are tender and browned around the edges. Cool, then peel the peppers, if wished, holding them over the baking dish. Whisk 2 tsp lemon juice with 1½ tbsp extra virgin olive oil in a salad bowl and season to taste. Add 115 g (4 oz) rocket or mixed red salad leaves and toss to coat. Pile the peppers and onions on top and drizzle over their cooking juices.

Plus points

• Herbalists recommend basil as a natural tranquilliser. It is also believed to aid digestion, ease stomach cramps and help to relieve the headaches associated with colds.

• Olives are a source of vitamin E, although they are usually not eaten in large enough quantities to make a significant contribution to the diet.

photo, page 193

Each serving provides   kcal 97, protein 2 g, fat 6 g (of which saturated fat 1 g), carbohydrate 10 g (of which sugars 9 g), fibre 3 g. Excellent source of niacin, vitamin A, vitamin B$_1$, vitamin B$_6$, vitamin C, vitamin E. Good source of folate.

Warm potato salad

Here tender new potatoes, cooked in their jackets, are combined with crunchy celery, spring onions and walnuts in a nutty dressing, then served warm. The salad is a delightful alternative to potato salads in creamy mayonnaise-based dressings, and goes well with cold meats or grilled fish, poultry, meat or vegetables.

Preparation time **10–20 minutes**   Cooking time **20–25 minutes**   *Serves 4*

450 g (1 lb) small new potatoes

50 g (1¾ oz) walnut pieces

3 celery sticks, thinly sliced

6 spring onions, thinly sliced

4 tbsp chopped parsley

sprigs of fresh flat-leaf parsley to garnish

Walnut balsamic dressing

2 tbsp walnut oil

1 tbsp balsamic vinegar

1 garlic clove, crushed (optional)

pinch of caster sugar

salt and pepper

1 Cut any large potatoes in half. Put the potatoes in a pan, cover with boiling water and bring back to the boil. Reduce the heat and simmer for 15–20 minutes or until the potatoes are just tender.

2 Meanwhile, make the dressing: whisk together the oil, vinegar, garlic, if using, sugar and seasoning.

3 Drain the potatoes and put them into a serving bowl. Add the walnuts, celery, spring onions and chopped parsley. Pour on the dressing and toss the ingredients together gently. Allow to cool slightly until just warm, then serve garnished with parsley.

Some more ideas

Use Jerusalem artichokes instead of new potatoes. Peel or scrub the artichokes, as preferred, and immediately put them in a saucepan of water with a slice of lemon or a little lemon juice added to prevent them from discolouring. Cook as for the new potatoes.

Add a peppery flavour with 55 g (2 oz) watercress or rocket leaves. Fresh coriander or basil can be used instead of parsley.

Replace half the quantity of potatoes with an equal weight of other root vegetables, such as young carrots and/or baby turnips. Cook the carrots and turnips with the potatoes.

Other oils can be used instead of walnut: try hazelnut, groundnut or pumpkin seed oil. For a creamy dressing, use 4 tbsp fromage frais instead of the oil.

Plus points

● Celery provides potassium, a mineral that is important for the regulation of fluid balance in the body, thus helping to prevent high blood pressure.

● Potatoes are a classic source of starchy carbohydrate for everyday meals. The preparation method makes a big difference to the amount of dietary fibre provided: new potatoes cooked in their skins offer a third more fibre than peeled potatoes. Cooking potatoes in their skins also preserves the nutrients found just under the skin.

● Walnuts have been shown to lower blood cholesterol.

Each serving provides   kcal 220, protein 4 g, fat 15 g (of which saturated fat 1 g), carbohydrate 19 g (of which sugars 2 g), fibre 2 g. Good source of vitamin B_6, vitamin C. Useful source of copper, folate, iron, potassium, vitamin B_1, vitamin E.

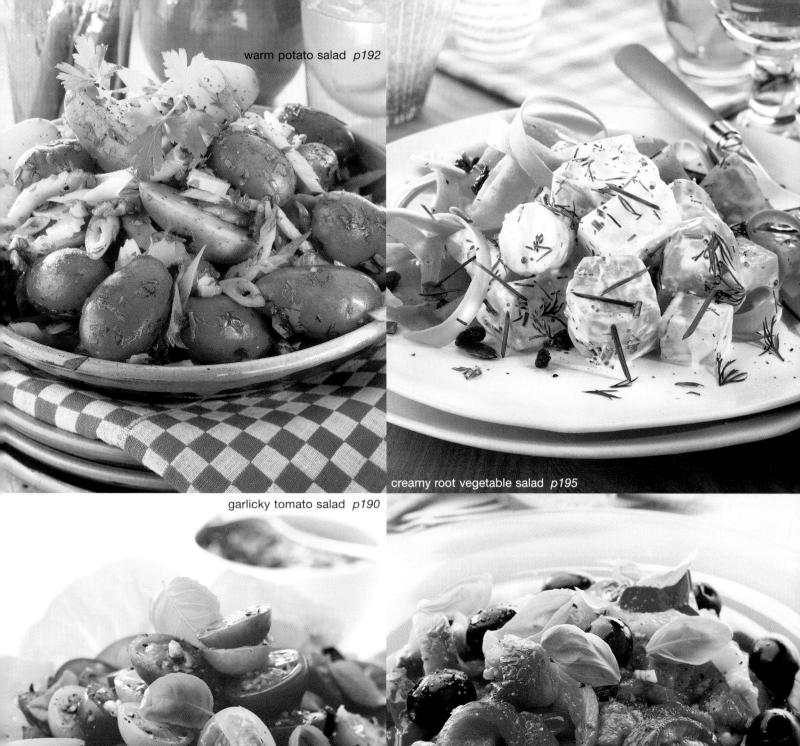
warm potato salad *p192*

creamy root vegetable salad *p195*

garlicky tomato salad *p190*

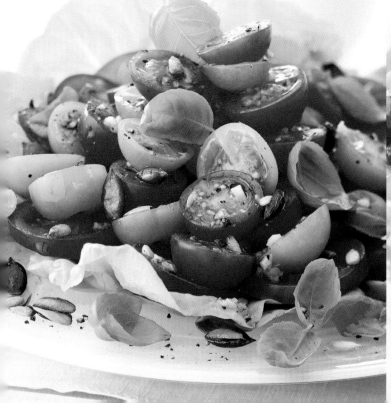

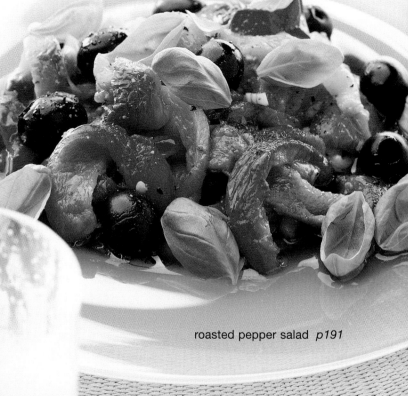
roasted pepper salad *p191*

Zesty tomato salad

Seek out the most delicious tomatoes available, preferably sun-ripened on the vine, and you will be rewarded with an incomparable flavour. Lemon, fresh coriander and mint add freshness and zest to the tomatoes in this tangy salad, which can easily be varied with other fresh herbs and flavourings such as onion and garlic.

Preparation time **10 minutes**   *Serves 4*

500 g (1 lb 2 oz) ripe tomatoes, sliced

pinch of caster sugar, or to taste

1 lemon

3 spring onions, thinly sliced

1 tbsp chopped fresh coriander

1 tbsp chopped fresh mint

sprigs of fresh mint to garnish

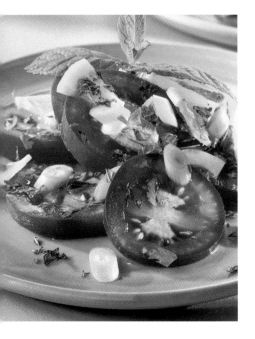

1 Place the tomatoes in a large shallow dish and sprinkle with the sugar. Cut the lemon in half lengthways. Set one half aside, then cut the other half lengthways into 4 wedges. Holding the wedges firmly together on a board, skin side up, thinly slice them across, including the peel. Discard the pips.

2 Arrange the pieces of thinly sliced lemon over the top of the tomatoes, then sprinkle with the spring onions, coriander and mint. Squeeze the juice from the remaining lemon half and sprinkle it over the salad. Serve immediately or cover and chill until ready to serve. Garnish with sprigs of mint just before serving.

Some more ideas

For a tomato salad with rosemary and basil, make a dressing by mixing together 1 tbsp each chopped fresh rosemary and basil, 1–2 garlic cloves, finely chopped, and 2 tsp raspberry vinegar or balsamic vinegar. Sprinkle the tomatoes with 3–4 pinches of sugar to emphasise their natural sweetness, and scatter over ½ red or white onion, thinly sliced. Sprinkle the dressing evenly over the tomatoes. Serve at once or cover and chill until ready to serve.

A tomato salad makes a delicious filling for baked potatoes and sweet potatoes. Bake 4 large potatoes until crisp and golden outside and floury inside, then split and fill with the tomato salad. Top with a spoonful of fromage frais or Greek-style yogurt and serve.

Tomato salads are good as omelette fillings. For each serving, make a plain omelette by lightly beating 2 eggs with 2 tbsp cold water and a little seasoning, then cooking in the minimum of olive oil in a very hot omelette pan until just set, lifting the edges to allow unset egg to run onto the hot pan. Spoon a quarter of the tomato salad over half of the set omelette and fold the other half over. Slide the omelette onto a warmed plate. Serve with a mixed green salad and crusty bread.

Plus points

• Vitamin C, found in raw tomatoes, is an antioxidant that helps to protect against cancer. Tomatoes also contain lycopene, another valuable anti-cancer agent, believed to be particularly useful in protecting against prostate cancer. Lycopene is enhanced by cooking, so canned tomatoes, tomato purée or paste and tomato ketchup are better sources than fresh tomatoes.

Each serving provides   kcal 25, protein 1 g, fat 0.5 g (of which saturated fat 0.1 g), carbohydrate 4 g (of which sugars 3 g), fibre 1 g. Excellent source of vitamin C. Good source of vitamin E. Useful source of folate, vitamin A.

Creamy root vegetable salad

It is easy to overlook root vegetables as a salad ingredient. Try this colourful mixture, tossed in a creamy, reduced-fat dressing, and discover a satisfying alternative to the ubiquitous mayonnaise-dressed potato salad. It makes a tempting light lunch or a delicious accompaniment to grilled meat or fish.

Preparation time **45 minutes, plus cooling and 2–3 hours chilling** *Serves 4*

300 g (10½ oz) small new or salad potatoes, cut into 2.5 cm (1 in) cubes

200 g (7 oz) celeriac, cut into 1 cm (½ in) cubes

170 g (6 oz) swede, cut into 1 cm (½ in) cubes

200 g (7 oz) sweet potato, cut into 2.5 cm (1 in) cubes

juice of ½ lemon

Mustard and herb dressing

1 tbsp reduced-fat mayonnaise

2 tbsp plain low-fat yogurt

1 tsp wholegrain mustard

2 tbsp snipped fresh chives

1 tbsp chopped fresh dill

freshly ground black pepper

To finish

4 carrots, about 250 g (9 oz) in total

4 tbsp currants

3 tbsp pumpkin seeds

1 tbsp orange juice

To garnish

snipped fresh chives and dill

1 Place the potatoes, celeriac and swede in a saucepan. Add boiling water to cover and bring back to the boil. Reduce the heat and simmer for 10 minutes or until tender.

2 Meanwhile, place the sweet potato in another pan. Cover with boiling water, bring back to the boil and simmer for 3 minutes.

3 Make the dressing while the vegetables are cooking. Mix the mayonnaise, yogurt and mustard together. Stir in the chives, dill and black pepper to taste.

4 Drain all the vegetables well and put them in a large mixing bowl. Add the lemon juice and the dressing, and toss lightly. Set the vegetables aside to cool, then cover and chill them for 2–3 hours.

5 To finish the salad, use a vegetable peeler to cut ribbon strips from the carrots. Mix the carrot strips with the currants and pumpkin seeds. Stir in the orange juice. Spread the carrot mixture in a large shallow serving bowl or place on individual plates.

6 Pile the chilled root vegetable salad on top of the carrot mixture. Garnish with a scattering of snipped chives and chopped dill, and serve.

Some more ideas

As an alternative to the carrot base, mix together 75 g (2½ oz) baby spinach leaves, 75 g (2½ oz) cos lettuce leaves, finely shredded, and 1 white onion, thinly sliced. Top with 75 g (2½ oz) sliced ready-to-eat dried apricots and 1 tbsp toasted sesame seeds, then sprinkle with the orange juice.

To vary the dressing for the root vegetables, replace the dill, chives and wholegrain mustard with 1 tbsp chopped fresh tarragon, 1 tbsp chopped parsley and 1 tsp Dijon mustard.

Plus points

• Root vegetables are generally good sources of fibre, and starchy ones provide complex carbohydrate.

• Carrots offer vitamin A as beta-carotene, which is essential for good night vision.

• Pumpkin seeds are rich in fibre and minerals, such as copper, iron and zinc.

photo, page 193

Each serving provides kcal 350, protein 7 g, fat 15 g (of which saturated fat 2 g), carbohydrate 50 g (of which sugars 30 g), fibre 7 g. Excellent source of vitamin A, vitamin B, vitamin E. Good source of folate, potassium, vitamin B$_1$, vitamin B$_6$. Useful source of calcium, copper, iron, niacin, zinc.

Melon, feta and orange salad

Here, the classic starter of melon and Parma ham is transformed into a tempting main-dish salad with the addition of feta cheese, cherry tomatoes, cucumber and oranges. Serve for lunch, with warm ciabatta bread to mop up the juices, or as a starter for 6 people.

Preparation time **20–25 minutes**   *Serves 4*

2 oranges

½ honeydew melon, peeled, seeded and sliced

115 g (4 oz) cherry tomatoes, halved

85 g (3 oz) stoned black olives

½ small cucumber, diced

4 spring onions, thinly sliced

6 slices of Parma ham, about 80 g (2¾ oz) in total, trimmed of all fat and cut into strips

75 g (3½ oz) feta cheese, roughly broken into pieces

Orange and basil dressing

½ tsp grated orange zest

4 tbsp orange juice

1 tbsp extra virgin olive oil

1 tsp toasted sesame oil

6 fresh basil leaves, shredded

cracked black pepper

1 Make the dressing first. Mix the orange zest and juice with the olive oil, sesame oil and basil in a large salad bowl. Season with salt and pepper to taste.

2 Cut the peel and pith away from the oranges with a sharp knife. Holding them over the salad bowl to catch the juice, cut between the membrane to release the orange segments. Add the segments to the bowl.

3 Add the melon, tomatoes, olives, cucumber, spring onions and Parma ham. Toss until the ingredients are well blended and coated in dressing. Scatter the feta cheese over the top and serve.

Some more ideas

Substitute Serrano ham from Spain or smoky Black Forest ham for the Parma ham.

As an alternative to honeydew melon, try other varieties such as Ogen or Charentais or a wedge of watermelon.

To make a **melon and fresh pineapple salad with cottage cheese**, mix the melon, tomato and cucumber with ½ pineapple, peeled, cored and chopped, and 3 shallots, thinly sliced. Make a lime dressing by mixing ½ tsp grated lime zest and 2 tbsp lime juice with

2 tbsp sunflower oil and 1 tsp clear honey. Season to taste. Stir the dressing into the melon mixture and pile onto 4 plates. Spoon 75 g (2½ oz) plain cottage cheese on top of each salad and scatter over roasted, chopped macadamia nuts, 50 g (1¾ oz) in total. Garnish generously with small sprigs of watercress.

Plus points

● Although feta cheese is high in fat and salt, it is an excellent source of calcium, and because it has a strong flavour a little goes a long way. Calcium in dairy products is much more easily absorbed by the body than calcium from other foods. Since the feta and ham provide a salty flavour, keep the sodium in this recipe low by avoiding extra salt.

● Only 1 in 4 people in the UK drink enough water or other fluid. Foods that have a high water content, such as melon and cucumber, are an easy way of increasing fluid intake.

Each serving provides kcal 220, protein 9 g, fat 12 g (of which saturated fat 5 g), carbohydrate 16 g (of which sugars 16 g), fibre 3 g. Excellent source of vitamin C. Good source of calcium, vitamin B_6, vitamin B_{12}. Useful source of folate, potassium, vitamin A, vitamin B_1, vitamin E.

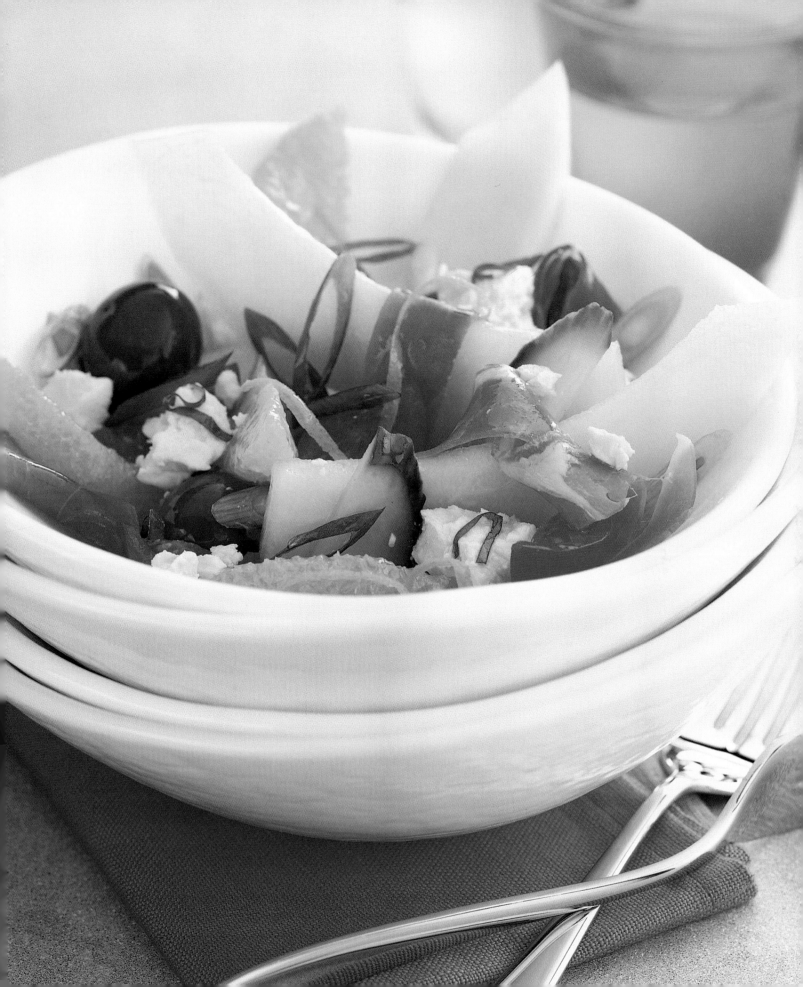

Golden mango salad

This mixture of salad leaves and herbs, each with its own robust flavour, marries well with the sweetness and smooth texture of mango. The result is a salad that is colourful and refreshing, ideal as a light starter or side dish. Serve with warm mixed-grain bread or rolls.

Preparation time **15 minutes**   *Serves 4*

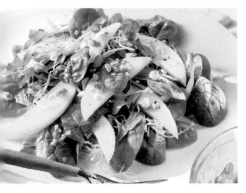

1 large ripe mango

200 g (7 oz) mixed baby spinach leaves, watercress and rocket or frisée

about 12 fresh basil leaves, coarsely shredded or torn

about 6 sprigs of fresh coriander, stalks discarded, then coarsely chopped

30 g (1 oz) cashew nuts or peanuts, toasted and coarsely chopped

Lime and ginger dressing

grated zest of 1 lime

2 tbsp lime juice

2 tsp finely chopped or grated fresh root ginger

1 tbsp toasted sesame oil

salt and pepper

1 Peel the mango. Cut the flesh from both sides of the stone and slice it thinly lengthways.

2 Mix the salad leaves on a platter, then sprinkle on the basil and coriander. Arrange the mango slices on and between the salad leaves.

3 Whisk the ingredients for the dressing together and spoon it over the salad. Sprinkle with the chopped cashew nuts or peanuts and serve.

Some more ideas

Thin strips of peeled cooked beetroot and cooked or raw celeriac are delicious additions to this salad.

Replace the nuts with spicy croûtons. Cut 2 slices of day-old bread into cubes and place in a polythene bag. Add a pinch of chilli powder, then hold the bag shut and shake well. Tip into a non-stick pan sprayed with oil and stir-fry until crisp and golden brown. Add to the salad just before serving.

For a completely fat-free dressing, mix 1 tbsp seasoned rice vinegar (the type sold for making Japanese sushi) with the ginger and lime zest and juice. Add 2 tbsp fresh orange juice. Or mix 2 tbsp each of orange juice, dry sherry and soy sauce for a punchy dressing.

A **mixed green salad** makes a versatile accompaniment for all meals or a useful base on which to serve ingredients such as fruit or smoked fish for a first course. Mix 225 g (8 oz) mixed salad leaves (cos, lamb's lettuce, Lollo Rosso, Little Gem, baby spinach or rocket) with about 45 g (1½ oz) mixed fresh herbs (basil, tarragon, chervil, flat-leaf parsley and mint), torn or coarsely chopped. Rub the inside of the salad bowl with a cut clove of garlic, if liked, then discard. Add the leaves and herbs to the bowl. For the dressing, whisk together 1 shallot, finely chopped, ½ tsp Dijon mustard, 2 tbsp white wine vinegar and 4 tbsp extra virgin olive oil with seasoning. Drizzle the dressing over the salad, then toss gently to coat the leaves.

Plus points

● Mango contains a wealth of carotenoids which protect against free radical attack and degenerative diseases. Mango also supplies iron, magnesium, potassium and vitamins E, C and B group.

● All the leaves provide minerals, such as potassium, calcium and iron. Raw spinach provides folate. All these minerals help to protect against cancer.

Each serving provides kcal 100, protein 3 g, fat 7 g (of which saturated fat 1.5 g), carbohydrate 6 g (of which sugars 3 g), fibre 2 g. Excellent source of vitamin C. Good source of vitamin A. Useful source of calcium, copper, folate, iron, vitamin B$_1$, vitamin E.

Mediterranean marinated salad

Inspired by Mediterranean cooking methods, this salad of roasted vegetables has a rich flavour cut by a piquant dressing. It is one of those any-time salads – ideal for a healthy mid-week meal with lots of crusty bread, some pasta or couscous; good as a dinner-party starter; or delicious with grilled fish, poultry or meat.

Preparation time about 1 hour, plus cooling and at least 4 hours marinating and 1 hour resting *Serves 4*

1 aubergine, cut into 1 cm (½ in) thick slices

1 red pepper, quartered lengthways and seeded

1 yellow pepper, quartered lengthways and seeded

4 baby courgettes, halved lengthways

1 tbsp extra virgin olive oil, or spray oil

1 garlic clove, crushed

4 canned anchovy fillets, drained and finely chopped

2 tbsp very finely chopped fresh rosemary

salt and pepper

sprigs of fresh rosemary to garnish (optional)

Honey mustard dressing

1 tbsp extra virgin olive oil

1 tbsp red wine vinegar

1 tsp runny honey

1 tsp Dijon mustard

1 Preheat the oven to 200°C (400°F, gas mark 6). Lay the aubergine slices in a single layer in a large roasting tin. Arrange the red and yellow peppers and courgettes around the aubergines, placing them cut sides up.

2 Brush or spray the vegetables lightly with the oil. Scatter the garlic, anchovies and chopped rosemary over the vegetables, and add seasoning to taste. Roast the vegetables for 25–30 minutes.

3 Cover the vegetables with foil and roast for a further 10–15 minutes or until they are tender. Transfer the cooked vegetables to a large dish, layering them neatly, then drizzle the cooking juices over them.

4 Whisk the dressing ingredients together and pour over the vegetables. Cover and leave to cool completely, then put the vegetable salad in the fridge to marinate for at least 4 hours.

5 Remove the salad from the fridge 1 hour before serving so it can return to cool room temperature. Garnish with sprigs of rosemary, if you wish.

Some more ideas

Replace the courgettes with 225 g (8 oz) plum tomatoes, halved, and use fresh thyme instead of rosemary. Roast the aubergines and peppers for 30 minutes, then add the tomatoes and roast for a further 15 minutes without covering with foil.

For a vegetarian version, omit the anchovies and add 2 tbsp chopped capers instead.

Plus points

* Aubergines are satisfyingly filling but low in calories – 100 g (3½ oz) contains just 15 kcal. They are renowned for absorbing oil when fried, but cooking them this way keeps the fat content very low.

* Rosemary is said to stimulate the nervous and circulatory systems, and soothe the digestive system.

* Courgettes provide vitamins B_1 and B_6.

* All of the vegetables in this dish are useful sources of fibre, and they provide lots of vitamins and minerals.

photo, page 201

Each serving provides kcal 140, protein 4 g, fat 10 g (of which saturated fat 1 g), carbohydrate 9 g (of which sugars 8 g), fibre 3 g. Excellent source of vitamin C. Good source of folate, vitamin A, vitamin B_6, vitamin E. Useful source of iron, niacin, potassium, vitamin B_{12}.

Mixed salad leaves with flowers and blueberries

This pretty summer salad is a delightful combination of edible flowers, salad leaves, alfalfa sprouts and juicy fresh blueberries. Some large supermarkets sell packs of edible flowers. Or you can pick them from your garden – just be sure to choose those that have not been sprayed with pesticides.

Preparation time **10–15 minutes**   *Serves 4*

1 small Oak Leaf lettuce, torn into bite-sized pieces

85 g (3 oz) rocket

85 g (3 oz) alfalfa sprouts

100 g (3½ oz) blueberries

30 g (1 oz) mixed edible flowers, including some or all of the following: nasturtiums, borage, violas or pansies, and herb flowers such as sage and rosemary

Honey mustard dressing

2 tbsp grapeseed oil

juice of 1 small lemon

1 tsp Dijon mustard

1 tsp clear honey

salt and pepper

1 To make the dressing, whisk the oil with the lemon juice, mustard, honey, and salt and pepper to taste in a large shallow salad bowl.

2 Add the lettuce and rocket and toss to coat with the dressing. Sprinkle the salad with the alfalfa sprouts and blueberries. Arrange the flowers on top and serve at once.

Some more ideas

Make a **flowery carrot salad**. Tear 1 batavia or Oak Leaf lettuce into bite-sized pieces and put into a shallow salad bowl. Add 2 carrots, cut into long thin ribbons with a swivel vegetable peeler, 2 oranges, peeled and divided into segments, and 75 g (2½ oz) blueberries. Make the dressing as in the main recipe, using orange juice instead of lemon. Drizzle it over the salad and garnish with mixed orange and yellow nasturtium flowers.

For a refreshingly **lemony leaf and raspberry salad**, mix 15 g (½ oz) sweet cicely leaves and a few lemon geranium leaves with 1 small Webb's Wonder or cos lettuce, torn into pieces. Scatter over 100 g (3½ oz) raspberries. For the dressing, whisk 2 tbsp extra virgin olive oil with the juice of 1 lemon

and seasoning to taste. Garnish the salad with 30 g (1 oz) mixed chive, sweet cicely and mint or viola flowers.

Try a **peppery salad with pears and wild garlic**. Separate 2 Little Gem lettuces into leaves and mix with 85 g (3 oz) rocket in a salad bowl. For the dressing whisk 2 tbsp extra virgin olive oil with the juice of 1 lemon and 3 tbsp chopped fresh chives. Add 1 ripe red Williams pear, cored and thinly sliced, and turn to coat with the dressing, then add the pear and dressing to the salad leaves and toss gently. Garnish with 30 g (1 oz) mixed wild garlic, chive and borage flowers.

Plus points

- Naturally sweet blueberries are rich in vitamin C and also contain antibacterial compounds thought to be effective against some gastrointestinal disorders and urinary infections such as cystitis.

- The nutritional value of petals and flower heads is very small as they are used in such tiny quantities, but you will get some essential oils and phytochemicals, particularly antioxidants, from some flowers, especially herb flowers.

Each serving provides   kcal 80, protein 2 g, fat 6 g (of which saturated fat 0.5 g), carbohydrate 5 g (of which sugars 5 g), fibre 2 g. Excellent source of niacin, vitamin B_2, vitamin B_6, vitamin C. Good source of vitamin E. Useful source of folate, vitamin A.

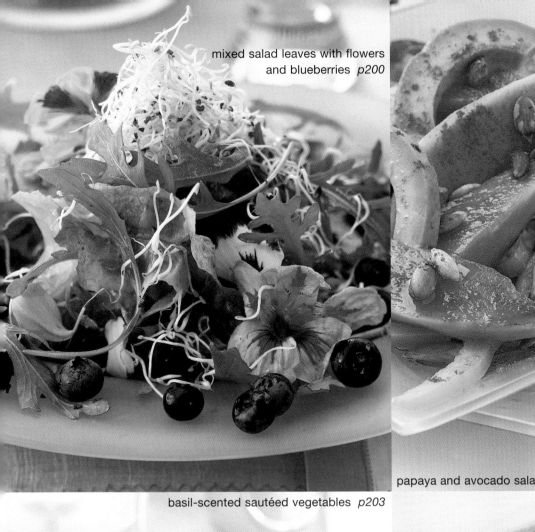
mixed salad leaves with flowers and blueberries *p200*

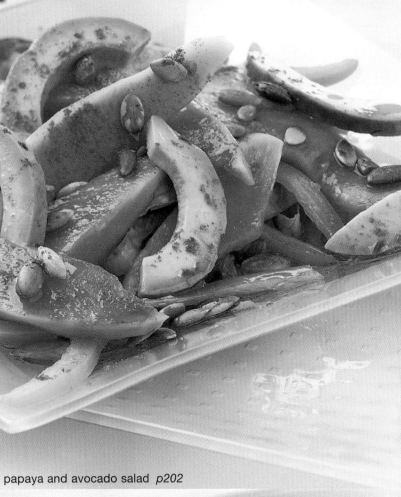
papaya and avocado salad *p202*

basil-scented sautéed vegetables *p203*
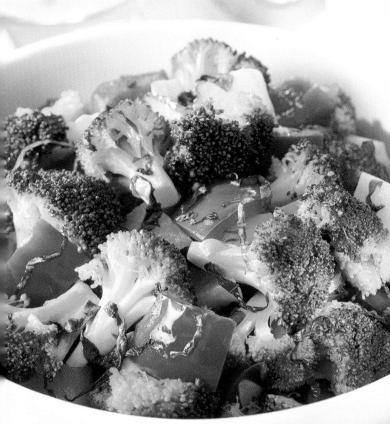

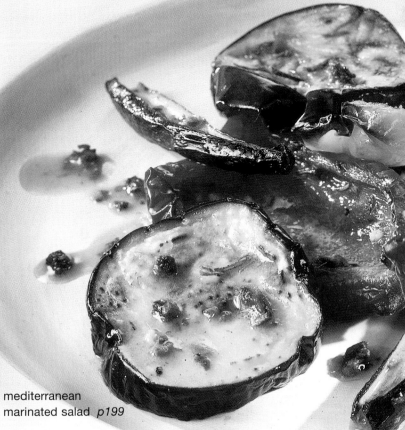
mediterranean marinated salad *p199*

Papaya and avocado salad

This refreshing salad with a hint of spice will convert anyone wary of mixing fruit with raw vegetables. Starting with a base of crisp lettuce, slices of orange or yellow pepper are layered with avocado and papaya. Toasted pumpkin seeds add protein and crunch. Serve with mixed grain or pumpkin bread for a light lunch.

Preparation time **12 minutes**   *Serves 4*

1 romaine or cos lettuce heart, about 170 g (6 oz)

2 spring onions, thinly sliced

1 large orange or yellow pepper, quartered and seeded

1 large avocado, about 200 g (7 oz)

1 large papaya, about 500 g (1 lb 2 oz)

6 tbsp pumpkin seeds

Spicy dressing

juice of ½ lime

1½ tbsp extra virgin olive oil

pinch of paprika

pinch of ground cumin

½ tsp light soft brown sugar

1 Shred the lettuce leaves and put them in a large shallow dish or 4 individual dishes. Sprinkle the spring onions over the lettuce.

2 Cut the pepper quarters across into thin strips and arrange them in the dish. Halve, stone and peel the avocado, and cut into 5 mm (¼ in) slices across the width. Peel, halve and seed the papaya, and cut into 5 mm (¼ in) slices across the width. Scatter the avocado and papaya slices over the pepper strips.

3 Whisk all the dressing ingredients together and pour over the salad. Heat a small heavy saucepan, add the pumpkin seeds and toss them in the pan to toast them lightly. Sprinkle the seeds over the salad and serve.

Some more ideas

For a **fennel, orange and melon salad**, thinly slice 1 small fennel bulb and mix with the segments from 2 oranges and ½ Galia or Ogen melon, cut into slivers. Arrange on a bed of rocket and scatter 8 halved black olives over the top.

For a **mango and avocado salad** with a chilli dressing, use mango instead of papaya, and a red pepper instead of orange or yellow; instead of paprika and cumin in the dressing, add a small fresh red or green chilli, seeded and finely chopped, and the grated zest of 1 lime. Top the salad with 100 g (3½ oz) toasted cashew nuts instead of pumpkin seeds.

Plus points

- Peppers are well known to be a rich source of vitamin C, and serving them raw in a salad makes more of this vitamin available than if they were cooked. They also contain high levels of beta-carotene and other members of the carotene family, such as capsanthin and zeaxanthin. All of these work as antioxidants, helping to prevent cancers, heart disease, strokes and cataracts.

- Papaya provides vitamin C and protective carotenes as well as calcium, iron and zinc.

- Pumpkin seeds have a lot to offer: protein, fibre, unsaturated fat, vitamin E and some B vitamins, as well as iron for healthy blood, magnesium for maintaining healthy body cells and zinc for growth and development.

photo, page 201

Each serving provides kcal 240, protein 2 g, fat 18 g (of which saturated fat 3 g), carbohydrate 17 g (of which sugars 17 g), fibre 5 g. Excellent source of vitamin A, vitamin C. Good source of vitamin B_6, vitamin E. Useful source of copper, iron, potassium, vitamin B_1, vitamin B_2.

Basil-scented sautéed vegetables

A large non-stick frying pan is ideal for sautéeing, the Western equivalent of stir-frying, based on quick cooking over high heat. This is a terrific method for preserving the colour of vegetables while bringing out their flavour to the full. Serve the vegetables with fish, poultry or meat, or toss them with freshly cooked noodles.

Preparation time **10 minutes**   Cooking time **7–8 minutes**   *Serves 4*

500 g (1 lb 2 oz) broccoli

1 tbsp extra virgin olive oil

3–4 large garlic cloves, thinly sliced (optional)

1 large or 2 small red peppers, seeded and cut into chunks

1 turnip, about 150 g (5½ oz), cut into bite-sized chunks

pinch of sugar

8 sprigs of fresh basil, stalks discarded, then finely shredded

salt

1 Cut the broccoli into small florets; trim and thinly slice the stalks. Heat the olive oil in a large non-stick frying pan or wok. Add the garlic, if using, the red pepper, turnip and slices of broccoli stalk. Sprinkle in the sugar and salt to taste. Cook for 2–3 minutes, turning frequently.

2 Add the broccoli florets and stir. Pour in 6 tbsp of water to provide a thin covering on the bottom of the pan. Cover and cook over a fairly high heat for 3–4 minutes. The broccoli should be just tender and bright green.

3 Stir in the basil, replace the lid and leave on the heat for a few more seconds. Serve immediately.

Some more ideas

Sugarsnap peas or mange-tout can be used instead of the broccoli. They will cook in 1–2 minutes and there is no need to add the water. Serve with lemon or lime wedges so that the juice can be squeezed over the vegetables.

As well as replacing the broccoli with sugarsnap peas, use yellow peppers in place of red. Omit the garlic. Substitute tiny parboiled new potatoes, halved, for the turnip

and sprinkle generously with fresh tarragon leaves rather than basil. This combination of sautéed vegetables is delicious with fish, especially grilled mackerel or salmon.

For a Far-Eastern flavour, replace the turnips with 8 canned water chestnuts, drained and quartered or halved, and add 1 tsp chopped fresh root ginger and ½ fresh green or red chilli, seeded and finely chopped, with the broccoli florets. Increase the quantity of sugar to 1–2 tsp. At the end of cooking, add 1 tbsp chopped fresh coriander with the basil.

Plus points

• This dish is loaded with ingredients that help to fight cancer and prevent heart disease. Broccoli, one of the brassicas, is a good source of the phytochemicals called glucosinolates. Red pepper is a rich source of the antioxidant beta-carotene which the body can convert into vitamin A.

• In addition to providing fibre, turnips contain the B vitamins niacin and B6, and are a surprisingly useful source of vitamin C.

photo, page 201

Each serving provides   kcal 90, protein 6 g, fat 4 g (of which saturated fat 1 g), carbohydrate 7 g (of which sugars 7 g), fibre 5 g. Excellent source of vitamin A, vitamin C. Good source of folate, vitamin E. Useful source of iron, niacin.

Sesame greens and bean sprouts

With a little inspiration and the availability of international ingredients, even the most humble vegetables can be elevated to feature in unusual, well-flavoured side dishes. This succulent stir-fry is full of flavour and crunch. It is ideal as part of an Oriental menu or equally delicious with plain grilled fish, poultry or meat.

Preparation time **10 minutes**   Cooking time **4–6 minutes**   *Serves 4*

30 g (1 oz) sesame seeds

2 tbsp sunflower oil

1 onion, chopped

2 garlic cloves, chopped

1 small Savoy cabbage, about 300 g (10½ oz), finely shredded

½ head of Chinese leaves, finely shredded

170 g (6 oz) bean sprouts

4 tbsp oyster sauce

salt and pepper

1 Heat a small saucepan and dry-fry the sesame seeds, shaking the pan frequently, until they are just beginning to brown. Turn the seeds out into a small bowl and set aside.

2 Heat the oil in a wok or large frying pan. Add the onion and garlic, and stir-fry for 2–3 minutes or until softened slightly. Add the cabbage and Chinese leaves and stir-fry over a fairly high heat for 2–3 minutes or until the vegetables are just beginning to soften. Add the bean sprouts and continue cooking for a few seconds.

3 Make a space in the centre of the pan. Pour in the oyster sauce and 2 tbsp of water, and stir until hot, then toss the vegetables into the sauce. Taste and add pepper, with salt if necessary (this will depend on the saltiness of the oyster sauce). Serve immediately, sprinkled with the toasted sesame seeds.

Some more ideas

Use 250 g (9 oz) red cabbage, finely shredded, instead of the Savoy cabbage, and add 3 cooked beetroot, chopped, with the bean sprouts. Red cabbage will require 2 minutes additional stir-frying, so add to the wok before the Chinese leaves. Use 1 tbsp clear honey with 2 tbsp soy sauce instead of the oyster sauce.

Finely shredded Brussels sprouts are crisp and full flavoured when stir-fried. Use them instead of the Savoy cabbage – slice the sprouts thinly, then shake the slices to loosen the shreds. Or use shredded spring greens. Toasted flaked almonds can be sprinkled over the vegetables instead of the sesame seeds.

Plus points

● As well as contributing distinctive flavour, sesame seeds are a good source of calcium and therefore useful for anyone who dislikes or does not eat dairy products, the main source of this mineral in the Western diet. Although the sesame seeds do bring the fat content up, most of this fat is unsaturated.

● Bean sprouts, along with other sprouted seeds, are rich in B vitamins and vitamin C. They also provide iron and potassium.

Each serving provides kcal 150, protein 5 g, fat 11 g (of which saturated fat 1 g), carbohydrate 9 g (of which sugars 5 g), fibre 4 g. Excellent source of folate, vitamin C. Good source of vitamin B$_{12}$. Useful source of calcium, iron, potassium, vitamin B$_1$.

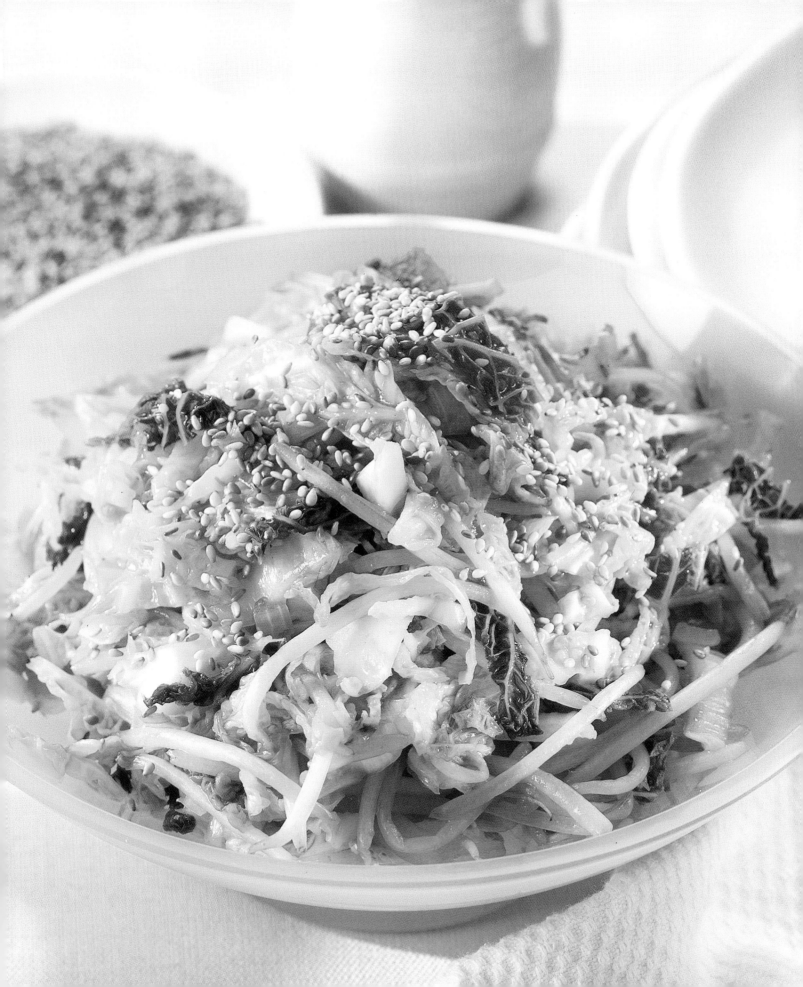

Roast root vegetables with herbs

Use this recipe as a basic guide for roasting single vegetables, such as potatoes or parsnips, as well as for a superb dish of mixed roots. Serve them in generous quantities with roast poultry or meat, but also remember that they are delicious with vegetarian main dishes and with lightly baked fish.

Preparation time **15–20 minutes**   Cooking time **30–35 minutes**   *Serves 4*

1 kg (2¼ lb) root vegetables, such as potatoes, sweet potatoes, carrots, parsnips, swede and kohlrabi

225 g (8 oz) shallots or pickling onions

2 tbsp extra virgin olive oil

1 tsp coarse sea salt

1 tsp cracked black peppercorns

few sprigs of fresh thyme

few sprigs of fresh rosemary

sprigs of fresh thyme or rosemary to garnish (optional)

1 Preheat the oven to 220°C (425°F, gas mark 7). Scrub or peel the vegetables, according to type and your taste. Halve or quarter large potatoes. Cut large carrots or parsnips in half lengthways, then cut the pieces across in half again. Cut swede or kohlrabi into large chunks (about the same size as the potatoes). Leave shallots or onions whole.

2 Place the vegetables in a saucepan and pour in enough boiling water to cover them. Bring back to the boil, then reduce the heat and simmer for 5–7 minutes or until the vegetables are lightly cooked, but not yet tender.

3 Drain the vegetables and place them in a roasting tin. Brush with the oil and sprinkle with the salt and peppercorns. Add the herb sprigs to the tin and place in the oven.

4 Roast for 30–35 minutes or until the vegetables are golden brown, crisp and tender. Turn the vegetables over halfway through the cooking. Serve hot, garnished with sprigs of thyme or rosemary, if liked.

Some more ideas

The vegetables can be roasted at the same time as a joint of meat or poultry. Allow 45 minutes at 200°C (400°F, gas mark 6), or longer at a lower temperature, if necessary.

Baby new vegetables can also be roasted. For example, try new potatoes, carrots, beetroot and turnips. As well as root vegetables, patty pan squash and asparagus are delicious roasted. Sprinkle with herbs and a little balsamic vinegar or lemon juice.

Quartered acorn squash is good roasted with mixed root vegetables.

Plus points

● Combining different root vegetables instead of serving roast potatoes alone provides a good mix of flavours and nutrients: as well as vitamin C from the potatoes and beta-carotene from the carrots, swedes are part of the brassica family, which offer cancer-fighting phytochemicals.

● All these vegetables provide plenty of flavour and satisfying bulk, so portions of meat can be modest. They also contribute dietary fibre.

Each serving provides kcal 200, protein 4 g, fat 7 g (of which saturated fat 1 g), carbohydrate 33 g (of which sugars 14 g), fibre 7 g. Excellent source of vitamin A, vitamin C. Good source of folate, vitamin B$_1$, vitamin B$_6$, vitamin E. Useful source of niacin, potassium.

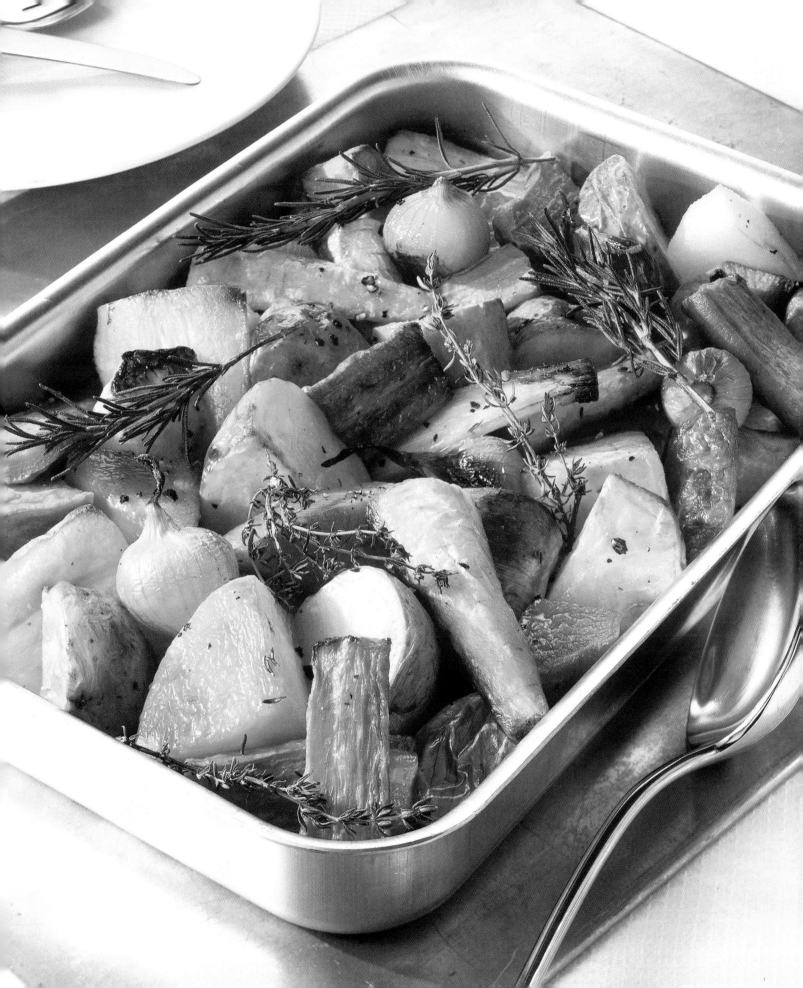

Sweet potato and celeriac purée

Mashes and purées are perennial favourites and an excellent way of boosting your daily intake of vegetables. They are so easy to eat that all the family will enjoy them in generous quantities. This sweet potato and celeriac purée is deliciously flavoured with apple and spices, and there are 2 more suggestions to tempt you.

Preparation time **15 minutes**   Cooking time **15–20 minutes**   *Serves 4*

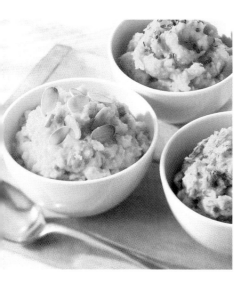

500 g (1 lb 2 oz) sweet potato

400 g (14 oz) celeriac

juice of 1 lemon

2 tbsp extra virgin olive oil

2 garlic cloves, finely chopped

1 tbsp coarsely grated fresh root ginger

½–1 tsp ground cumin

1 Golden Delicious apple, peeled, cored and finely chopped

1 tbsp coriander seeds, roughly crushed

1 Cut the sweet potato and celeriac into similar-sized chunks and place in a large saucepan. Add half the lemon juice, then pour in boiling water to cover the vegetables and bring back to the boil. Reduce the heat and simmer gently for 15–20 minutes or until the vegetables are tender.

2 Meanwhile, heat the oil in a small saucepan. Add the garlic, ginger and cumin, and cook for 30 seconds. Stir in the apple and remaining lemon juice and cook for 5 minutes or until the apple begins to soften.

3 Toast the crushed coriander seeds in a small dry pan, stirring occasionally, until they are fragrant.

4 Drain the vegetables well, then mash them. Stir in the apple mixture and sprinkle with the toasted coriander seeds. Serve piping hot.

Some more ideas

For a **creamy root vegetable purée**, use 3 carrots, 3 parsnips and 1 small swede, about 900 g (2 lb) in total. Cut into similar-sized chunks and place in a large saucepan. Pour in boiling water to cover and bring back to the boil. Reduce the heat and simmer for 20–25 minutes or until the vegetables are tender. Drain well. Add 5 tbsp 0% fat Greek-style yogurt and mash until smooth, or purée in a food processor. Stir in 4 spring onions, finely chopped, and season to taste.

For a **chilli-spiced split pea purée**, rinse 225 g (8 oz) yellow split peas in cold water, drain and place in a saucepan. Add 2 whole garlic cloves (if liked) and pour in boiling water to cover the peas generously. Bring to the boil, then reduce the heat and simmer for about 1 hour or until tender. Drain well. Mash the peas with about 5 tbsp semi-skimmed milk and 30 g (1 oz) butter using a vegetable masher, or purée in a food processor. Stir in 2 small fresh red chillies, seeded and finely chopped; 4 tbsp chopped fresh coriander or parsley; 8 sprigs of fresh basil, tough stalks discarded, then shredded. Season to taste.

Plus points

- Sweet potatoes are an excellent source of beta-carotene, an antioxidant that helps to protect against free radical damage, which can age us and increase the risk of heart disease and cancer. Sweet potatoes also provide good amounts of vitamin C and potassium, and contain more vitamin E than any other vegetable.

Each serving provides kcal 163, protein 3 g, fat 3.5 g (of which saturated fat 0.5 g), carbohydrate 32 g (of which sugars 12 g), fibre 7 g. Excellent source of vitamin A, vitamin C, vitamin E. Good source of folate. Useful source of potassium, vitamin B_1, vitamin B_6.

Pork and pear salad with pecans

This is a simple yet substantial salad of new potatoes, crunchy red and white radishes, peppery watercress and juicy pears, topped with slices of roast pork and finished with a scattering of toasted pecan nuts. The dressing is delicately flavoured with ginger juice, squeezed from fresh root ginger.

Preparation time **35 minutes**   *Serves 4*

55 g (2 oz) pecan nuts

900 g (2 lb) even-sized new potatoes, scrubbed

1 small mooli (Japanese white radish), about 170 g (6 oz), peeled and thinly sliced

115 g (4 oz) red radishes, cut into quarters

2 ripe but firm dessert pears

1 Oak Leaf lettuce, separated into leaves

100 g (3½ oz) watercress, tough stalks discarded

340 g (12 oz) roast pork loin, fat removed and thinly sliced

Mustard and ginger dressing

30 g (1 oz) fresh root ginger, peeled and finely chopped

2 tsp wholegrain mustard

2 tsp white wine vinegar

1 tbsp groundnut oil

1 tbsp hazelnut oil

salt and pepper

1 Heat a frying pan and toast the pecan nuts over a moderate heat for 6–7 minutes. Cool, then chop roughly. Set aside.

2 Cook the potatoes in a saucepan of boiling water for 15 minutes or until tender. Drain. When cool enough to handle, cut into quarters and place in a mixing bowl.

3 To make the dressing, first put the ginger in a garlic crusher and press to squeeze out the juice (this will have to be done in 3 or 4 batches). You need 2 tsp of this ginger juice. Put the ginger juice, mustard, vinegar, groundnut and hazelnut oils, and seasoning to taste, in a screwtop jar. Shake well to mix. Pour about a third of the dressing over the warm potatoes and toss gently to coat. Leave to cool.

4 Meanwhile, in another bowl, toss the mooli and red radishes with half of the remaining dressing, to prevent them from browning. Halve the pears lengthways and scoop out the cores, then cut into long wedges. Toss with the mooli and radishes.

5 Arrange the lettuce leaves and watercress in a shallow salad bowl. Add the mooli mixture to the potatoes and gently mix together. Pile onto the middle of the salad leaves, and arrange the pork slices on top.

6 Stir the toasted pecans into the remaining dressing and drizzle over the top of the salad. Serve immediately.

Some more ideas

Instead of pears, use other fresh fruit such as 2 peaches or 4 apricots, or 30 g (1 oz) chopped ready-to-eat dried apricots soaked in a little orange or apple juice to soften them.

For a **pork and apple salad with hazelnuts**, replace the pears with red-skinned dessert apples. Instead of mooli and red radishes, cut 150 g (5½ oz) each celeriac and carrots into 5 cm (2 in) long matchstick strips. Finish with toasted hazelnuts instead of pecans.

Plus points

• Pork provides many B vitamins – excellent amounts of B_{12} and good amounts of B_1 and B_6 – and it is a good source of zinc.

• Radishes offer useful amounts of fibre and vitamin C and, in common with other members of the cruciferous family, they contain phytochemicals that may help to protect against cancer. Most of the enzymes responsible for the hot taste are found in the skin – if you find the taste overpowering, peeling will help to reduce the heat.

Each serving provides kcal 511, protein 37 g, fat 20.5 g (of which saturated fat 4 g), carbohydrate 48 g (of which sugars 14 g), fibre 6 g. Excellent source of folate, niacin, vitamin B_1, vitamin B_6, vitamin B_{12}, zinc. Good source of copper, potassium, selenium, vitamin B_2. Useful source of calcium, iron, vitamin A.

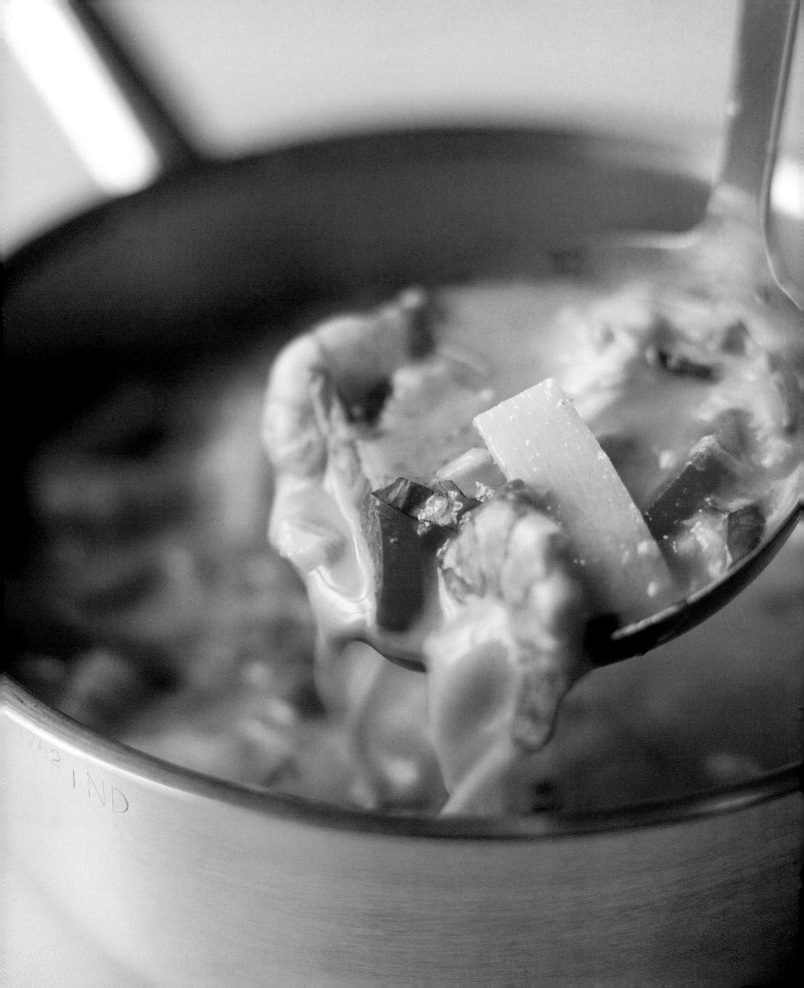

Soups and stews

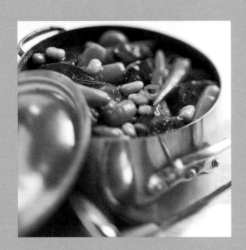

Chicken stock

After roasting a chicken, the bones can be used to make a delicious stock. The flavour from the bones seeps into the simmering stock, creating a rich home-made base for soups or meat dishes. Small bits of meat may come off the bones, flavouring the stock even more.

Preparation time **10 minutes**   Cooking time **about 2 hours**   *Makes about 1.4 litres (2½ pints)*

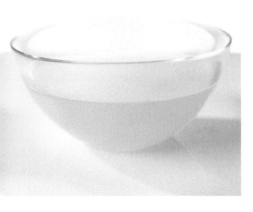

1 chicken carcass or the bones from 4 chicken pieces, cooked or raw, or 1 raw chicken leg quarter, about 250 g (8½ oz)

1 onion, quartered

1 large carrot, roughly chopped

1 celery stick, cut into chunks

1 bay leaf

1 sprig of parsley, stalk bruised

1 sprig of fresh thyme

8 black peppercorns

½ tsp salt

1 Break up the chicken carcass or bones; leave the leg joint whole. Place in a large saucepan. Add the onion, carrot and celery. Pour in 2 litres (3½ pints) water and bring to the boil over a high heat, skimming off any scum from the surface.

2 Add the bay leaf, parsley, thyme, peppercorns and salt. Reduce the heat, cover and simmer gently for 2 hours.

3 Strain the stock through a sieve into a heatproof bowl, discarding the bones or joint and vegetables. Cool and chill the stock, then skim off any fat that sets on the surface.

Some more ideas

To make turkey stock, use a turkey carcass. For game stock, use the carcass from 1–2 cooked game birds.

Plus points

• Canned chicken broth and chicken bouillon are very high in sodium. By making your own natural stock, the amount of salt added can be controlled. Even though it may take a little time to prepare the home-made stock, it is a much healthier choice.

• Canned chicken broth and bouillon powder also may contain monosodium glutamate (MSG), which is a powdered flavour enhancer derived from glutamic acid. Many people are sensitive to MSG and experience headaches and dizziness after consuming the additive.

Note: Home-made stocks, such as this one, contain some calories (approximately 33 kcal per pint) and a small amount of fat (3–4 g per 500 ml/1 pint), but also contribute beneficial nutrients.

Quick chicken soup

This bright and easy recipe is perfect for a quick lunch or supper. Red pepper, sweetcorn and a sprinkling of fresh greens bring colour and texture to a simple chicken soup base, and adding a little sherry makes it taste just that bit more special. With seeded bread rolls it makes a tasty light meal.

Preparation time **10 minutes**   Cooking time **about 15 minutes**   *Serves 4*

900 ml (1½ pints) boiling water

2 chicken stock cubes, crumbled

1 red pepper, seeded and cut into fine strips

125 g (4½ oz) frozen sweetcorn

225 g (8 oz) skinless boneless chicken breasts (fillets), cut into short 1 cm (½ in) strips

125 g (4½ oz) purple sprouting broccoli, cut into small pieces, or spring greens, finely shredded

2 tbsp medium sherry

3 tbsp snipped fresh chives

3 tbsp chopped fresh tarragon

salt and pepper

1 Pour the water into a large saucepan. Add the stock cubes and whisk over a high heat until the stock boils. Add the red pepper strips and sweetcorn. Bring back to the boil, then add the chicken strips and immediately reduce the heat to low. Cover and simmer gently for 5 minutes.

2 Uncover the pan and bring the soup back to the boil. Sprinkle the sprouting broccoli or spring greens into the soup, but do not stir them in. Leave the broccoli or greens to cook on the surface of the soup, uncovered, for 3–4 minutes until just tender.

3 Take the pan off the heat. Stir in the sherry, chives, tarragon and seasoning to taste. Serve at once.

Some more ideas

A generous amount of fresh tarragon gives this soup a powerful flavour. For a delicate result use 1 tbsp tarragon or use chervil instead.

Use Savoy cabbage or curly kale instead of the greens. Trim off any very thick stalks before shredding the cabbage or kale.

To give the soup a Chinese flavour, omit the salt and marinate the chicken strips in a mixture of 2 tbsp soy sauce, 2 tbsp rice wine or dry sherry and 2 tsp grated fresh root ginger for 10 minutes while you prepare the vegetables. Use pak choy instead of purple sprouting broccoli or spring greens. Slice the thick white stalks lengthways and the green tops across into ribbon strips. Add the white strips in step 2 and cook for 1 minute, then add the green tops and 2 chopped spring onions. Cook for 2–3 minutes.

Fine strips of lean boneless pork can be used instead of chicken.

Add 75 g (2½ oz) dried thin egg noodles to make the soup more substantial. Crush the noodles and stir them into the soup in step 2 and bring to the boil before adding the greens.

Plus points

• Sweetcorn adds carbohydrate and dietary fibre to the soup. Green vegetables are also a good source of fibre, which is thought to reduce the risk of cancer of the colon.

• In this fast recipe, cutting fresh broccoli in small pieces and greens in fine strips means they cook quickly to retain as much of their vitamin C as possible.

• Red pepper is an excellent source of vitamin C, as well as beta-carotene and bioflavonoids.

photo, page 215

Each serving provides   kcal 140, protein 16 g, fat 4 g (of which saturated fat 1 g), carbohydrate 10 g (of which sugars 5 g), fibre 2 g. Good source of vitamin A, vitamin C. Useful source of niacin, vitamin B$_6$.

Chicken and potato chowder

The simple, delicious flavours of this soup will make it popular with all the family. Try it for lunch at the weekend, served with plenty of crusty bread and fresh fruit to follow.

Preparation time **20 minutes**   Cooking time **about 50 minutes**   *Serves 4*

1 tbsp extra virgin olive oil

2 lean smoked back bacon rashers, rinded and finely chopped

1 chicken thigh, about 140 g (5 oz), skinned

2 onions, finely chopped

500 g (1 lb 2 oz) potatoes, peeled and diced

750 ml (1¼ pints) chicken stock, preferably home-made (see page 212)

leaves from 4 sprigs of fresh thyme or ½ tsp dried thyme

300 ml (10 fl oz) semi-skimmed milk

salt and pepper

chopped parsley, or a mixture of chopped parsley and fresh thyme, to garnish

1 Heat the oil in a large saucepan. Add the bacon, chicken and onions, and cook over a low heat for 3 minutes. Increase the heat and cook for a further 5 minutes, stirring the ingredients occasionally and turning the chicken once, until the chicken is pale golden.

2 Add the potatoes and cook for 2 minutes, stirring all the time. Pour in the stock, then add the thyme and seasoning to taste. Bring to the boil. Reduce the heat, cover the pan and leave to simmer for 30 minutes.

3 Using a draining spoon, transfer the chicken to a plate. Remove and chop the meat and discard the bone. Return the chicken to the soup. Stir in the milk and reheat the soup gently without boiling.

4 Ladle the soup into bowls and garnish with chopped parsley or parsley and thyme. Serve at once.

Some more ideas

For a smooth result, purée the soup in a blender or food processor before reheating in step 3.

Garlic is delicious in potato soups – add 2–3 chopped garlic cloves with the potatoes.

A pinch of grated nutmeg could also be stirred in with, or instead of, the thyme.

Boost the vitamin C and iron content with watercress. Add 75 g (2½ oz) watercress sprigs and the juice of 1 lemon with the chopped cooked chicken and purée the soup until smooth. Stir in the milk, adding an extra 150 ml (5 fl oz). Reheat the soup and serve, swirling 1 tbsp single cream in each bowl.

For a **winter vegetable soup** use 800 g (1¾ lb) mixed diced leeks (white and pale green parts), carrot and swede instead of the onions and potatoes. Finely chop the green tops from the leeks, and add them to the soup with the milk at the end of cooking.

Plus points

• Potatoes undeservedly have a reputation for being fattening. In fact, they are rich in complex carbohydrate and low in fat, making them satisfying without being highly calorific. They also provide useful amounts of vitamin C and potassium, and good amounts of fibre.

• Onions contain a phytochemical called allicin, that is thought to help to reduce the risk of cancer and also of blood clots forming, helping to prevent coronary heart disease.

Each serving provides   kcal 220, protein 12 g, fat 6 g (of which saturated fat 2 g), carbohydrate 30 g (of which sugars 9 g). Good source of calcium, potassium, vitamin B_1, vitamin B_6, vitamin B_{12}, vitamin C. Useful source of copper, iron, niacin, vitamin B_2, zinc.

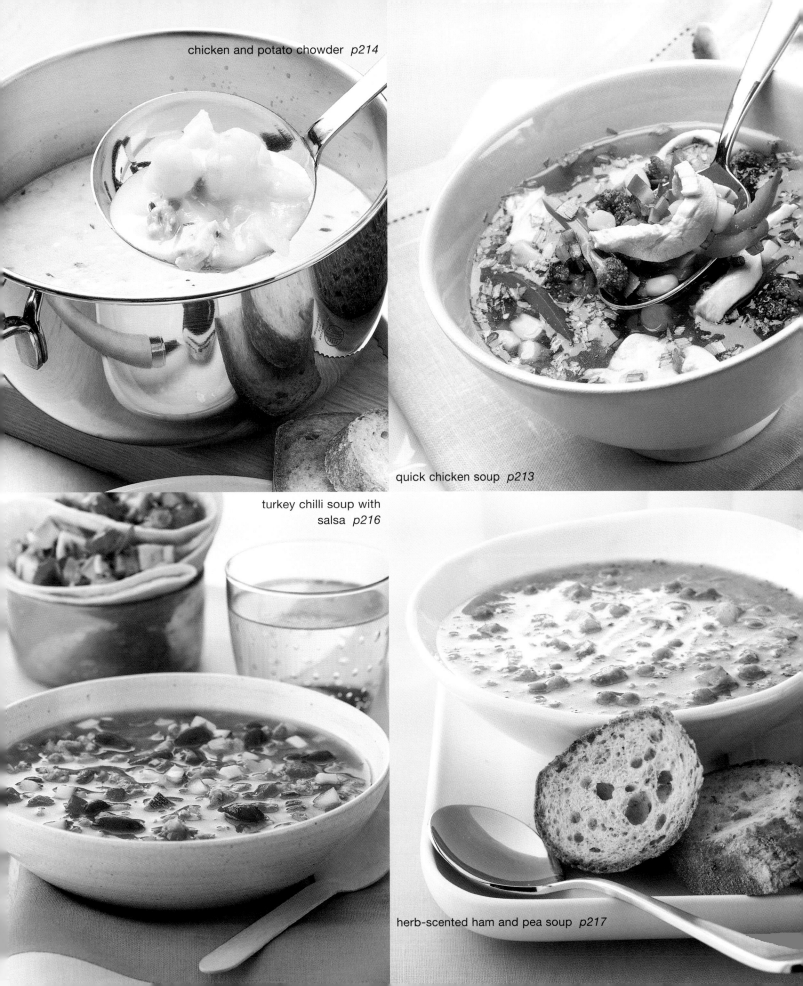

chicken and potato chowder *p214*

quick chicken soup *p213*

turkey chilli soup with salsa *p216*

herb-scented ham and pea soup *p217*

Turkey chilli soup with salsa

This colourful soup is inspired by the spicy and complex flavours of chilli con carne. Full of delicious vegetables and served with tortillas and a refreshing salsa, it makes a healthy main course that is fun to eat.

Preparation time **35 minutes**   Cooking time **50 minutes**   *Serves 6*

2 tsp extra virgin olive oil

450 g (1 lb) minced turkey

1 onion, finely chopped

2 celery sticks, finely chopped

1 red or yellow pepper, seeded and finely chopped

3 garlic cloves, finely chopped

1 can chopped tomatoes, about 400 g

1 litre (1¾ pints) turkey or chicken stock, preferably home-made (see page 212)

¼ tsp ground coriander

¼ tsp ground cumin

¼ tsp dried oregano

½ tsp chilli powder, or to taste

200 g (7 oz) courgettes, diced

150 g (5½ oz) fresh or frozen sweetcorn, thawed if necessary

1 can borlotti or kidney beans, about 400 g, drained and rinsed

salt and pepper

12 flour tortillas to serve (1 packet, about 312 g)

Avocado salsa

2 tbsp fresh lime juice

2 avocados

1 Heat the oil in a large saucepan over a high heat. Add the turkey and cook for about 4 minutes, stirring occasionally, until lightly browned. Reduce the heat to moderate and add the onion, celery, pepper and garlic. Continue cooking, stirring often, for about 2 minutes or until the onion begins to soften. Stir in the tomatoes with the juice from the can, the stock, coriander, cumin, oregano and chilli powder. Bring to the boil, then reduce the heat to low, cover the pan and simmer for 20 minutes.

2 Preheat the oven to 160°C (325°F, gas mark 3). Add the courgettes, sweetcorn and borlotti or kidney beans to the soup. Bring back to the boil, then reduce the heat to low and cover the pan again. Simmer the soup for a further 10 minutes or until the courgettes are just tender.

3 Meanwhile, wrap the stack of tortillas tightly in foil and heat in the oven for about 10 minutes or until warmed through and soft.

4 To make the salsa, place the lime juice in a bowl. Halve, stone, peel and dice the avocados, then add to the bowl and toss them in the lime juice. Gently mix in the tomatoes, spring onions and rocket, adding seasoning to taste. Take care not to break up the diced avocados.

5 Season the soup with a little salt and pepper to taste. Ladle the soup into warm bowls and serve. Spoon the salsa on top of the soup or eat it, wrapped in the warm tortillas, as an accompaniment.

Plus points

● Beans and pulses are a good source of dietary fibre, particularly soluble fibre which can help to reduce high blood cholesterol and blood glucose levels. They also provide useful amounts of vitamin B_1 and iron.

● Vitamin C from the salsa will help the body to absorb iron from the beans.

● Avocados are rich in vitamin B_6, which is vital for making the 'feel-good' hormone serotonin. They also provide the antioxidant vitamin E which can help to protect against heart disease.

photo, page 215

Each serving provides   kcal 400, protein 28 g, fat 11 g (of which saturated fat 2 g), carbohydrate 51 g (of which sugars 10 g), fibre 8 g. Excellent source of vitamin A, vitamin C. Good source of vitamin B_1, vitamin B_2, vitamin B_6 and vitamin B_{12}. Useful source of folate, iron, niacin, selenium, vitamin E.

Herb-scented ham and pea soup

A hint of cream makes this fresh green soup seem delightfully indulgent. The high proportion of peas fills the soup with vitamins and fibre, while a modest amount of lean cooked ham adds protein and depth of flavour. Serve with crusty bread for a satisfying starter or add a sandwich and enjoy it for lunch.

Preparation time **about 15 minutes**   Cooking time **about 1 hour**   *Serves 4*

1 tbsp extra virgin olive oil

1 onion, chopped

1 small carrot, diced

2 garlic cloves, sliced

1 leek, chopped

1 celery stick, diced

2 tbsp chopped parsley

1 potato, peeled and diced

100 g (3½ oz) lean boiled or baked ham, diced

500 g (1 lb 2 oz) shelled fresh or frozen peas

½ tsp dried herbes de Provence, or to taste

1 litre (1¾ pints) vegetable stock, preferably home-made light (see page 224), or a mix-ture of half stock and half water

3 large lettuce leaves, finely shredded

2 tbsp whipping cream

salt and pepper

1 Heat the oil in a saucepan. Add the onion, carrot, garlic, leek, celery, parsley, potato and ham. Stir well, then cover the pan, reduce the heat and sweat the vegetables for about 30 minutes or until they are softened. Stir the vegetables occasionally so that they cook evenly.

2 Add the peas, herbes de Provence and stock, or stock and water. Bring to the boil, then reduce the heat to moderately high and cook until the peas are just tender – allow about 10 minutes for fresh peas or 5 minutes for frozen. Add the lettuce and cook gently for a further 5 minutes.

3 Purée half to two-thirds of the soup in a blender, then stir the purée back into the rest of the soup. Alternatively, use a hand-held blender to partly purée the soup in the pan. Reheat the soup gently, if necessary, and taste and adjust the seasoning. Ladle the soup into warm bowls. Swirl a little cream into each portion and serve at once.

Some more ideas

For a more substantial soup, add a generous spoonful of freshly cooked rice or vermicelli to each bowl.

For a **split pea soup**, use 140 g (5 oz) dried split peas (yellow or green) instead of fresh or frozen peas. Add 125 g (4½ oz) peeled, diced celeriac, ¼ tsp ground cumin and a few shakes of chilli sauce, such as Tabasco, to the vegetables and ham in step 1. Increase the volume of stock to 1.5 litres (2¾ pints), and simmer for 1–1½ hours or until the peas are tender. Omit the lettuce and whipping cream. Purée all the soup until smooth. Add pepper to taste and reheat.

Plus points

• Throughout history garlic has been used to treat everything from athlete's foot to colds and flu. Scientific facts now give credence to the folklore – for example, allicin, the compound that gives garlic its characteristic smell and taste, is known to act as a powerful antibiotic and it also has anti-viral and anti-fungal properties.

• Peas are a good source of the B vitamins B_1 B_6, and niacin, and they provide useful amounts of folate and vitamin C. As a good source of soluble fibre, they are useful for anyone with high cholesterol levels.

photo, page 215

Each serving provides   kcal 250, protein 16 g, fat 17 g, fat 8 g (of which saturated fat 3 g), carbohydrate 30 g (of which sugars 7 g), fibre 8 g. Excellent source of folate, vitamin A, vitamin B_1, vitamin B_6, vitamin C. Good source of iron, potassium, zinc. Useful source of calcium, copper, niacin.

Fish soup with pepper polenta

Good stock provides the flavour base for this delicate broth. If you are not making your own low-salt stock, try a high-quality commercial stock sold chilled, rather than a stock cube, but still keep added salt to the minimum. The polenta accompaniment is prepared in advance, so the soup is simple to cook at the last minute.

Preparation and cooking time **about 1½ hours**, plus **about 1½ hours** cooling and **10–20 minutes** infusing   *Serves 4*

900 ml (1½ pints) fish stock

1 bay leaf

1 sprig of parsley

1 sprig of fresh thyme

2 celery sticks, thinly sliced

1 bulb of fennel, quartered lengthways and thinly sliced

2 carrots, halved lengthways and thinly sliced

zest of 1 lemon, finely shredded or coarsely grated

1 shallot, finely chopped

1 garlic clove, finely chopped

1 fresh red chilli, halved and seeded (optional)

225 g (8 oz) monkfish fillet, cut into bite-sized chunks

225 g (8 oz) skinless white fish fillet, such as cod or haddock, cut into bite-sized chunks

salt and pepper

leaves from the fennel bulb, herb fennel or fresh dill to garnish

Pepper polenta sticks

2 red peppers, halved lengthways and seeded

½ tsp salt

200 g (7 oz) instant polenta

45 g (1½ oz) Parmesan cheese, freshly grated

1 Prepare the polenta sticks in advance. Preheat the grill to high. Place the pepper halves on the grill rack, cut sides down, and grill for 10 minutes or until the skin is charred all over. To make them easy to peel, transfer them to a polythene bag and leave to stand for 15 minutes or until cool enough to handle. Peel the peppers and cut lengthways into 5 mm (¼ in) wide strips. Set aside.

2 Cook the polenta with the salt according to the instructions on the packet. Continue to cook, stirring constantly, until it is thick.

3 Sprinkle a plastic chopping board or tray with water and turn the polenta out onto it. Use a wet palette knife to spread out the polenta into a rectangle about 1 cm (½ in) thick. Arrange the strips of pepper diagonally on top, gently pressing them into the polenta. Wet a sharp knife and use this to trim and neaten the edges of the polenta rectangle. Leave to cool.

4 Preheat the oven to 200°C (400°F, gas mark 6) and grease a baking tray. Sprinkle the Parmesan cheese over the polenta and cut it into 16 sticks. Transfer the polenta sticks to the baking tray and bake for 15 minutes or until the cheese is melted and bubbling. Leave to cool for 2 minutes, then transfer to a wire rack and leave to cool completely.

5 For the soup, pour the stock into a saucepan. Tie the bay leaf, parsley and thyme together into a bouquet garni and add to the pan with celery, fennel, carrots, lemon zest, shallot, garlic and chilli, if using. Heat gently until boiling, then leave to simmer for 5 minutes or until the vegetables are slightly tender. Cover the pan and remove it from the heat. Leave to stand for 10–20 minutes so the flavours can infuse the liquid.

Each serving provides kcal 370, protein 29 g, fat 6 g, (of which saturated fat 2 g), carbohydrate 47 g (of which sugars 10 g). Excellent source of vitamin A, vitamin C. Good source of folate, potassium, vitamin B_{12}. Useful source of selenium, vitamin B_1.

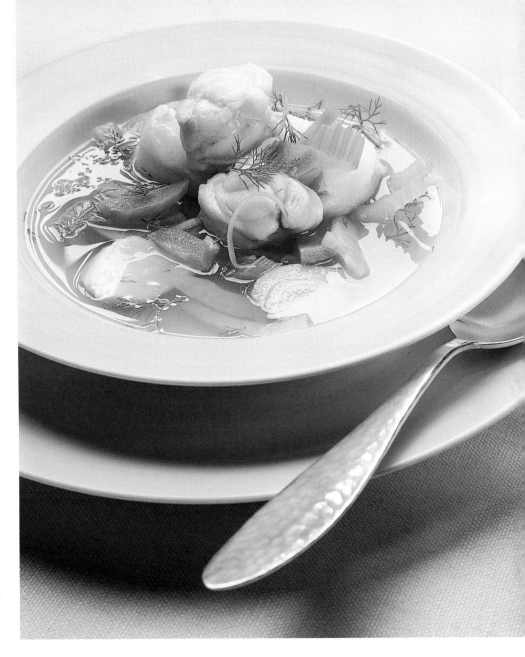

6 Remove and discard the bouquet garni and chilli halves. Bring the liquid back to the boil. Reduce the heat, add the monkfish and white fish, and poach for about 4 minutes or until all the fish chunks are opaque and will flake easily. Season with salt and pepper to taste.

7 Transfer the polenta sticks to a serving plate. Ladle the soup into warmed bowls and sprinkle with the fennel leaves or dill. Serve at once.

Another idea

For **mushroom polenta**, cook 170 g (6 oz) sliced mushrooms with 1 crushed garlic clove and 1 tbsp chopped shallot in 1 tbsp extra virgin olive oil for about 5 minutes. Add 1 tbsp snipped fresh chives and spread over the polenta sticks. Sprinkle 2 tbsp freshly grated Parmesan cheese over the mushrooms and brown under the grill instead of baking.

Plus points

● Celery and fennel provide potassium. Celery also acts as a diuretic, helping to reduce fluid and salt retention.

● Like other white fish, cod, haddock and monkfish are very low in fat and calories.

Hearty mussel soup

This soup tastes fabulous. The diced potatoes absorb the flavours from the herbs and vegetables to make a mellow complement to the mussels. Warm soda bread is an ideal partner, delicious for dunking and mopping up the last of the soup. To complete the meal, serve a light, fruity dessert for a refreshing, vitamin-packed finale.

Preparation time **30 minutes**   Cooking time **40–50 minutes**   *Serves 4*

1 kg (2¼ lb) mussels in shells, scrubbed

2 tbsp extra virgin olive oil

1 onion, finely chopped

2 garlic cloves, finely chopped

2 leeks, thinly sliced

3 celery sticks, thinly sliced

2 carrots, diced

400 g (14 oz) potatoes, peeled and cut into small cubes

900 ml (1½ pints) vegetable stock, preferably home-made light (see page 23)

150 ml (5 fl oz) dry white wine

1 tbsp lemon juice

1 bay leaf

1 sprig of fresh thyme

4 tbsp chopped parsley

2 tbsp snipped fresh chives

salt and pepper

1 Prepare the mussels: discard any broken shells or shells that do not close when tapped. Put the wet mussels into a clean saucepan and cover tightly. Cook over medium heat for 4 minutes, shaking the pan occasionally. Check that the mussels have opened – if not, cover and cook for a further 1–2 minutes. Drain the mussels, reserving the juices that have come from the shells. Reserve a few mussels in their shells for garnish; remove the remainder from their shells and set aside. Discard the shells and any unopened mussels.

2 Heat the oil in the rinsed-out saucepan. Add the onion, garlic, leeks, celery and carrots, and cook gently for 5–10 minutes, stirring frequently, until the vegetables are softened but not browned. Add the potatoes, stock, wine, reserved juices from the mussels, lemon juice, bay leaf, thyme and salt and pepper to taste. Bring to the boil, then reduce the heat to low. Cover the pan and simmer the soup gently for 20–30 minutes or until all the vegetables are tender.

3 Remove the bay leaf and thyme, then add the shelled mussels, parsley and chives to the pan. Heat gently for about 1 minute. Do not allow the soup to boil or cook for any longer than this or the mussels will become tough and shrink.

4 Ladle the soup into warm bowls and garnish with the reserved mussels in shells. Serve at once, while piping hot.

Another idea

Cooked fresh mussels are available in most supermarkets, usually vacuum packed and displayed in chiller cabinets. Use 300 g (10½ oz) shelled mussels. Alternatively, use 2 cans mussels in brine, each about 250 g, or 4 cans smoked mussels in vegetable oil, each about 85 g. Drain the canned mussels and pat dry before adding them to the soup.

Plus points

• Like other shellfish, mussels are a good low-fat source of protein. They are an extremely good source of vitamin B_{12} and provide useful amounts of copper, iodine, iron, phosphorus and zinc.

• Vitamin C from the potatoes, parsley and chives aids the absorption of iron from the mussels.

• Celery is said to have a calming effect on the nerves.

photo, page 223

Each serving provides   kcal 260, protein 17 g, fat 8 g (of which saturated fat 1 g), carbohydrate 24 g (of which sugars 7 g). Excellent source of vitamin A. Good source of folate, vitamin B_6, vitamin B_{12}, vitamin C. Useful source of vitamin B_1, vitamin B_2, selenium.

King prawn bisque

This classic seafood soup is ideal for a special first course. A last-minute addition of chopped red pepper brings a delightful flourish of flavour, texture and extra vitamins instead of the fat in the traditional swirl of cream.

Preparation time **about 45 minutes**, plus cooling   Cooking time **about 35 minutes**   *Serves 6*

450 g (1 lb) raw king prawns, without heads

4 tbsp dry white wine

4 slices of lemon

4 black peppercorns, lightly crushed

2 sprigs of parsley, stalks bruised

1 bulb of fennel

1 tsp lemon juice

15 g (½ oz) butter

1 tbsp sunflower oil

1 shallot, finely chopped

45 g (1½ oz) fine white bread-crumbs, made from day-old slices of bread

pinch of paprika

1 red pepper, seeded and finely diced

salt and pepper

chopped leaves from the fennel bulb, or herb fennel, to garnish

1 Peel the prawns and set aside. Place the shells in a large saucepan. Pour in 1.2 litres (2 pints) cold water and add the white wine, lemon slices, peppercorns and parsley. Bring to the boil, then reduce the heat and simmer for 20 minutes. Skim off any scum that rises to the surface during cooking.

2 Use a small sharp knife to make a shallow slit along the curved back of each prawn. With the tip of the knife remove the black vein and discard it. Cover and chill the prawns until required.

3 Allow the prawn-shell stock to cool slightly, then pick out and discard the lemon slices. Line a sieve with muslin and place it over a large bowl or measuring jug. Process the stock in a blender or food processor until the shells are finely ground, then strain through the muslin-lined sieve. Discard the residue from the shells.

4 Coarsely chop 85 g (3 oz) of the fennel, and finely chop the remainder of the bulb. Place the finely chopped fennel in a bowl, add the lemon juice and toss well, then cover closely with cling film and set aside.

5 Melt the butter with the oil in the rinsed-out saucepan. Add the coarsely chopped fennel and the shallot. Cook, stirring frequently, over a moderate heat for about

8 minutes or until the vegetables are soft but not browned. Stir in the breadcrumbs, paprika and stock. Bring slowly to the boil, then reduce the heat so that the soup simmers. Add the prawns and continue simmering for 3 minutes.

6 Use tongs or a draining spoon to remove 6 prawns for garnishing the soup. Set them aside. Season the soup with salt and pepper to taste and simmer for a further 15 minutes.

7 Purée the soup in a blender or food processor until smooth. Return to the pan and add the finely chopped fennel and the red pepper. Reheat the soup until piping hot. Serve garnished with the reserved prawns and chopped fennel leaves.

Plus points

● Prawns are a good source of low-fat protein. They are an excellent source of vitamin B_{12}, selenium and phosphorus.

● Making the stock with the prawn shells gives the bisque a full flavour, and at the same time boosts its calcium content.

photo, page 223

Each serving provides kcal 165, protein 8 g, fat 6 g (of which saturated fat 2 g), carbohydrate 9 g (of which sugars 3 g), fibre 1 g. Excellent source of phosphorus, selenium, vitamin A, vitamin B_6, vitamin B_{12}, vitamin C. Good source of copper, iron, zinc. Useful source of calcium, folate, potassium, vitamin B_2.

Piquant cod chowder

A variety of vegetables ensures that this wonderful soup is as healthy as it is delicious. The broth can be prepared a day in advance, ready for adding the fish at the last minute, which is useful when cooking mid-week meals. Planning ahead like this means a healthy dinner can be on the table in minutes.

Preparation time **about 20 minutes**   Cooking time **about 40 minutes**   *Serves 4*

2 sprigs each of parsley and fresh thyme

1 bay leaf

7.5 cm (3 in) piece of celery stick

1 can chopped tomatoes, about 400 g

750 ml (1¼ pints) fish stock

4 tbsp medium cider

1 large onion, chopped

400 g (14 oz) waxy potatoes, cut into large chunks

225 g (8 oz) carrots, thickly sliced

225 g (8 oz) courgettes, thickly sliced

225 g (8 oz) green beans, cut into short lengths

1 yellow or red pepper, seeded and sliced

550 g (1¼ lb) cod fillet, skinned and cut into large pieces

salt and pepper

To garnish

2 tbsp finely chopped parsley

1 tbsp snipped fresh chives

finely shredded zest of 1 lemon

1 Tie the parsley, thyme and bay leaf with the celery to make a bouquet garni. Put the bouquet garni in a large saucepan. Add the tomatoes and their juice, the stock, cider and onion, stir and bring to the boil. Reduce the heat to low, half cover the pan and simmer for 15 minutes.

2 Add the potatoes and carrots. Increase the heat to moderate and cook, covered, for 15 minutes or until the vegetables are almost tender. Stir in the courgettes, green beans and yellow or red pepper and continue simmering, covered, for 5 minutes or until all the vegetables are tender. Discard the bouquet garni.

3 Season with salt and pepper to taste, then add the cod to the gently simmering broth. Cover and cook gently for 3–5 minutes or until the fish is opaque, just firm and flakes easily. Do not allow the broth to boil rapidly or the fish will overcook and start to break up.

4 For the garnish, mix the parsley, chives and lemon zest together. Ladle the fish and vegetables into warm bowls, then add the broth. Sprinkle the garnish over the top and serve at once.

Some more ideas

Ring the changes by using different vegetables – broccoli florets, sliced leeks, sweetcorn, peas and green peppers are all suitable. Add them instead of the courgettes, green beans and yellow pepper in step 2.

Plus points

• Serving wholemeal rolls with the soup will add to the dietary fibre provided by all the vegetables.

• Green beans are a good source of fibre and they also provide valuable amounts of folate.

• One serving of this soup can provide 3 of the recommended 5 portions of fruit and vegetables a day.

Each serving provides   kcal 290, protein 33 g, fat 2.5 g (of which saturated fat 0.5 g), carbohydrate 35 g (of which sugars 16 g), fibre 7 g. Excellent source of vitamin B_6, vitamin B_{12}, vitamin C. Good source of folate, iron, potassium, vitamin A. Useful source of calcium, niacin, selenium.

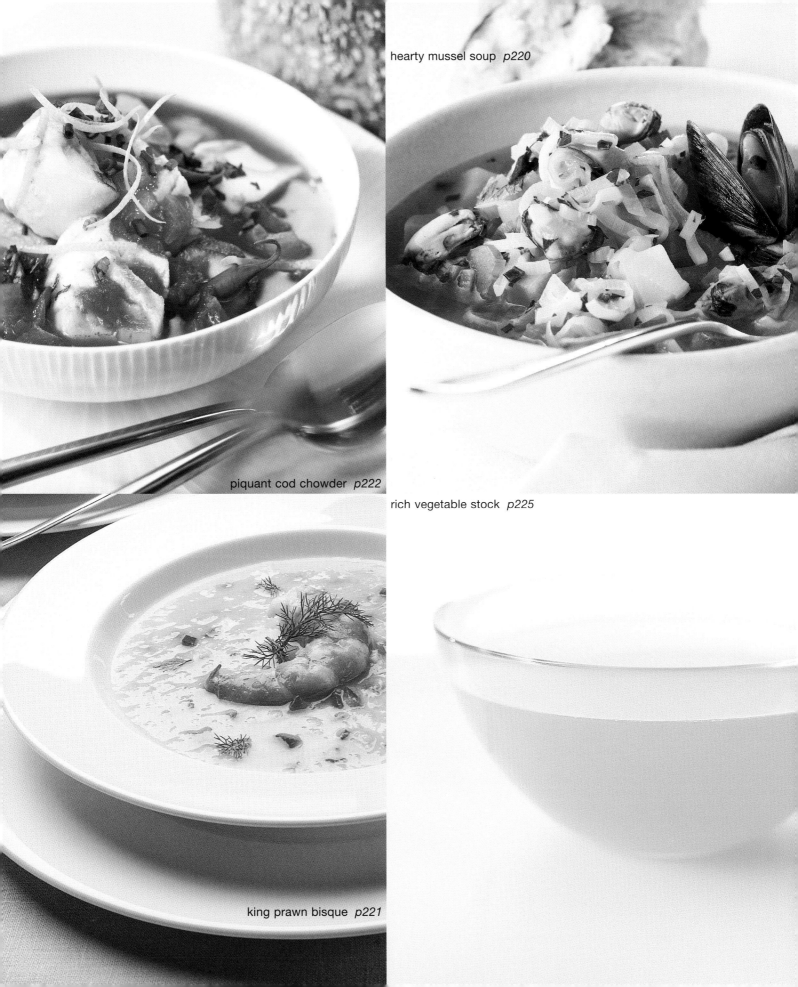

hearty mussel soup *p220*

piquant cod chowder *p222*

rich vegetable stock *p225*

king prawn bisque *p221*

Light vegetable stock

This light stock is suitable for vegetarian dishes and for fish, poultry or meat recipes when a delicate flavour is required.

Preparation time **15 minutes**   Cooking time **about 1 hour**   *Makes about 1.7 litres (3 pints)*

1 tbsp sunflower oil

225 g (8 oz) leeks, chopped

1 large onion, chopped

1 large bay leaf

several sprigs of fresh thyme

several sprigs of parsley, stalks bruised

225 g (8 oz) carrots, diced

3 large celery sticks with any leaves, diced

½ tsp salt

5 black peppercorns

1 Heat the oil in a large heavy-based saucepan or stockpot. Add the leeks and onion, stir well and reduce the heat to low. Cover with a tight-fitting lid and leave the vegetables to sweat for about 20 minutes, shaking the pan occasionally but without lifting the lid.

2 Add the bay leaf, thyme, parsley, carrots, celery and salt. Pour in 2 litres (3½ pints) cold water and increase the heat to high. Bring slowly to the boil, skimming the surface of the liquid to remove any scum.

3 As soon as the water boils and all the scum has been removed, add the peppercorns and reduce the heat to low. Cover and simmer for 35 minutes.

4 Strain the stock into a large, heatproof bowl and set it aside to cool. Use at once or cool and then chill until required.

Plus point

- Because this stock is mild and has a light flavour, it works well when used as a cooking liquid for rice and pasta and adds useful nutrients to the meal.

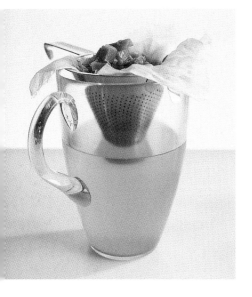

Note: Home-made stocks, such as these, contain some calories (approximately 33 kcal per pint) and a small amount of fat (3–4 g per 500 ml/1 pint), but also contribute beneficial nutrients.

Rich vegetable stock

This stock is excellent in meat soups and casseroles, and is ideal for hearty vegetarian recipes. It is easy to prepare and can be stored in the refrigerator for several days for use in a variety of dishes.

Preparation time **55 minutes**   Cooking time **55 minutes**   *Makes about 1.7 litres (3 pints)*

125 g (4½ oz) whole wheat grains

1 tbsp sunflower oil

125 g (4½ oz) dark flat mushrooms, chopped

2 onions, chopped

3 carrots, chopped

3 celery sticks, chopped

1 sprig of parsley, stalk bruised

1 sprig of fresh thyme

1 sprig of fresh marjoram

2 bay leaves

8 black peppercorns

½ tsp salt

1 Preheat the oven to 180ºC (350ºF, gas mark 4). Put the wheat in a roasting tin and roast for 30 minutes or until the grains are dark brown.

2 Heat the oil in a large heavy-based saucepan over a low heat. Add the mushrooms and onions and stir to coat them in the oil. Cover the pan and sweat the vegetables for 5 minutes, shaking the pan occasionally.

3 Stir in the roasted wheat, carrots and celery. Pour in 2 litres (3½ pints) water, increase the heat to high and bring to the boil, skimming off any scum that rises to the surface.

4 Reduce the heat. Add the parsley, thyme, marjoram, bay leaves, peppercorns and salt. Cover the pan and simmer for 45 minutes.

5 Strain the stock through a fine sieve into a heatproof bowl. Use at once or leave to cool, then chill until required.

Some more ideas

Try making herb cubes by adding 1 teaspoon dried herbs (basil, thyme, oregano) to each cube before adding the stock. Store the cubes in the freezer and add them to tomato sauce, soups or pasta dishes as needed.

Plus points

● Freeze the stock in an ice cube tray, then use the cubes individually as needed in place of oil when sautéing vegetables. This eliminates the need for oil and adds flavour to the vegetables as they cook.

photo, page 223

Wild mushroom broth with herby ciabatta croutons

Mixtures of fresh wild mushrooms, widely available in supermarkets, are good for making a quick soup that tastes really special. Instead of thickening or puréeing the soup, serving it as a light broth allows the individual flavours of the mushrooms, vegetables and herbs to be fully appreciated.

Preparation time **10 minutes**   Cooking time **about 20 minutes**   *Serves 6*

3 tbsp extra virgin olive oil

1 small onion, finely chopped

1 small bulb of fennel, finely chopped

1 garlic clove, chopped

500 g (1 lb 2 oz) mixed fresh mushrooms, such as chanterelles (girolles), horns of plenty, oysters and chestnuts, roughly chopped

900 ml (1½ pints) boiling water

1½ vegetable stock cubes, crumbled, or 1 tbsp vegetable bouillon powder or paste

8 thin slices ciabatta bread

2 tbsp chopped parsley

2 tbsp chopped fresh mint

salt and pepper

1 Heat 2 tbsp of the oil in a large saucepan. Add the onion and fennel and cook over a high heat for 5 minutes, stirring frequently, until slightly softened. Stir in the garlic and mushrooms. Continue to cook, stirring frequently, for a further 5 minutes. Pour in the boiling water and stir in the stock cubes, powder or paste. Bring back to the boil, then reduce the heat and simmer the soup, uncovered, for 10 minutes.

2 Meanwhile, preheat the grill. Brush the slices of ciabatta bread lightly on both sides with the remaining 1 tbsp oil and toast them under the grill for about 1 minute on each side or until golden. Cut the bread into cubes and place in a bowl. Add the parsley and mint and toss well.

3 Taste the soup and add seasoning if necessary. Ladle the soup into bowls. Sprinkle with the parsley and mint croutons and serve at once.

Some more ideas

For a rich and creamy version of this soup, thicken with a yolk and cream liaison. Whisk 1 egg yolk with 2 tbsp single cream until lightly mixed. When the soup is cooked and croutons prepared, remove the pan from the heat and stir a ladleful of soup into the liaison.

Pour the mixture into the pan and stir over a low heat for about 30 seconds. Do not allow the soup to get too hot and start to simmer or the egg yolk will curdle. Serve at once.

Use 3 diced celery sticks instead of fennel.

Dried wild mushrooms can be used for this soup, although it will take a bit longer to make. Use 1 packet of dried porcini, about 15 g, and 225 g (8 oz) chestnut mushrooms. Soak the porcini in some of the boiling water for 15 minutes and add them to the soup with the water. Cook the chestnut mushrooms in step 1 with the garlic.

Plus points

● In Asian cultures mushrooms are renowned for their ability to boost the immune system, and the Chinese have put them to medicinal use for over 6000 years. Mushrooms are a useful source of the B vitamins B$_6$, folate and niacin, as well as copper.

● Brushing slices of bread with oil and toasting under the grill before cutting them into cubes is a good way to make low-fat, crisp croutons.

Each serving provides   kcal 95, protein 3 g, fat 5 g (of which saturated fat 1 g), carbohydrate 10 g, (of which sugars 1 g), fibre 1 g. Excellent source of copper, vitamin B$_1$. Good source of niacin, vitamin B$_6$, vitamin C. Useful source of folate.

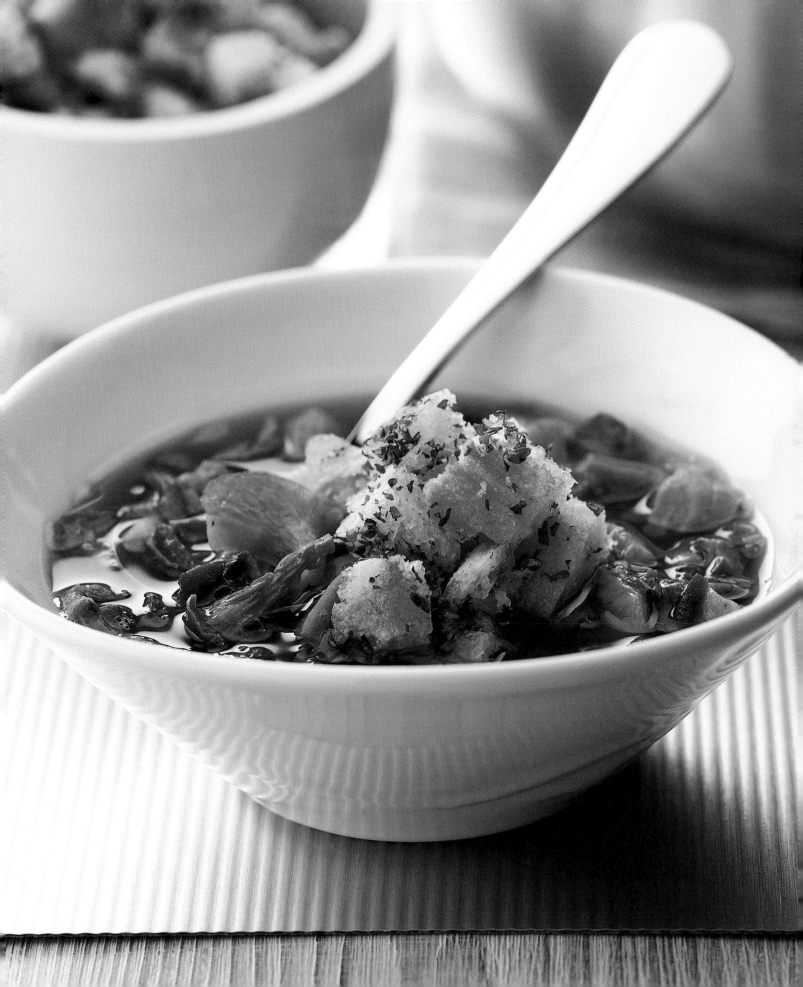

Classic gazpacho

This traditional Spanish soup is full of wonderfully fresh flavours and packed with vitamins as all the vegetables are raw. Cool and refreshing, it is the ideal choice for a simple lunch or midsummer supper, with some seeded country-style bread or rolls. Or serve it as a light starter on a warm evening.

Preparation time **20 minutes**   Chilling time **2 hours**   *Serves 4*

500 g (1 lb 2 oz) full-flavoured tomatoes, quartered and seeded

¼ cucumber, peeled and coarsely chopped

1 red pepper, seeded and coarsely chopped

2 garlic cloves

1 small onion, quartered

1 slice of bread, about 30 g (1 oz), torn into pieces

2 tbsp red wine vinegar

½ tsp salt

2 tbsp extra virgin olive oil

500 ml (17 fl oz) tomato juice

1 tbsp tomato purée

To serve

1 red pepper

4 spring onions

¼ cucumber

2 slices of bread, toasted

1 Mix all the ingredients in a large bowl. Ladle batches of the mixture into a blender and purée until smooth. Pour the soup into a large clean bowl, cover and chill for 2 hours.

2 Prepare the vegetables to serve with the soup towards the end of the chilling time. Seed and finely dice the red pepper; thinly slice the spring onions; and finely dice the cucumber. Cut the toasted bread into small cubes to make croutons. Place these vegetables and croutons in separate serving dishes.

3 Taste the soup and adjust the seasoning, then ladle it into bowls. Serve at once, offering the accompaniments so that they can be added to taste as the soup is eaten.

Some more ideas

In very hot weather, add a few ice cubes to the soup just before serving, to keep it well chilled. This will also slightly dilute it.

To make a **fresh green soup**, use 500 g (1 lb 2 oz) courgettes instead of tomatoes and cucumber. Add 450 ml (15 fl oz) vegetable stock, preferably home-made (see page 224), instead of the tomato juice.

Use a green pepper instead of a red one. Add 15 g (½ oz) fresh basil leaves and 85 g (3 oz) pitted green olives. Mix, purée and chill the soup as above. Serve with a diced green pepper instead of red.

Plus points

● Up to 70 per cent of the water-soluble vitamins – B and C – can be lost in cooking. In this classic soup the vegetables are eaten raw, which means they retain maximum levels of vitamins and minerals.

● Peppers have a naturally waxy skin that helps to protect them against oxidation and prevents loss of vitamin C during storage. As a result their vitamin C content remains high even several weeks after harvesting.

photo, page 231

Each serving provides kcal 215, protein 6 g, fat 9 g (of which saturated fat 1.5 g), carbohydrate 30 g (of which sugars 17 g), fibre 5 g. Excellent source of niacin, potassium, vitamin A, vitamin B$_1$, vitamin B$_6$, vitamin C.

Tomato and red pepper warmer

Sweet red peppers and passata make a beautiful red soup that is sophisticated yet simple to prepare. Swirled with crème fraîche and accompanied by hot pesto bread, it makes a splendid special-occasion starter. For a mid-week supper, garnish the soup with fresh herbs instead of crème fraîche and serve with wholemeal bread.

Preparation time **25 minutes**   Cooking time **25 minutes**   *Serves 6*

1 long French loaf

3 tbsp pesto

1 tbsp extra virgin olive oil

1 onion, coarsely chopped

1 garlic clove, chopped

675 g (1½ lb) red peppers (3–4 peppers, depending on size), seeded and coarsely chopped

300 ml (10 fl oz) vegetable stock, preferably home-made light or rich (see page 224)

300 ml (10 fl oz) passata

1 tsp chopped fresh thyme or ½ tsp dried thyme

¼ tsp ground cinnamon

1 tsp sugar

salt and pepper

To garnish

6 tbsp half-fat crème fraîche

6 sprigs of fresh basil

1 Preheat the oven to 180°C (350°F, gas mark 4). Cut the French loaf across in half so that it will fit into the oven. Cut each half into 3.5 cm (1½ in) thick slices, leaving the slices attached at the base. Hold the slices apart and spread each one thinly with pesto, then press them back together. Wrap the bread in foil and set aside.

2 Heat the oil in a saucepan. Add the onion and garlic and fry gently for 5 minutes or until softened but not browned. Stir in the peppers and cook for a further 5 minutes, stirring occasionally. Pour in the stock and remove from the heat.

3 Place the bread in the oven to heat for 15 minutes. Meanwhile, purée the soup in a blender until smooth. Return the soup to the pan and stir in the passata, thyme, cinnamon and sugar. Heat the soup gently without allowing it to boil. Season to taste.

4 Ladle the soup into warm bowls and garnish each portion with a spoonful of crème fraîche and a sprig of basil. Serve with the hot pesto bread.

Some more ideas
Plain low-fat yogurt or fromage frais can be used instead of crème fraîche.

For a spicy version, add 1 seeded and finely chopped fresh red chilli with the onion, or a dash of Tabasco or other chilli sauce with the final seasoning.

For a **tomato and carrot soup**, use 675 g (1½ lb) diced carrots instead of the red peppers. After the stock is added, cover the pan and simmer the carrots for 10 minutes or until they are tender. Finish as in the main recipe, omitting the sugar.

Plus points
• Red peppers are an excellent source of vitamin C – weight for weight they contain over twice as much vitamin C as oranges. They also provide good amounts of carotenoids and bioflavonoids – both antioxidants that help to protect against heart disease and cancer.

• Tomatoes contain lycopene, a carotenoid compound and a valuable antioxidant that is thought to help protect against prostate cancer. Lycopene is enhanced by cooking and so is most readily available in processed tomato products, such as canned tomatoes, tomato purée and passata.

photo, page 231

Each serving provides   kcal 300, protein 8 g, fat 8 g (of which saturated fat 2 g), carbohydrate 44 g (of which sugars 11 g), fibre 4 g. Excellent source of vitamin A, vitamin C. Good source of folate, vitamin B_1. Useful source of niacin.

Garden of Eden soup

An assortment of vegetables cooked in tomato juice and stock makes a simple, satisfying soup that tastes terrific. For this recipe you can take advantage of frozen vegetables, such as broccoli, beans and peas. They cut down on preparation time, and are just as nutritious as fresh vegetables.

Preparation time **10 minutes**   Cooking time **about 20 minutes**   *Serves 4*

300 ml (10 fl oz) boiling water

1 vegetable stock cube, crumbled, or 2 tsp vegetable bouillon powder or paste

1 litre (1¾ pints) tomato juice

2 garlic cloves, crushed

4 spring onions, finely chopped

1 large potato, scrubbed and diced

1 large carrot, diced

100 g (3½ oz) frozen broccoli florets

100 g (3½ oz) white cabbage, finely shredded or coarsely chopped

55 g (2 oz) frozen cut green beans

55 g (2 oz) frozen peas

55 g (2 oz) frozen broad beans

8 large sprigs of fresh basil

salt and pepper

1 Pour the boiling water into a saucepan. Stir in the stock cube, powder or paste, the tomato juice, garlic, spring onions, potato and carrot. Bring to the boil, then reduce the heat and cover the pan. Simmer the soup for about 10 minutes, stirring occasionally.

2 Use a sharp knife to cut any large frozen broccoli florets into smaller pieces, then add them to the soup with the cabbage, green beans, peas and broad beans. Bring the soup back to the boil, then reduce the heat slightly, but keep the soup simmering rapidly. Cook for about 5 minutes or until the vegetables are just tender but still crisp.

3 Taste and season the soup, then ladle it into warm bowls. Use scissors to snip half the basil into shreds and scatter over the soup, discarding the tough ends of the sprigs. Add a whole sprig of basil to each portion and serve at once.

Some more ideas

Instead of weighing out 4 types of frozen vegetables, use 250 g (8½ oz) frozen mixed vegetables. There are many different mixtures for simmering or stir-frying; all are great for making quick soups.

For a hearty soup, add 1 can borlotti beans, about 400 g, drained and rinsed, with the frozen vegetables. Before serving, swirl 1 tsp pesto into each bowl of soup and sprinkle with 1 tsp lightly toasted pine nuts.

The soup can be varied according to the fresh or frozen vegetables you have in the house. For example, try 1 peeled sweet potato with, or instead of, the ordinary potato and add 1 peeled and diced turnip.

Plus points

• This is a good example of a 'cold-start' recipe, in which the vegetables are added straight to the liquid without being cooked in fat. The resulting soup is virtually fat free.

• Different fruit and vegetables contain different phytochemicals, so it is important to eat a variety. This soup includes a good mixture of vegetables.

Each serving provides kcal 135, protein 7 g, fat 1 g (of which saturated fat 0 g), carbohydrate 25 g (of which sugars 14 g), fibre 6 g. Excellent source of vitamin A, vitamin C. Good source of vitamin B₆. Useful source of iron.

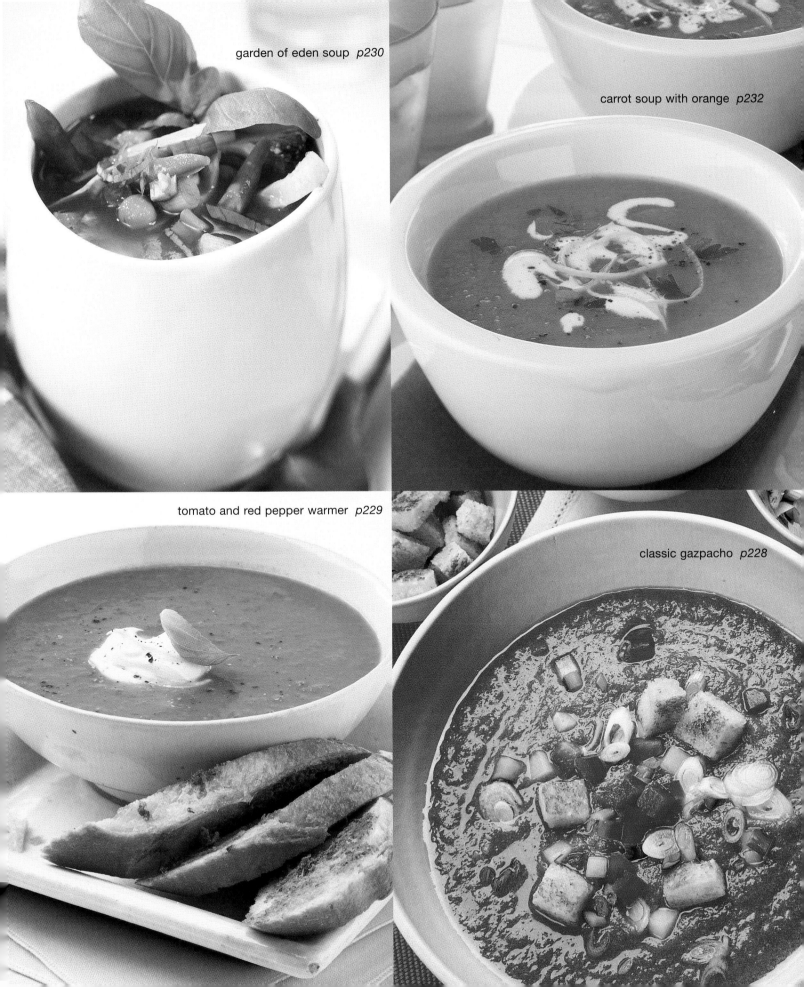

garden of eden soup *p230*

carrot soup with orange *p232*

tomato and red pepper warmer *p229*

classic gazpacho *p228*

Carrot soup with orange

Thickening soup with potato gives a velvety smooth result without adding the fat used in other traditional methods. Served either hot or chilled, this soup is ideal as a dinner-party starter all through the year.

Preparation time **15–20 minutes**   Chilling time **4 hours** (if served cold)   Cooking time **about 25 minutes**   *Serves 4*

1 litre (1¾ pints) vegetable stock, preferably home-made (see page 224)

500 g (1 lb 2 oz) carrots, finely diced

100 g (3½ oz) potato, peeled and finely diced

100 g (3½ oz) leeks, chopped

2 strips of pared orange zest

4 tbsp orange juice, or to taste

salt and pepper

To garnish

4 tbsp single cream

2 tbsp coarsely chopped fresh flat-leaf parsley

1 strip of pared orange zest, cut into fine shreds

1 Pour the stock into a large saucepan and add the carrots, potato, leeks and orange zest. Bring to the boil over a high heat, skimming the surface as necessary, then reduce the heat to moderate and leave the soup to bubble for about 20 minutes or until all the vegetables are very tender.

2 Remove and discard the strips of orange zest. Purée the soup in a blender or food processor until smooth.

3 If serving the soup hot, return it to the rinsed-out saucepan. Reheat and add the orange juice, then adjust the seasoning. Ladle the soup into bowls and add a spoonful of cream to each, drizzling it over the surface. Sprinkle with the parsley and shredded orange zest and serve at once.

4 To serve the soup chilled, leave to cool, then chill for at least 4 hours. When ready to serve, stir in the orange juice, then adjust the seasoning. Garnish and serve as for the hot soup.

Some more ideas

To make a filling **broccoli soup**, replace the carrots with 500 g (1 lb 2 oz) broccoli florets. Sprinkle each serving with a little grated nutmeg and top with about 1 tbsp crumbled blue cheese, such as Stilton. Omit the cream.

Make a **green bean soup** using this basic recipe. Replace the carrots with 450 g (1 lb) green beans, trimmed and chopped. Omit the orange zest and add 30 g (1 oz) finely chopped fennel, about ¼ bulb. Depending on the choice of beans, this soup may need sieving to remove fibres after puréeing the mixture – this is particularly important if using runner beans. Serve sprinkled with finely chopped fresh fennel leaves (from the bulb) or dill.

Plus points

* Making soup is an excellent way of preserving all the water-soluble vitamins – the B group and vitamin C – which are otherwise lost when the cooking water from vegetables is discarded.

* This low-fat soup is made with leeks instead of the usual onion. Leeks are a useful source of several water-soluble vitamins, including vitamin C and folate.

photo, page 231

Each serving provides kcal 100, protein 2 g, fat 4 g (of which saturated fat 2 g), carbohydrate 16 g (of which sugars 12 g), fibre 4 g. Excellent source of vitamin A, vitamin E. Good source of vitamin C. Useful source of folate, potassium, vitamin B_1, vitamin B_6.

Chunky vegetable soup

Although this is a hearty soup, laden with vegetables, it has a delicate flavour. Home-made stock is best, but you can use a good-quality bought stock (chilled or from a cube or powder); if using a cube or powder, do not add additional salt at the beginning of cooking as you may find these products provide enough salty seasoning.

Preparation time **15 minutes**   Cooking time **about 1 hour**   *Serves 4*

1 tbsp sunflower oil

1 small onion, chopped

1 small leek, thinly sliced

1 large carrot, thinly sliced

1 bulb of fennel, sliced

225 g (8 oz) swede, cubed

225 g (8 oz) potato, peeled and cubed

1 bay leaf

several sprigs of fresh thyme

several sprigs of parsley

600 ml (1 pint) vegetable stock, preferably home-made (see page 224)

1 can chopped tomatoes, about 400 g

salt and pepper

fennel leaves (from the bulb, above) or snipped fresh chives, to garnish

1 Heat the oil in a large saucepan. Add the onion and cook for about 5 minutes, stirring occasionally, or until softened but not browned.

2 Add the leek, carrot, fennel, swede and potato, and cook for a further 5 minutes or until slightly softened. Tie the bay leaf, thyme and parsley sprigs together into a bouquet garni. Add to the pan, together with the stock and tomatoes with their juice. Season to taste and bring to the boil, then cover the pan and reduce the heat. Simmer gently for 45 minutes or until all the vegetables are tender.

3 Remove the bouquet garni and check the seasoning. Sprinkle the soup with snipped fennel leaves or chives and serve piping hot. Mixed-grain or wholemeal bread are delicious with this soup.

Some more ideas

For a hearty winter's chowder-type soup, simply add more vegetables. Try celeriac, turnips and parsnips. Shredded white or green cabbage is also good – add green cabbage halfway through the simmering. Cool and chill any leftovers and reheat them next day, when the soup will taste even better.

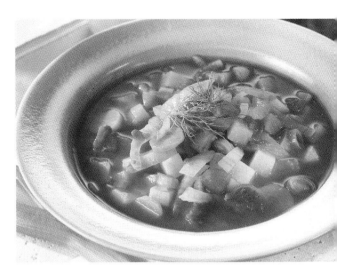

Pearl barley adds a delightful nutty texture, and its low Glycaemic Index is an added benefit. Stir 55 g (2 oz) pearl barley into the softened vegetables, just before adding the stock and tomatoes.

Plus points

• In these days of refrigerated transport and all-year-round variety, it is easy to forget the importance of traditional vegetables, such as swedes and potatoes, as a source of vitamin C. At one time, these roots were very important in preventing scurvy during winter months. Eaten frequently, they contribute a useful amount of vitamin C, the antioxidant properties of which are important in the prevention of cancer and heart disease.

Each serving provides   kcal 130, protein 4 g, fat 4 g (of which saturated fat 1 g), carbohydrate 20 g (of which sugars 10 g), fibre 5 g. Excellent source of vitamin A, vitamin C, vitamin E. Good source of folate, vitamin B$_1$, vitamin B$_6$. Useful source of copper, iron, niacin, potassium.

Artichoke soup with caraway

Looking like knobbly new potatoes, Jerusalem artichokes have a distinctive, yet delicate, flavour that goes well with other root vegetables, particularly in a smooth-textured soup. Sweetly aromatic caraway seeds complement the vegetable flavours and transform an unassuming, familiar dish into something rather special.

Preparation time **about 15 minutes**   Cooking time **about 40 minutes**   *Serves 6*

1 tbsp lemon juice

500 g (1 lb 2 oz) Jerusalem artichokes

15 g (½ oz) butter

1 celery stick, chopped

1 small onion, chopped

2 carrots, chopped

1 garlic clove, chopped

1.2 litres (2 pints) chicken stock, preferably home-made (see page 212)

1 tsp caraway seeds

150 ml (5 fl oz) semi-skimmed milk

4 tbsp single cream

salt and pepper

To garnish

1 small carrot

2–3 tbsp chopped parsley

1 Add the lemon juice to a bowl of cold water. Peel and slice the artichokes, adding them to the water as soon as they are cut. (Artichokes discolour quickly once peeled and exposed to air.)

2 Melt the butter in a large saucepan. Drain the artichokes and add them to the saucepan with the celery, onion, carrots and garlic. Cover the pan and sweat the vegetables gently for 10 minutes or until softened.

3 Stir in the stock and caraway seeds. Bring to the boil, then reduce the heat and cover the pan. Simmer for about 20 minutes or until the vegetables are tender. Cool the soup slightly, then purée it in a blender until smooth or press it through a fine sieve. Alternatively, use a hand-held blender to purée the soup in the pan.

4 Return the soup to the pan, if necessary. Stir in the milk and cream and season to taste with salt and pepper. Reheat the soup very gently without allowing it to boil. Meanwhile, cut the carrot for garnish into short, fine julienne or matchstick strips. Serve the soup hot, garnishing each portion with carrot strips and a little chopped parsley.

Some more ideas

Use vegetable stock, preferably home-made rich (see page 225) instead of chicken stock.

For **celeriac and parsnip soup**, use 500 g (1 lb 2 oz) peeled and chopped celeriac instead of Jerusalem artichokes, and 2 chopped parsnips instead of carrots. Omit the celery.

Bacon is delicious with artichokes and other root vegetables. Cook 115 g (4 oz) rinded and chopped smoked back bacon in the butter, then remove with a draining spoon and set aside. Add the vegetables and continue as in the recipe. Sprinkle the bacon over the soup instead of carrot, together with wholemeal toast cut into croutons and chopped parsley.

Plus points

- Jerusalem artichokes are a useful winter vegetable. Combining them with familiar roots, such as carrots, is a good way of introducing them to children and bringing variety to the diet.

- Jerusalem artichokes contain compounds called fructoligosaccarides – a type of dietary fibre that stimulates friendly bacteria in the gut while inhibiting harmful bacteria.

Each serving provides   kcal 103, protein 4 g, fat 5 g (of which saturated fat 3 g), carbohydrate 14 g (of which sugars 5 g), fibre 4 g. Good source of vitamin A, vitamin C. Useful source of calcium, potassium, vitamin B_1.

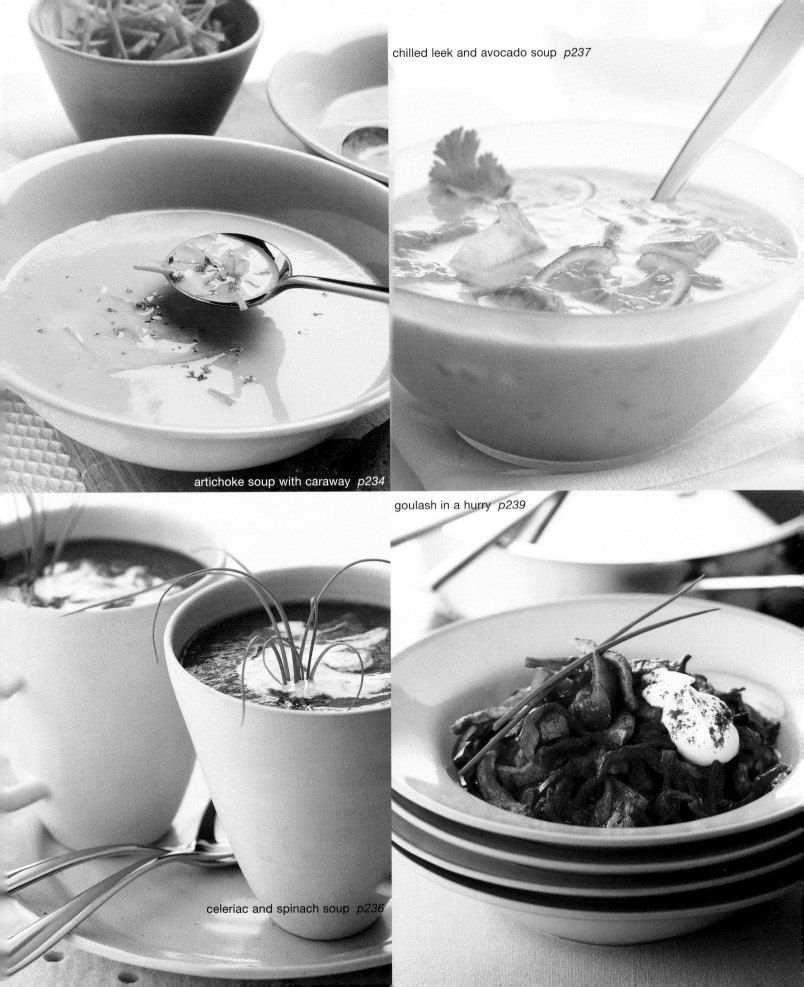

chilled leek and avocado soup *p237*

artichoke soup with caraway *p234*

goulash in a hurry *p239*

celeriac and spinach soup *p236*

Celeriac and spinach soup

Celeriac makes a rich soup with lots of flavour and a creamy texture. Young leaf spinach complements the celeriac beautifully, bringing colour and a light, fresh taste in the final minutes of cooking.

Preparation time **10 minutes**   Cooking time **about 20 minutes**   *Serves 4*

2 tbsp extra virgin olive oil

1 large onion, thinly sliced

1 garlic clove, crushed

1 celeriac, about 600 g (1 lb 5 oz), peeled and grated

1 litre (1¾ pints) boiling water

1 vegetable stock cube, crumbled, or 2 tsp vegetable bouillon powder or paste

500 g (1 lb 2 oz) young leaf spinach

grated nutmeg

salt and pepper

To garnish

4 tbsp 0% fat Greek-style yogurt

fresh chives

1 Heat the oil in a large saucepan. Add the onion and garlic, and cook for about 5 minutes or until the onion is softened but not browned. Add the celeriac. Pour in the boiling water and stir in the stock cube, powder or paste. Bring to the boil over a high heat, then reduce the heat and cover the pan. Cook the soup gently for 10 minutes or until the celeriac is tender.

2 Add the spinach to the soup and stir well. Increase the heat and bring the soup to the boil, then remove the pan from the heat. Leave the soup to cool slightly before puréeing it, in batches, in a blender or food processor until smooth. Alternatively, you can purée it in the pan using a hand-held blender. The soup will be fairly thick.

3 Reheat the soup, if necessary, then stir in a little grated nutmeg, salt and pepper to taste. Ladle the soup into warm bowls. Swirl a spoonful of cream into yogurt portion and garnish with fresh chives, then serve at once.

Some more ideas

Crispy bacon makes a delicious garnish for the soup. While the soup is cooking, grill 4 rinded lean back bacon rashers until crisp and golden. Drain on kitchen paper, then crumble or chop the rashers into small pieces. Omit salt from the recipe.

For a **hearty winter soup** substitute shredded spring greens for the spinach.

For a more substantial dish, add a poached egg to each bowl of soup.

To make a delicious **potato and watercress** version of this soup, use peeled and diced potatoes instead of celeriac, and watercress instead of spinach. Add extra stock or semi-skimmed milk if the puréed soup is too thick.

Plus points

- Celeriac, a relative of celery, complements both the flavour and texture of spinach, making the most of the modest amount of yogurt used to enrich the soup. It also provides potassium.

- Onions have many health benefits. They contain sulphur compounds, which give onions their characteristic smell and make your eyes water. These compounds transport cholesterol away from the artery walls.

photo, page 235

Each serving provides   kcal 140, protein 6 g, fat 8.5 g (of which saturated fat 2 g), carbohydrate 9 g (of which sugars 7 g), fibre 9 g. Excellent source of folate, vitamin A. Good source of calcium, iron, vitamin B$_6$, vitamin C. Useful source of vitamin E.

Chilled leek and avocado soup

Coriander and lime juice accentuate the delicate avocado flavour in this refreshing soup. It is simple yet interesting, and ideal for a summer's dinner-party first course or a light lunch. Do not add the avocado too soon – not only will it discolour slightly, but its flavour will mellow and lose the vital freshness.

Preparation time **15-20 minutes**   Cooking time **25 minutes**   *Serves 4*

1 tbsp extra virgin olive oil

450 g (1 lb) leeks, halved lengthways and thinly sliced

1 garlic clove, finely chopped

750 ml (1¼ pints) vegetable or chicken stock, bought chilled or made with a stock cube or bouillon powder

1 large ripe avocado

125 g (4½ oz) plain low-fat yogurt

1 tbsp lime juice

2 tbsp chopped fresh coriander

salt and pepper

To garnish

8–12 ice cubes (optional)

slices of lime

sprigs of fresh coriander

1 Heat the oil in a saucepan, add the leeks and garlic, and cook for 10 minutes, stirring frequently, until the leeks are slightly softened but not coloured. Pour in the stock and bring to the boil. Cover the pan, reduce the heat and simmer for 10 minutes or until the leeks are cooked.

2 Remove the soup from the heat and let it cool slightly, then purée it in a blender or food processor. Alternatively the soup can be puréed in the saucepan with a hand-held blender. Pour the soup into a bowl and leave it to cool, then chill well.

3 Just before serving the soup, prepare the avocado. Halve the avocado and discard the stone. Scoop the flesh from the peel and press through a fine stainless-steel or nylon sieve. The avocado can also be puréed in a blender or food processor until smooth, adding a little of the chilled soup to thin the purée and ensure it is completely smooth.

4 Stir the avocado purée into the soup together with the yogurt, lime juice and coriander. Add seasoning to taste, then ladle the soup into 4 bowls. Float 2–3 ice cubes in each bowl, if you wish, then add slices of lime and sprigs of coriander. Serve at once.

Some more ideas

This soup is also good hot. Purée the hot soup with the avocado and stir in half-fat crème fraîche instead of yogurt.

For a soup with Mexican flavours, cook 1–2 seeded and finely chopped fresh green chillies with the leeks.

For a simple no-cook avocado soup, blend 2 avocados with 450 ml (15 fl oz) vegetable stock, then add the yogurt and lime juice, and season to taste.

To make **vichyssoise**, the chilled leek and potato soup, use 1 litre (1¾ pints) stock and cook 2 peeled, sliced potatoes with the leeks. Omit the avocado, coriander and lime juice.

Plus points

• Half an avocado provides a quarter of the recommended daily intake of vitamin B_6 and useful amounts of vitamin E and potassium. Although avocados are high in fat, they contain the healthier, mono-unsaturated type.

• Leeks provide useful amounts of folate, which is important for proper blood cell formation and development of the nervous system in an unborn baby.

photo, page 235

Each serving provides kcal 170, protein 5 g, fat 14 g (of which saturated fat 3 g), carbohydrate 7 g (of which sugars 5 g), fibre 4 g. Good source of potassium, vitamin B_6, vitamin C, vitamin E. Useful source of folate, vitamin A, vitamin B_1.

Golden lentil soup

This velvety-smooth soup owes its rich colour to a combination of lentils, parsnips and carrots. With dry sherry and a horseradish-flavoured cream adding to the flavour, it is a perfect dinner-party first course. Serve it with crunchy melba toast or oatcakes.

Preparation time **about 15 minutes**   Cooking time **about 1½ hours**   *Serves 4*

15 g (½ oz) butter, plus 1 tsp olive oil

1 large onion, finely chopped

450 g (1 lb) parsnips, cut into small cubes

340 g (12 oz) carrots, cut into small cubes

150 ml (5 fl oz) dry sherry

85 g (3 oz) red lentils

1.2 litres (2 pints) vegetable stock, preferably home-made light or rich (see page 224)

salt and pepper

fresh chives to garnish

To serve

2 tsp grated horseradish

6 tbsp half-fat crème fraîche

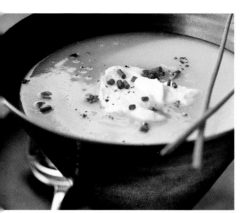

1 Melt the butter and olive oil in a large saucepan. Add the onion, stir well and cover the pan. Sweat the onion over a gentle heat for 10 minutes or until softened. Stir in the parsnips, carrots and sherry. Bring to the boil, then cover the pan again and leave to simmer very gently for 40 minutes.

2 Add the lentils, stock, and salt and pepper to taste. Bring to the boil, then reduce the heat and cover the pan. Simmer for a further 15–20 minutes or until the lentils are tender. Purée the soup in a blender until smooth or use a hand-held blender to purée the soup in the pan. Return the soup to the pan if necessary, and reheat it gently until boiling. If it seems a bit thick, add a little stock or water.

3 Stir the grated horseradish into the crème fraîche. Snip some of the chives for the garnish and leave a few whole. Ladle the soup into warm bowls and top each portion with a spoonful of the horseradish cream. Scatter snipped chives over the top and add a few lengths of whole chive across the top of each bowl. Serve at once.

Some more ideas

Use celeriac instead of parsnips, and swede instead of carrots. Prepare and cook the soup as in the main recipe. Dry white vermouth or white wine can be added in place of the sherry for a lighter flavour.

For a lower-fat version, top each portion with 1 tsp creamed horseradish instead of the horseradish and crème fraîche mixture, and scatter chopped parsley over the soup.

Plus points

• Lentils are a good source of protein and an excellent source of fibre. High-fibre foods are bulky and make you feel full for longer, so are very satisfying. When eaten regularly, lentils can help to lower blood glucose levels.

• Root vegetables have long been enjoyed as an excellent source of vitamins and minerals during the winter months.

• Children who are reluctant to sample plain cooked vegetables will not even realise they are eating them in this tasty, colourful soup.

Each serving provides kcal 207, protein 6 g, fat 6 g (of which saturated fat 2 g), carbohydrate 25 g (of which sugars 11 g), fibre 6 g. Excellent source of vitamin A. Good source of folate, potassium, vitamin B$_1$, vitamin B$_6$. Useful source of calcium, iron.

Goulash in a hurry

This short-cut version of classic Hungarian goulash is rich and delicious. Strips of lean pork, shredded red cabbage and green pepper cook quickly and taste excellent with the traditional flavourings of paprika and caraway seeds. Serve rice or noodles and a simple green salad alongside, to complete the meal.

Preparation time **10 minutes**   Cooking time **about 20 minutes**   *Serves 4*

2 tbsp extra virgin olive oil

1 large onion, finely chopped

2 garlic cloves, crushed

3 thick lean pork loin steaks, about 300 g (10½ oz) total weight, cut into thin strips

1 tbsp plain flour

1 can tomatoes, about 800 g

120 ml (4 fl oz) extra dry white vermouth

2 tbsp paprika

1 tsp caraway seeds

1 tsp caster sugar

1 pork or chicken stock cube, crumbled

1 large green pepper, seeded and chopped

200 g (7 oz) red cabbage, finely shredded

salt and pepper

To serve

4 tbsp Greek-style yogurt

paprika

fresh chives

1 Heat the oil in a large frying pan or saucepan. Add the onion, garlic and pork, and cook over a high heat for about 3 minutes or until the meat has changed colour and become firm and the onion is slightly softened. Meanwhile, blend the flour with 4 tbsp juice from the canned tomatoes to make a smooth paste; set aside.

2 Add the vermouth, paprika, caraway seeds and sugar to the pan and stir, then add the tomatoes with the rest of their juice, breaking them up as you mix them in. Stir in the stock cube, and the flour and tomato juice mixture. Bring to the boil, stirring, and cook until the juices thicken.

3 Stir in the green pepper and red cabbage until both are thoroughly coated in the cooking juices. Reduce the heat, cover the pan and simmer the goulash for about 15 minutes or until the meat is cooked and the vegetables are just tender, but still slightly crisp.

4 Taste the goulash and season with salt and pepper, if necessary. Ladle the goulash into bowls and top each portion with a spoonful of Greek-style yogurt and a sprinkle of paprika. Garnish with chives and serve.

Some more ideas

To make a **vegetarian goulash**, omit the pork and cabbage. Cut 1 aubergine into chunks and add to the softened onion and garlic in step 1 with 6 halved sun-dried tomatoes, 2 thickly sliced celery sticks and 2 thickly sliced courgettes. Follow the main recipe, using a vegetable stock cube. Simmer for 25 minutes, then stir in 1 can chickpeas, about 400 g, and 1 can red kidney beans, about 200 g, both well drained. Cook for a further 5 minutes.

Halved small new potatoes are good in the vegetarian version, above. Add them with the other vegetables and leave out the canned red kidney beans.

Plus points

● Several studies have shown that eating garlic can reduce the risk of heart attack and stroke by making the blood less sticky and likely to clot. Garlic can also help to reduce high blood pressure.

● Onions share garlic's healthy properties and they are also a natural decongestant. Using onions as the basis for everyday dishes contributes to good eating.

photo, page 235

Each serving provides   kcal 270, protein 21 g, fat 12 g (of which saturated fat 3 g), carbohydrate 16 g (of which sugars 12 g), fibre 4 g. Excellent source of vitamin B$_{12}$, vitamin C. Good source of vitamin B$_1$, vitamin B$_6$. Useful source of folate, iron, niacin, selenium, zinc.

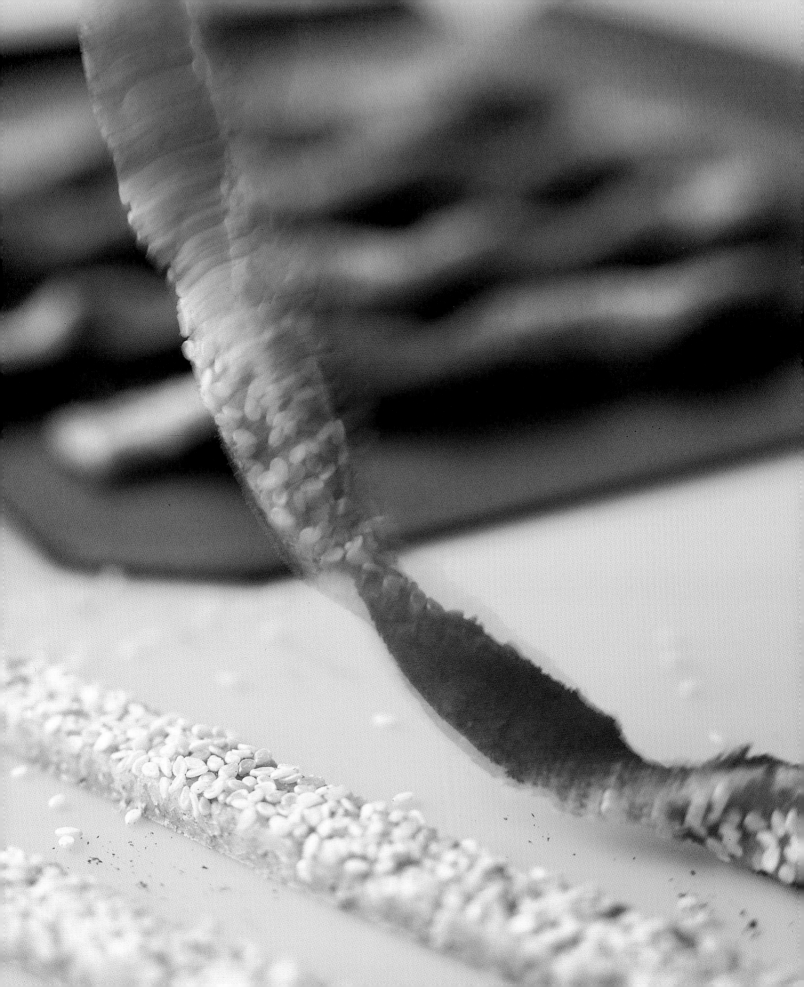

Breads and snacks

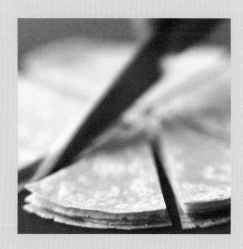

Blackcurrant teabread

Tart blackcurrants make an excellent summer teabread that is fruity without being too sweet, while mint adds a fresh, herbal note. If you have a glut of blackcurrants, make a few loaves and freeze for up to 2 months.

Preparation time **20 minutes**   Cooking time **1¼ hours**   *Makes 1 large loaf (cuts into about 12 slices)*

340 g (12 oz) self-raising flour

1 tsp baking powder

50 g (1¾ oz) unsalted butter, cut into small pieces

100 g (3½ oz) light muscovado sugar

150 g (5½ oz) fresh blackcurrants

3 tbsp chopped fresh mint

150 ml (5 fl oz) orange juice, or as needed

1 Preheat the oven to 180°C (350°F, gas mark 4). Grease and line a 900 g (2 lb) loaf tin. Sift the flour and baking powder into a bowl, then rub in the butter with your fingertips until the mixture resembles fine breadcrumbs. Stir in the sugar, and make a well in the centre.

2 Put the blackcurrants and mint into the well in the dry ingredients and pour in the orange juice. Gradually stir the dry ingredients into the liquid until everything is thoroughly combined. The mixture should be soft, so add 1–2 tbsp more orange juice if necessary.

3 Turn the mixture into the prepared tin and smooth the top. Bake for about 1¼ hours or until risen, brown and firm to the touch. If the loaf looks as though it is browning too much after about 50 minutes, place a piece of foil loosely over the top.

4 Leave the teabread to cool in the tin for 5 minutes, then turn it out onto a wire rack to cool completely. This teabread is best left overnight before serving, and can be kept in an airtight tin for up to 3 days.

Some more ideas

Make blueberry teabread by substituting fresh blueberries for the blackcurrants.

For **cranberry pecan teabread**, substitute roughly chopped fresh cranberries for the blackcurrants. Replace the mint with ½ tsp ground cinnamon, sifting it with the flour, and stir in 100 g (3½ oz) pecan nuts with the sugar.

Plus points

• Blackcurrants are an excellent source of vitamin C – weight for weight, they contain 4 times as much vitamin C as oranges. They also provide useful amounts of potassium, and are rich in a group of phytochemicals called bioflavonoids, which may help to protect against heart disease.

• The oils menthol, menthone and menthyl acetate, responsible for the characteristic flavour of mint, are believed to have powerful antiseptic properties. Naturopaths prescribe mint to help to relieve toothache, stress headaches and digestive problems.

photo, page 245

Each serving provides   (one slice) kcal 170, protein 3 g, fat 4 g (of which saturated fat 2 g), carbohydrate 32 g (of which sugars 11 g), fibre 1 g. Good source of vitamin C. Useful source of potassium, vitamin B_1.

Light rye bread

Rye flour is lower in gluten than wheat, so it produces a close-textured, moist loaf. Caraway seeds are a traditional seasoning, complementing the nutty flavour of rye to make an excellent bread that goes well with fish – particularly smoked mackerel, grilled kippers and pickled herrings – and soft cheeses.

Preparation time **20 minutes, plus about 1 hour rising**   Cooking time **40–45 minutes**   *Makes 1 small loaf (24 thin slices)*

300 g (10½ oz) rye flour

100 g (3½ oz) strong white (bread) flour

½ tsp salt

1 tsp caster sugar

1 sachet easy-blend dried yeast, about 7 g

2 tsp caraway seeds

2 tbsp extra virgin olive oil

200 ml (7 fl oz) tepid water

1 Sift the rye flour, white flour, salt and sugar into a bowl, and stir in the yeast and caraway seeds. Stir the olive oil into the tepid water, then pour this over the flour mixture. Mix the ingredients together with a wooden spoon at first, then with your hand, to make a stiff, but sticky and slightly grainy dough.

2 Turn the dough out onto a floured work surface and knead for about 10 minutes or until smooth. The dough should be very firm. Shape it into an oval loaf about 18 cm (7 in) long, and place it on a greased baking sheet. Cover loosely with cling film and leave to rise in a warm place for about 1 hour or until almost doubled in size. It will be slightly cracked on top.

3 Towards the end of the rising time, preheat the oven to 200°C (400°F, gas mark 6). Uncover the loaf and bake for 40–45 minutes or until it is lightly browned and sounds hollow when tapped on the base.

4 Transfer to a wire rack and leave to cool. Once cold, place the loaf in a polythene bag and leave overnight (this allows the crust to soften). After this, the loaf can be kept for up to 2 days.

Some more ideas

To make dark rye bread, stir 2 tbsp molasses or black treacle into the water with the oil.

Substitute wholemeal flour for the white flour.

For a lighter loaf, use 200 g (7 oz) rye flour and 200 g (7 oz) strong white (bread) flour.

Cumin or fennel seeds also taste good in rye bread. Toast 1 tbsp of the seeds in a small, heavy-based frying pan over a moderate heat for 1–2 minutes or until they are aromatic. Remove from the heat, then leave to cool. Add to the flour instead of the caraway seeds.

For **orange and caraway rye bread**, add the grated zest of 1 large orange and 2 tbsp light muscovado sugar to the flour with the seeds, and substitute sunflower oil for the olive oil.

Plus points

• Making a variety of breads from different types of flour means that there is always an interesting loaf to complement a meal. This will help to increase the intake of starchy carbohydrates.

• Caraway seeds are said to stimulate the production of saliva and aid digestion.

photo, page 245

Each serving provides   (one slice) kcal 65, protein 1.5 g, fat 1 g (of which saturated fat 0 g), carbohydrate 13 g (of which sugars 0 g), fibre 1.5 g.

Sesame cheese twists

These crisp cheese sticks are delicious served fresh and still warm from the oven. Enriched with egg yolks and well flavoured with freshly grated Parmesan cheese, they are made with a combination of wholemeal and plain flour, so that they are substantial without being at all heavy.

Preparation time **10–15 minutes**   Cooking time **15 minutes**   *Makes 40 sticks*

85 g (3 oz) plain wholemeal flour, preferably stoneground

85 g (3 oz) plain white flour, plus extra for rolling

¼ tsp salt

45 g (1½ oz) butter

45 g (1½ oz) Parmesan cheese, freshly grated

1 large egg

2 tbsp semi-skimmed milk

1 tsp paprika

1 tbsp sesame seeds

1 Preheat the oven to 180°C (350°F, gas mark 4). Sift the flours and salt into a bowl, tipping in the bran left in the sieve. Rub in the butter until the mixture resembles fine breadcrumbs. Stir in the Parmesan cheese.

2 Whisk the egg and milk together. Reserve 1 tsp of this mixture, and stir the rest into the dry ingredients to make a firm dough. Knead on a lightly floured surface for a few seconds or until smooth.

3 Sprinkle the paprika over the floured surface, then roll out the dough on it to form a square slightly larger than 20 cm (8 in). Trim the edges to make them straight. Brush the dough with the reserved egg mixture and sprinkle over the sesame seeds. Cut the square of dough in half, then cut into 10 cm (4 in) sticks that are about 1 cm (½ in) wide.

4 Twist the sticks and place on a large baking sheet lined with baking parchment. Press the ends of the sticks down so that they do not untwist during baking.

5 Bake for 15 minutes or until lightly browned and crisp. Cool on the baking sheets for a few minutes, then serve warm, or transfer to a wire rack to cool completely. The sticks can be kept in an airtight tin for up to 5 days.

Another idea

For **blue cheese and walnut biscuits**, mash 30 g (1 oz) blue cheese, such as Stilton or Danish blue, with 55 g (2 oz) reduced-fat spread. Sift over 45 g (1½ oz) plain wholemeal flour, 30 g (1 oz) self-raising white flour and 30 g (1 oz) ground rice, tipping in the bran left in the sieve. Add 15 g (1 oz) chopped toasted walnuts. Rub together, then knead lightly to form a dough. Shape into a roll about 12 cm (5 in) long. Wrap in cling film and chill for about 30 minutes. Cut into slices, arrange on a baking sheet lined with baking parchment and bake in a preheated 190°C (375°F, gas mark 5) oven for 15 minutes. Transfer to a wire rack to cool. Makes about 16 biscuits.

Plus points

• Sesame seeds are a good source of calcium as well as providing iron and zinc.

• Wholemeal flour has a lot to offer: dietary fibre, B vitamins and vitamin E, together with iron, selenium and magnesium. Stoneground wholemeal flour has slightly more B vitamins than factory-milled wholemeal flour, because stonegrinding keeps the grain cool. Milling with metal rollers creates heat, which spoils some of the nutrients.

Each serving provides (two sticks) kcal 32, protein 1 g, fat 2 g (of which saturated fat 1 g), carbohydrate 3 g (of which sugars 0.1 g), fibre 0.3 g.

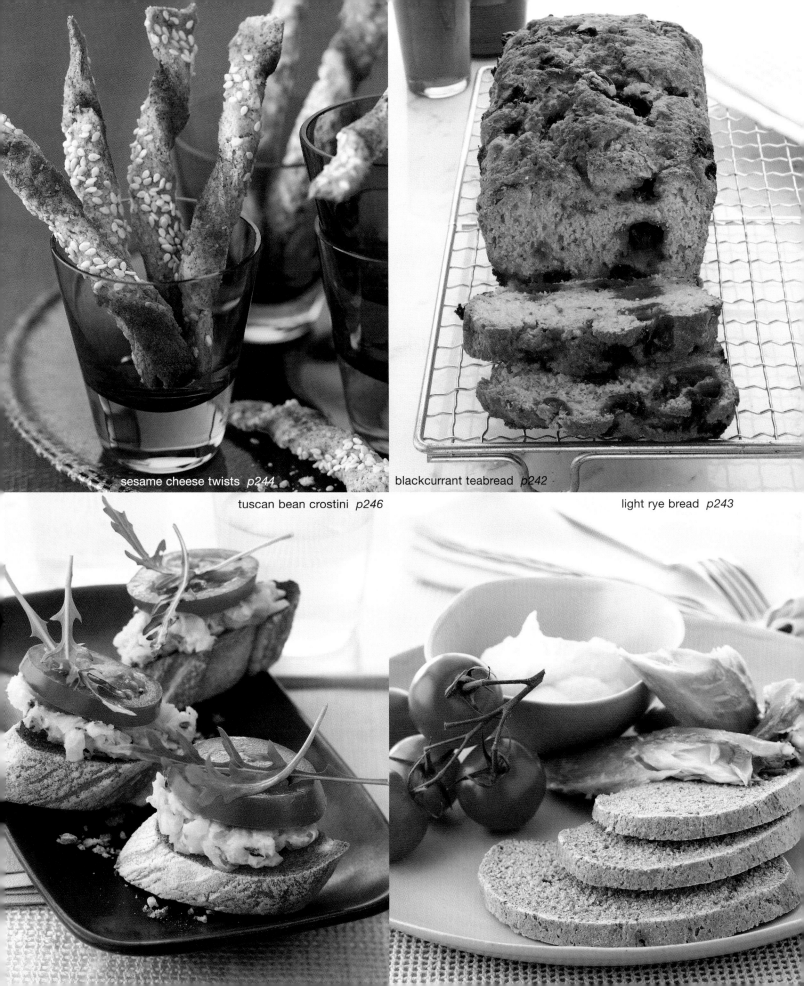

sesame cheese twists *p244*

blackcurrant teabread *p242*

tuscan bean crostini *p246*

light rye bread *p243*

Tuscan bean crostini

Here's a delicious snack to be enjoyed hot or cold – toasted slices of baguette topped with a creamy white bean purée flavoured with garlic and thyme, and finished with colourful slices of tomato and leaves of rocket.

Preparation and cooking time **about 25 minutes**   *Makes 22 crostini*

2 tsp extra virgin olive oil

1 small onion, finely chopped

1 garlic clove, crushed

1 can cannellini beans, about 400 g, drained and rinsed

2 tbsp crème fraîche

1 tbsp chopped fresh thyme

1 thin baguette, about 250 g (8½ oz)

3 plum tomatoes, thinly sliced

salt and pepper

rocket or sprigs of fresh herbs, to garnish

1 Heat the oil in a small frying pan, add the onion and garlic, and cook gently for about 10 minutes or until softened, stirring occasionally.

2 Meanwhile, place the cannellini beans in a bowl and mash with a potato masher or fork. Remove the pan of onion and garlic from the heat and stir in the mashed beans, crème fraîche and thyme. Season with salt and pepper to taste and mix well. Keep warm while preparing the toasts.

3 Preheat the grill to high. Remove the crusty ends off the baguette and cut the loaf into 22 equal slices, each about 1.5 cm (¾ in) thick. Toast the slices on both sides under the grill. (The toasts can be left to cool and then kept in an airtight tin; when ready to serve, top with the bean mixture, cooled to room temperature, and garnish.)

4 Thickly spread some bean mixture over each toast, top with a tomato slice and garnish with rocket or fresh herb sprigs.

Some more ideas

Instead of cannellini beans, use other canned pulses, such as butter beans or chickpeas.

Top the bean mixture with grilled courgette slices, lightly cooked button mushrooms or halved cherry tomatoes.

Herbs such as fresh basil, oregano, sage or parsley can be used in place of the thyme.

Use different types of bread, such as ciabatta, pugliese, wholemeal or granary.

Make **tuna crostini**. Drain and flake 1 can tuna in spring water, about 400 g. Mix with 1½ tbsp each mayonnaise and plain low-fat yogurt, 2 tbsp chopped fresh chives and pepper to taste. Spread each slice of toast with ½ tsp tomato relish or chutney, top with the tuna mixture and garnish with tiny watercress sprigs or rocket leaves.

Plus points

● Cannellini beans belong to the same family as the haricot bean and have a similar floury texture when cooked. Though an excellent source of dietary fibre, beans can produce side effects such as bloating and wind. These can be minimised by ensuring that canned beans are thoroughly rinsed before use.

● Crème fraîche is a cream that has been allowed to mature and ferment so that it thickens slightly and develops a tangy taste. Because of its rich texture, only a little is needed to give a creamy finish.

photo, page 245

Each serving provides **(one toast)** kcal 62, protein 2 g, fat 2 g (of which saturated fat 1 g), carbohydrate 9 g (of which sugars 1 g), fibre 1 g.

Goat's cheese toasts

Indulge your guests with these tasty morsels, made by topping toasted slices of crusty baguette with slices of plum tomato and tangy goat's cheese, sprinkled with pine nuts and fresh herbs. Choose your favourite type of goat's cheese: delicate or strong in flavour, soft or firm in texture.

Preparation time **15 minutes**   Cooking time **4–5 minutes**   *Makes 16 toasts*

1 baguette, about 280 g (10 oz), cut into 2.5 cm (1 in) slices

4 tbsp passata

2 tbsp sun-dried tomato paste

4 plum tomatoes, about 250 g (8½ oz) in total

140 g (5 oz) goat's cheese

1d tbsp extra virgin olive oil

15 g (½ oz) pine nuts

few sprigs of fresh thyme or oregano, plus extra to garnish

1 Preheat the grill to moderate. Place the baguette slices on a rack in the grill pan and lightly toast on both sides.

2 Mix together the passata and tomato paste and spread a little on top of each toast, covering the surface completely.

3 Slice the tomatoes lengthways, discarding a slim slice from the curved edges, to give 4 flat slices from each tomato. Lay a slice of tomato on top of each toast.

4 Place 1 small slice of firm goat's cheese or about 1 tsp of soft goat's cheese on top of each tomato slice, and drizzle over a little olive oil. Scatter on a few pine nuts and thyme or oregano leaves.

5 Grill for 4–5 minutes or until the cheese is beginning to melt and the pine nuts are golden. Serve the toasts hot, garnished with sprigs of thyme or oregano.

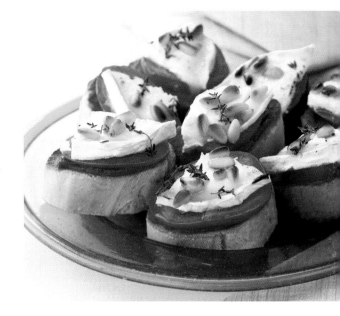

Another idea

Make **fruity goat's cheese toasts**. Instead of the tomato topping, mix together 2 tbsp each of cranberry sauce and mango, peach or another fruit chutney. Spread this over the toasts, top with the goat's cheese and scatter over a few flaked almonds, then grill as in the main recipe.

Plus points

● Pine nuts, used in Middle Eastern rice dishes and stuffings and an important ingredient in Italian pesto sauce, are rich in a variety of minerals including magnesium, potassium, iron, zinc and copper.

● Goat's cheese is a tasty source of protein and calcium, as well as B vitamins (B_1, B_6, B_{12} and niacin) and phosphorus. A medium-fat goat's cheese contains about half the fat of Cheddar cheese.

Each serving provides   (one toast) kcal 89, protein 3 g, fat 4 g (of which saturated fat 1 g), carbohydrate 11 g (of which sugars 1 g), fibre 0.5 g. Useful source of vitamin E.

Baked potato skins with smoked salmon and fresh dill

Potato skins are usually deep-fried, but brushing with a mixture of olive oil and butter and then baking gives just as good a flavour and crisp texture. Here the potato skins are topped with a herby fromage frais, smoked salmon and dill filling, to make a really special and nutritious snack to enjoy with drinks.

Preparation and cooking time **1¾–2 hours**   *Serves 8*

8 small baking potatoes, about 200 g (7 oz) each

2 tbsp extra virgin olive oil

20 g (¾ oz) butter

125 g (4½ oz) smoked salmon

1 tbsp lemon juice

150 g (5½ oz) fromage frais

1 tbsp capers, drained and chopped

2 tbsp chopped fresh dill

salt and pepper

small sprigs of fresh dill to garnish

1 Preheat the oven to 200ºC (400ºF, gas mark 6). Scrub the potatoes and dry them with kitchen paper. Thread them onto metal skewers – this helps them to cook more quickly. Brush the skin of the potatoes with 1 tbsp of the oil, then sprinkle with a little salt. Arrange on a baking tray and bake for 1–1¼ hours or until tender.

2 Remove the potatoes from the skewers and cut them in half lengthways. Scoop out the flesh, leaving a layer of potato next to the skin about 1 cm (½ in) thick. (Use the scooped-out flesh for fish cakes or mash to make a savoury pie topping.) Cut each piece in half lengthways again, and place flesh side up on a large, clean baking tray.

3 Melt the butter with the remaining 1 tbsp oil and season with salt and pepper to taste. Lightly brush this mixture over the flesh side of the potato skins. Return to the oven and bake for a further 12–15 minutes or until golden and crisp.

4 Meanwhile, cut the smoked salmon into fine strips and sprinkle with the lemon juice. Mix together the fromage frais, capers and chopped dill in a bowl, and stir in the salmon.

5 Allow the potato skins to cool for 1–2 minutes, then top each with a little of the salmon and fromage frais mixture. Garnish each with a small sprig of dill, and serve while the potato skins are still warm.

Plus points

● Baking potatoes in their skins helps to retain their vitamins and minerals – many nutrients are found just beneath the skin. Eating the skins also boosts the intake of dietary fibre.

● Salmon is an oily fish and a rich source of essential omega-3 fatty acids, a type of polyunsaturated fat that is thought to help protect against heart disease. Smoking the salmon doesn't destroy the beneficial oils.

● Capers, the pickled buds of a shrub mostly grown in southern Europe, are commonly used to add a salt-sour taste, and can reduce the need for salt in a dish.

Each serving provides   kcal 162, protein 7 g, fat 7 g (of which saturated fat 3 g), carbohydrate 18 g (of which sugars 2 g), fibre 2.5 g. Useful source of folate, niacin, potassium, vitamin B_1, vitamin B_6, vitamin B_{12}, vitamin C.

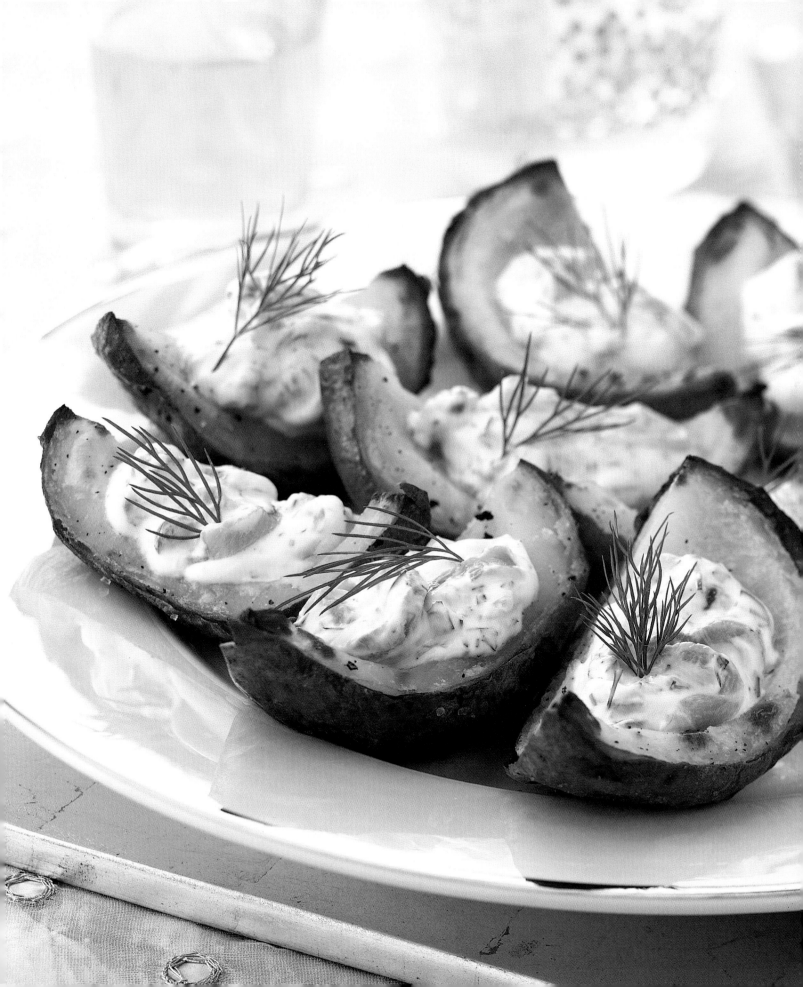

Caramelised onion tartlets

Croustades – made from thin slices of bread pushed into bun tins, brushed with melted butter and baked to crisp – are a great alternative to pastry for savoury tartlets. These are filled with a mixture of onions and sun-dried tomatoes. Both the croustades and filling can be prepared ahead, then warmed and assembled for serving.

Preparation time **20 minutes**   Cooking time **35 minutes**   *Makes 12 tartlets*

spray oil, plus 1 tbsp butter, melted

12 thin slices white bread

1 tbsp extra virgin olive oil

2 large onions, about 450 g (1 lb) in total, thinly sliced

30 g (1 oz) sun-dried tomatoes packed in oil, drained and roughly chopped

2 tsp finely chopped fresh thyme

30 g (1 oz) walnut pieces

salt and pepper

1 Preheat the oven to 230°C (450°F, gas mark 8). Lightly spray 12 deep bun tins with a little of the spray oil. Using a 7.5 cm (3 in) pastry cutter, cut a disc from each slice of bread. Flatten each bread disc with a rolling pin, then press into the buttered bun tins to line them evenly, curving the edge of the bread slightly to make large scallop shapes.

2 Brush the bread cases with the melted butter and bake for 8–10 minutes or until crisp and golden. Set aside in a warm place until ready to fill. (If made ahead, keep the bread cases in an airtight tin.)

3 Heat the oil in a large heavy pan with a well-fitting lid. Add the onions and stir well. Cover with the lid and cook over a low heat for 20 minutes or until the onions are very soft.

4 Remove the lid, turn up the heat and cook rapidly, stirring, until the onions turn a dark golden brown. Remove from the heat and stir in the sun-dried tomatoes and thyme. Season with salt and pepper to taste. (If made ahead, cool the filling and keep in the fridge, then reheat just before filling the bread cases.)

5 Divide the onion filling among the croustades, then scatter the chopped walnuts over the top. Serve hot.

Another idea
Use filo pastry cases instead of croustades. Spray the bun tins with spray oil, then cut 270 g (9½ oz) filo pastry into 9 cm (3½ in) squares (you will need 48 squares). Press 4 squares, at different angles, into each bun tin, then brush with the melted butter. Bake in a preheated 220°C (425°F, gas mark 7) oven for 4–5 minutes or until crisp and golden.

Plus point
• Eating walnuts in moderate but regular amounts may help to reduce blood cholesterol levels and guard against heart disease and cancer. This is because of the antioxidant nutrients found in walnuts: copper, selenium, vitamin E and zinc.

photo, page 253

Each serving provides   kcal 115, protein 4 g, fat 4 g (of which saturated fat 1 g), carbohydrate 19 g (of which sugars 3 g), fibre 1 g. Good source of vitamin E. Useful source of copper, selenium, vitamin B$_1$.

Tortilla chips with fresh mango and tomato salsa

Here is a fresh-tasting, colourful salsa that is rich in vitamins and valuable antioxidants. It is a perfect dip for crunchy, home-made tortilla chips, quickly baked rather than deep-fried for a healthy, low-fat result. Either corn tortillas or flour tortillas can be used to make the chips.

Preparation and cooking time **40 minutes, plus cooling**   *Serves 6*

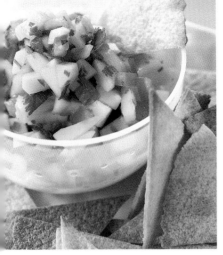

8 corn tortillas, about 300 g
(10½ oz) in total

Mango and tomato salsa

2 ripe mangoes, about 800 g
(1¾ lb) in total

1 large ripe tomato, about
200 g (7 oz)

grated zest and juice of 1 lime

1 medium-hot fresh green chilli,
seeded and finely chopped

1 garlic clove, crushed

2 tbsp chopped fresh coriander

1 tbsp snipped fresh chives

salt and pepper

1 Peel the mangoes and cut the flesh away from the central stone. Chop the flesh into small pieces and place in a large bowl. Chop the tomato into small pieces and add to the mango.

2 Add the lime zest and juice, chilli, garlic, coriander and chives. Stir, then season with salt and pepper to taste. Spoon into a serving bowl, cover and set aside in a cool place while preparing the tortilla chips.

3 Preheat the oven to 160°C (325°F, gas mark 3). Cut each tortilla into wedges using kitchen scissors. Spread out the wedges on a large baking sheet and bake for 15 minutes or until crisp and firm. Transfer to a wire rack and leave to cool.

4 To serve, place the bowl of salsa on one side of a large serving platter and scatter the tortilla chips next to it.

Some more ideas

Instead of the corn tortillas, use 4 large or 8 small flour tortillas (also called wraps), about 325 g (11 oz) in total.

Make a fresh **peach salsa** by using 4 ripe peaches instead of the mangoes. There is no need to skin the peaches. Just cut them in half, remove the stone and chop them.

For **nachos**, prepare the tortilla chips and leave to cool, then make a melted cheese dip. Finely chop 3 spring onions, 2 green peppers and 1 medium-hot fresh green chilli, seeded, and put into a shallow ovenproof dish. Sprinkle over ¼ tsp cumin seeds and season to taste with salt and pepper. Cut 200 g (7 oz) low-fat soft cheese into small cubes and scatter over the vegetables. Bake in a preheated 190°C (375°F, gas mark 5) oven for 10–15 minutes or until the cheese has melted. Scatter a little finely shredded Little Gem lettuce over the top, and serve hot, with the tortilla chips.

Plus points

● Fresh mangoes contain the antioxidant vitamin C, but the amount can vary considerably – in 100 g (3½ oz) mango flesh there can be as little as 10 mg vitamin C or as much as 180 mg.

● Chillies are another source of vitamin C, containing more, weight for weight, than citrus fruit such as oranges and lemons.

Each serving provides kcal 214, protein 5 g, fat 1 g (of which saturated fat 0.1 g), carbohydrate 50 g (of which sugars 20 g), fibre 5 g. Excellent source of vitamin A, vitamin C, vitamin E. Useful source of calcium, iron, niacin, potassium, vitamin B_1, vitamin B_6, zinc.

Piquant crab dip with crudités

This creamy dip is based on ingredients that can be kept in the storecupboard, so can be rustled up quickly if guests drop by unexpectedly. It is served with celery and cucumber sticks as well as juicy pineapple wedges, all of which add important nutrients to this snack. Breadsticks are another good dipper.

Preparation time **15 minutes**   *Serves 4*

2 celery sticks, about 125 g (4½ oz) in total

½ cucumber, about 125 g (4½ oz)

1 small pineapple, about 340 g (12 oz)

Crab dip

1 can white crab meat, about 120 g, drained

2 tbsp reduced-fat mayonnaise

2 tbsp plain low-fat yogurt

1 tsp tomato purée

grated zest of 1 lime

30 g (1 oz) sun-dried tomatoes packed in oil, drained and finely chopped

30 g (1 oz) gherkins, finely chopped

a few drops of Tabasco sauce, or to taste

1 To make the dip, put the crab meat, mayonnaise, yogurt, tomato purée, lime zest, sun-dried tomatoes and gherkins in a bowl and stir together thoroughly. Season with Tabasco sauce to taste. Place the dip in a small serving bowl, cover and chill while preparing the crudités.

2 Cut the celery and cucumber into chunky sticks. Remove the crown of leaves from the pineapple (wash and keep the leaves for garnish, if you like). Cut the flesh into wedges, leaving the skin on, then cut away the core.

3 Arrange the celery, cucumber and pineapple on a platter with the bowl of dip. Garnish with the pineapple leaves, if liked, and serve.

Some more ideas

Use the crab dip to fill the hollows in 2 halved and stoned avocados, piling up the dip over the surface. Scatter a little diced cucumber and red pepper over the top, and serve with salad leaves and bread as a light lunch.

Make a **smoked mackerel dip**. Mix 125 g (4½ oz) skinless smoked mackerel fillet with the mayonnaise and yogurt, then flavour with 1 tsp horseradish sauce, the grated zest of 1 lemon and 30 g (1 oz) chopped watercress.

Garnish with sprigs of watercress. This is delicious served with medium-thick slices of crisp red and green apple as crudités.

For canapés, serve the crab dip or smoked mackerel dip on rounds of cucumber, cut about 1 cm (½ in) thick. Garnish the canapés with thin julienne strips of radish or little watercress leaves.

Plus points

● Crab is a good source of phosphorus, a mineral needed for the development and maintenance of healthy bones. Phosphorus also plays an important role in releasing energy from food.

● Celery, first grown as a medicinal herb, only became a popular vegetable in the late 17th century. It provides potassium, and green celery sticks and leaves contain the antioxidant beta-carotene.

Each serving provides kcal 157, protein 8 g, fat 9.5 g (of which saturated fat 1 g), carbohydrate 12 g (of which sugars 11 g), fibre 2 g. Excellent source of vitamin E. Good source of copper, vitamin C, zinc. Useful source of calcium, potassium.

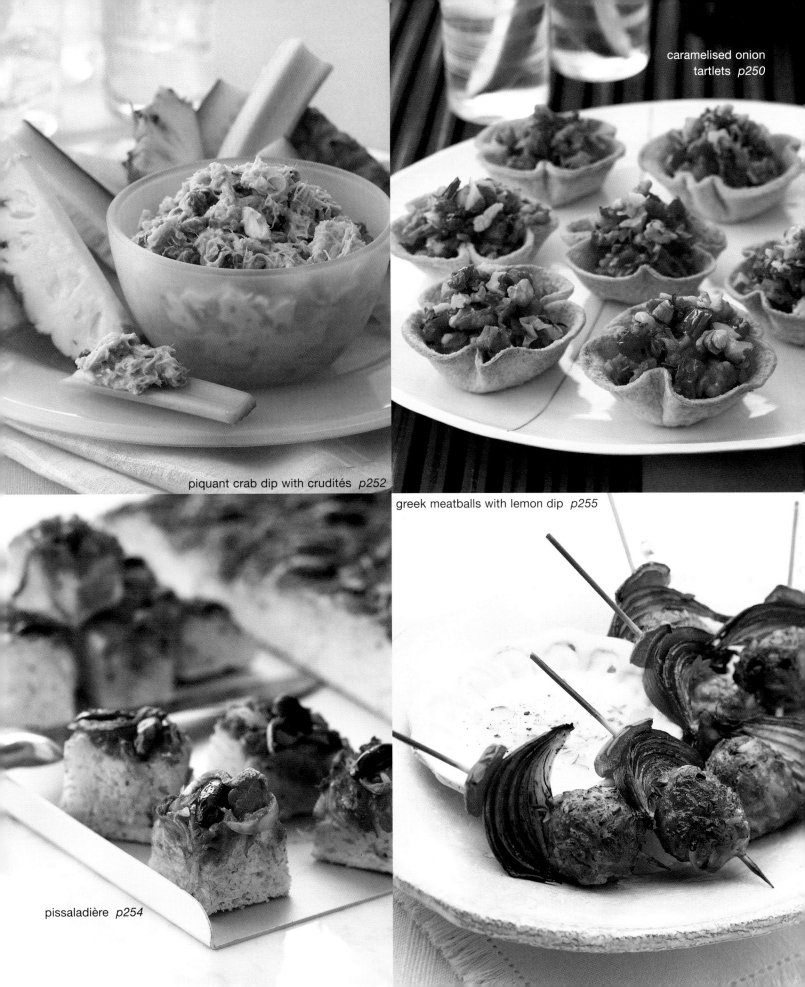

caramelised onion tartlets *p250*

piquant crab dip with crudités *p252*

pissaladière *p254*

greek meatballs with lemon dip *p255*

Pissaladière

Pissaladière is a Provençal relative of Italian pizza. The thick bread base, enriched with olive oil, is topped with a flavoursome tomato and onion mixture, then decorated with a lattice of anchovies and black olives. Serve warm or cool, cut in bite-sized squares for canapés, or into 16 larger snack-sized squares.

Preparation time **1½ hours, plus 1 hour rising**   Cooking time **40 minutes**   *Makes 64 bite-sized squares*

Dough

450 g (1 lb) strong (bread) flour, plus extra for kneading

1 tsp salt

1 sachet easy-blend dried yeast, about 7 g

3 tbsp extra virgin olive oil

300 ml (10 fl oz) hand-hot water

Topping

3 tbsp extra virgin olive oil

4 onions, about 750 g (1 lb 10 oz) in total, thinly sliced

2 garlic cloves, crushed

1 can chopped tomatoes in rich tomato juice, about 400 g

2 tbsp tomato purée

1 tbsp chopped fresh oregano

2 cans anchovy fillets, about 50 g each, drained and halved lengthways

16 stoned black olives, about 55 g (2 oz) in total, quartered

pepper

1 For the dough, sift the flour and salt into a bowl, then stir in the yeast. Make a well in the centre and pour in the oil and water. Gradually mix the dry ingredients into the liquids, using a spoon at first and then your hand, to make a soft, slightly sticky dough.

2 Turn the dough out onto a lightly floured surface and knead for 10 minutes or until the dough is smooth and springy. Place in a lightly oiled bowl, cover with cling film and leave in a warm place to rise for about 45 minutes or until doubled in size.

3 Meanwhile, make the topping. Heat the oil in a large saucepan, add the onions and garlic, and cook over a low heat for about 40 minutes or until very soft and lightly golden but not browned. Add the tomatoes with their juice, the tomato purée, oregano and pepper to taste, and cook gently for a further 10 minutes, stirring ocasionally. Remove from the heat and leave to cool.

4 When the dough has risen, knock it back and knead again gently. Roll it out on a floured surface to a 30 cm (12 in) square and place on a lightly oiled baking sheet.

5 Preheat the oven to 200°C (400°F, gas mark 6). Spread the onion mixture evenly over the dough square, then make a criss-cross pattern on top with the anchovy fillets. Place the olive quarters in the squares. Leave the pissaladière to rise at room temperature for about 15 minutes.

6 Bake the pissaladière for about 30 minutes or until the crust is golden and firm, then reduce the oven temperature to 190°C (375°F, gas mark 5) and bake for a further 10 minutes. Allow to cool slightly before cutting into squares for serving.

Plus points

• This pissaladière is made with a thick bread base, providing generous starchy carbohydrate. As white flour by law must contain added iron, calcium, vitamin B_1 and niacin, the bread base can also make a contribution to the intake of these nutrients.

• Canned tomatoes are a nutritious store-cupboard ingredient as the canning process does not destroy the lycopene content but rather enhances it. Lycopene is a phyto-chemical with powerful antioxidant properties.

photo, page 253

Each serving provides   (one square) kcal 44, protein 1.5 g, fat 1.5 g (of which saturated fat 0.2 g), carbohydrate 6.5 g (of which sugars 1 g), fibre 0.5 g.

Greek meatballs with lemon dip

These little meatballs, made from a mixture of minced lamb and rice, flavoured with thyme, lemon and nutmeg, are grilled on sticks for easy eating. The classic Greek egg and lemon dipping sauce served alongside has a tangy flavour, which is a perfect complement for the meatballs.

Preparation time **25 minutes**   Cooking time **20–25 minutes**   *Makes 24 kebabs*

30 g (1 oz) long-grain rice

2 small red onions

400 g (14 oz) lean minced lamb

1 small onion, very finely chopped

1 garlic clove, crushed

1 tbsp chopped fresh thyme

½ tsp freshly grated nutmeg

finely grated zest of 1 lemon

1 large red pepper, seeded and cut into 24 small squares

extra virgin olive oil for brushing

salt and pepper

Egg and lemon dip

1½ tsp arrowroot

juice of 2 small lemons

100 ml (3½ fl oz) lamb or chicken stock

1 small egg

2 tsp chopped fresh thyme

salt and pepper

1 Place the rice in a pan, cover with cold water and bring to the boil. Cook for 10 minutes or according to the packet instructions. Drain and set aside.

2 Soak 24 long wooden cocktail sticks in warm water for about 10 minutes, then drain. Preheat the grill to moderate.

3 Cut each red onion into 12 thin wedges, keeping them still attached at the root end.

4 Combine the minced lamb, finely chopped onion, cooked rice, garlic, thyme, nutmeg and lemon zest in a bowl, and season with salt and pepper to taste. Mix well together using your hands. Shape the meat mixture into 24 small balls.

5 Thread a meatball, 1 piece of pepper and 1 onion wedge onto each cocktail stick. Arrange in one layer on a rack in the grill pan. (The kebabs can be prepared 3–4 hours ahead and then kept in the fridge, covered with cling film.) Brush lightly with oil and grill for 15–18 minutes, turning occasionally, until golden brown and thoroughly cooked.

6 Meanwhile, make the dip. Mix the arrowroot with about half of the lemon juice, then stir in the rest. Heat the stock in a small saucepan until boiling, then stir in the arrowroot and lemon juice mixture. Bring back to the boil, stirring constantly, then remove from the heat.

7 Put the egg in a bowl and whisk lightly. Slowly pour in the hot stock mixture in a thin, steady stream, whisking constantly. Return to the pan and whisk over a low heat for about 4 minutes or until the sauce is smooth and thick. Do not boil or the egg may curdle and spoil the texture. Stir in the chopped thyme, and season with salt and pepper to taste.

8 Serve the meatball skewers with the hot lemon sauce.

Some more ideas

Use green or yellow instead of red pepper, or replace it with wedges of bulb fennel.

For a quick and easy lemon-mint dip, stir the grated zest of 1 lemon and 2 tbsp chopped fresh mint into 200 g (7 oz) Greek-style yogurt.

Plus points

● Minced lamb can have quite a high fat content, but because these meatballs are grilled, much of the excess fat is drained off.

● Making the meatballs with a mixture of lamb and rice means less meat is used than normal, and healthy starchy carbohydrates are added with the rice.

photo, page 253

Each serving provides   **(two kebabs)** kcal 72, protein 8 g, fat 3 g (of which saturated fat 0.2 g), carbohydrate 4 g (of which sugars 2 g), fibre 0.4 g. Useful source of vitamin A, vitamin C.

Gingered crab filo parcels

These Oriental-style, triangular parcels of crisp, light filo pastry enclose a ginger-flavoured filling of crab, water chestnuts and sweetcorn. They look and taste wonderful, and are really easy to make. Prepare them ahead for a party, then bake just before serving with a sweet chilli dipping sauce.

Preparation time **45–50 minutes**   Cooking time **12–13 minutes**   *Makes 18 parcels*

1 can white meat crab, about 170 g, drained

1 can water chestnuts, about 225 g, drained and coarsely chopped

1 can sweetcorn, about 200 g, drained

4 spring onions, chopped

1 tbsp finely chopped fresh root ginger

1 fresh red chilli, seeded and finely chopped

2 tbsp Chinese cooking wine or dry sherry

2 tbsp groundnut oil

1 tbsp toasted sesame oil

6 sheets filo pastry, about 50 x 30 cm (20 x 12 in) each, about 225 g (8 oz) in total

1 tbsp sesame seeds

salt and pepper

To serve

spring onions

Thai sweet chilli dipping sauce

1 Preheat the oven to 200°C (400°F, gas mark 6). Combine the crab, water chestnuts, sweetcorn, spring onions, ginger, red chilli and Chinese cooking wine or sherry in a bowl, and season with salt and pepper to taste. Mix together the groundnut and sesame oils in a cup.

2 Roll up the 6 sheets of filo pastry loosely, rolling from a short side. Using a sharp knife, cut the roll across evenly into 3. Cover 2 of these shorter rolls with cling film to prevent them from drying out. Unravel the third roll, remove one of the strips and set the rest aside, covered.

3 Lay the strip of filo flat on the work surface, with a short end nearest to you, and brush with a little of the oil mixture. Place a heaped teaspoon of the crab mixture near the bottom, towards the right-hand corner of the short end, and fold the pastry diagonally over it. Continue folding diagonally, over and over, until you reach the end of the strip, making a neat triangular parcel. Place on a baking sheet, seam side down.

4 Repeat with remaining strips of filo, uncovering them only when needed, until all of the crab mixture is used. (The parcels can be prepared in advance; cover the baking sheets with cling film and keep in the fridge. The baking time may need to be increased to 15 minutes if the parcels are very cold.)

5 Lightly brush the tops of the parcels with any remaining oil mixture and sprinkle with the sesame seeds. Bake for 12–13 minutes or until crisp and golden.

6 Transfer the parcels to a wire rack and cool slightly. Meanwhile, shred the tops of the spring onions for garnishing, to form 'brushes'. Serve the parcels warm, on a tray garnished with the spring onion brushes and a little dish of Thai sweet chilli dipping sauce to accompany.

Some more ideas

For **prawn filo parcels**, use 125 g (4½ oz) chopped cooked peeled prawns in place of the crab meat.

To make **mini spring rolls** with a vegetable filling, mix together 200 g (7 oz) bean sprouts, 1 grated carrot, 1 can sliced bamboo shoots, about 220 g, drained and chopped, 4 chopped spring onions and 125 g (4½ oz) chopped mushrooms. Heat 1 tbsp groundnut oil in a large pan, add 1 tbsp finely chopped fresh root ginger and 2 crushed garlic cloves,

Each serving provides   (one dumpling) kcal 79, protein 3 g, fat 3 g (of which saturated fat 0.5 g), carbohydrate 11 g (of which sugars 1 g), fibre 0.5 g.

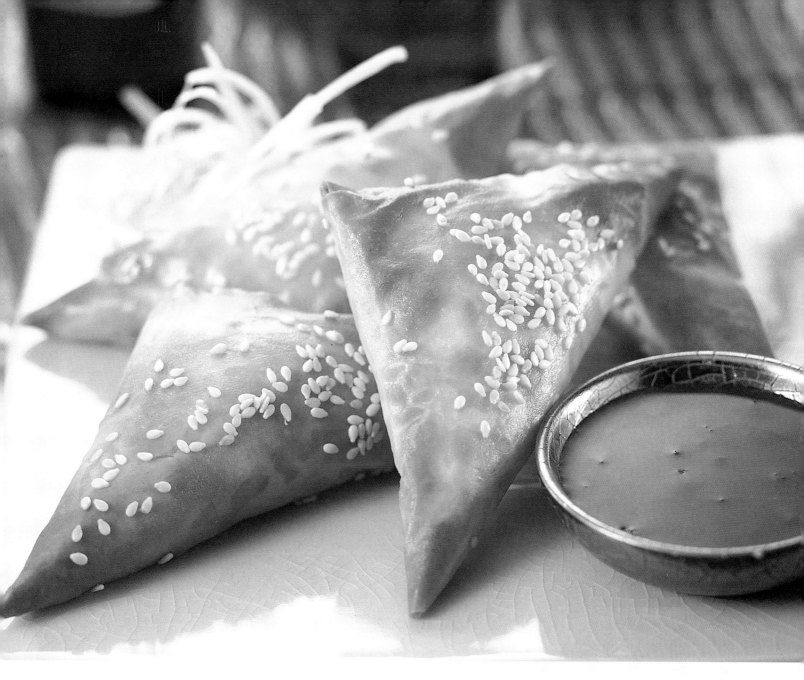

and stir-fry for 30 seconds. Add the vegetable mixture and stir-fry for 1 minute. Sprinkle over 1 tbsp light soy sauce and 1 tbsp Chinese cooking wine or dry sherry, and stir-fry for 1 minute, then cool. Cut the filo pastry into strips as in the main recipe. Mix together 2 tbsp groundnut oil

and 1 tbsp toasted sesame oil. Lightly brush a strip of filo with a little of the oil mixture, then place a heaped teaspoon of filling on the centre base. Fold in the sides and roll up to make a little cigar shape. Repeat with the remaining filo and filling. Finish and bake as in the main recipe.

Plus points

- Using filo for these parcels keeps the fat content low. This is because only a light brushing of oil is needed to stick the pastry edges together and to give a golden brown sheen and crisp texture, and the parcels are baked rather than deep fried.

- Ginger is believed to aid digestion and help to stimulate the circulation. It is also used as an antiseptic, to help to relieve the symptoms of colds as well as morning and travel sickness.

Smoked turkey and apricot bites

Dried apricots moistened with orange juice, then wrapped in smoked turkey rashers make a tasty snack to pass round with drinks, as well as an interesting garnish for a festive roast chicken or turkey. Take care when grilling turkey rashers – they cook more quickly than bacon and, because they contain no fat, will dry out if overcooked.

Preparation time **10 minutes**   Cooking time **2 minutes**   *Makes 24 bites*

24 ready-to-eat dried apricots

juice of 1 orange

2 tsp marmalade

2 tsp wholegrain mustard

6 smoked turkey rashers, about 150 g (5½ oz) in total

1 tsp extra virgin olive oil

chopped fresh flat-leaf parsley to garnish (optional)

1 Place the apricots in a small bowl, sprinkle over the orange juice and toss so that they are moistened all over (this will prevent them from burning under the grill).

2 Mix the marmalade with the mustard. Spread each turkey rasher with a little of the mustard mixture, then, using scissors, cut it in half lengthways. Cut each piece in half again, this time across the middle, to make a total of 24 strips of turkey.

3 Preheat the grill to moderate. Drain the apricots. Wrap a strip of turkey around each apricot and secure it with a wooden cocktail stick.

4 Arrange the turkey bites on the grill pan, then brush each with a little oil. Grill for 1 minute on each side or until the turkey is just cooked.

5 Pile the bites in a small shallow bowl and sprinkle with chopped parsley, if using. Serve hot.

Some more ideas

Instead of the mustard and marmalade mixture, spread the turkey rashers with a little pesto sauce.

To make **smoked turkey and banana chutney bites**, cut 3 medium-sized bananas into chunky pieces (8 pieces each) and toss in a little lemon or lime juice to prevent them from discolouring. Wrap each piece in a strip of turkey rasher that has been spread with a little mango chutney, then grill for 1 minute on each side. Serve hot.

For **pineapple and Black Forest ham bites**, peel a small pineapple, about 900 g (2 lb) with the leaves. Cut into quarters lengthways and trim away the woody core. Cut each quarter across into 8 to make 32 pieces in total. Cut 8 slices of Black Forest ham in half lengthways, then cut each piece across in half. Wrap a strip of ham around each wedge of pineapple and secure with a cocktail stick. Serve as soon as possible.

Plus points

• Ready-to-eat dried apricots are one of the richest fruit sources of iron and a useful source of calcium.

• Turkey rashers offer an excellent lower-fat alternative to bacon: 100 g (3½ oz) contains 1.6 g fat and 99 kcals, whereas the same weight of back bacon contains 21 g fat and 249 kcals.

photo, page 261

Each serving provides (one turkey bite) kcal 75, protein 3 g, fat 0.5 g (of which saturated fat 0.1 g), carbohydrate 15 g (of which sugars 15 g), fibre 2.5 g. Useful source of copper, potassium.

Spicy date, apple and ricotta dip

The natural sweetness of dates makes them an excellent sweetener in desserts, cakes and chutneys. Here they are cooked until smooth and pulpy with apple and aromatic spices to create a dip to serve with fruit and vegetable pieces. Alternatively, use this as an unusual topping for toast, scones or sweet crostini made with fruited bread.

Preparation time **15–20 minutes, plus cooling**   *Serves 4*

3 green cardamom pods

1 Bramley cooking apple, about 225 g (8 oz), peeled and roughly chopped

125 g (4½ oz) stoned dried dates, roughly chopped

½ tsp ground cinnamon

250 g (9 oz) ricotta cheese

To serve

crudités such as wedges of red and green-skinned apples, carrot, celery and cucumber sticks, wedges of pineapple, seedless grapes and slices of carambola

1 Lightly crush the cardamom pods with the flat side of a chef's knife to split them open, then remove the seeds. Discard the pods and crush the seeds with the side of the knife. (This can be done with a pestle and mortar.)

2 Put the apple, dates, crushed cardamom seeds and cinnamon in a saucepan with 200 ml (7 fl oz) water. Bring to the boil over a moderate heat, stirring occasionally. Turn down the heat and simmer for 10 minutes or until the apples are cooked and the dates are pulpy. Stir the mixture occasionally during cooking.

3 Remove from the heat and leave to cool. When the apple mixture is cold, beat in the ricotta cheese. Keep, covered, in the fridge until needed. (The dip will keep for 3–4 days.)

4 Serve in a shallow bowl or dish surrounded by an assortment of fruit and vegetable crudités.

Another idea

To make a **date, apple and orange dip**, omit the ricotta cheese and instead beat in the grated zest and juice of 1 large orange. Pile into a bowl and serve surrounded with chunky wedges of apple and pear, and sticks of celery and carrot.

Plus points

● Ricotta is an Italian cheese made from the whey drained off when making cheeses such as mozzarella. It has a high moisture content, which makes it lower in fat and calories than many other soft, creamy cheeses.

● In common with all cheeses, ricotta is a good source of calcium, and it contains vitamins A and D. Less of these vitamins are present in low-fat cheeses such as ricotta – vitamin D is fat-soluble, so the less fat in the cheese, the less vitamin D – but the amounts are still useful.

● The apple and dried dates provide useful amounts of fibre.

● Both cinnamon and cardamom are spices that can help to relieve indigestion. Also, cinnamon acts as a nasal decongestant.

photo, page 261

Each serving provides   (dip alone) kcal 195, protein 7 g, fat 7 g (of which saturated fat 4 g), carbohydrate 27 g (of which sugars 27 g), fibre 2 g. Useful source of calcium, niacin, vitamin A, vitamin B$_{12}$, vitamin C.

Date and walnut flapjacks

Flapjacks are a favourite sweet for lunchboxes as well as for coffee or teatime. The modern streamlined version here uses less butter than usual, and adds dates for natural sweetness as well as walnuts and sunflower seeds for extra texture. The result is both nutritious and delicious.

Preparation time **15 minutes**   Cooking time **20 minutes**   *Makes 16 flapjacks*

100 g (3½ oz) unsalted butter

3 tbsp sunflower oil

55 g (2 oz) light muscovado sugar

3 tbsp clear honey

grated zest of 1 orange

2 tbsp orange juice

100 g (3½ oz) dried stoned dates, chopped

75 g (2½ oz) walnut pieces, chopped

250 g (8½ oz) porridge oats

30 g (1 oz) sunflower seeds

1 Preheat the oven to 180°C (350°F, gas mark 4). Lightly grease a shallow non-stick baking tin measuring 28 x 18 x 2.5 cm (11 x 7 x 1 in), or a 20 cm (8 in) square tin. If you do not have a non-stick tin, lightly grease an ordinary baking tin, then line the bottom with baking parchment.

2 Place the butter, oil, sugar, honey, and orange zest and juice in a heavy-based saucepan and heat gently, stirring until the butter has melted. Remove the pan from the heat and stir in the dates and walnuts. Then stir in the oats, making sure they are evenly coated with the butter mixture.

3 Turn the mixture into the prepared tin, pressing it down firmly and evenly. Sprinkle the sunflower seeds over the top and press down so they are lightly embedded in the surface.

4 Bake for 20 minutes or until deep golden around the edges. Remove from the oven and allow to cool slightly in the tin, then mark out 16 pieces on the top surface with a sharp knife.

5 Leave to cool completely, still in the tin, before cutting into bars along the marked lines. The flapjacks can be kept in an airtight container for up to 1 week.

Some more ideas

Sprinkle the top with pumpkin seeds instead of the sunflower seeds.

Other dried fruits, such as dried cranberries or plump juicy raisins, can be added to the flapjack mixture, in addition to the dates, or add 2 tbsp good-quality mincemeat.

Substitute desiccated coconut for 30 g (1 oz) of the muscovado sugar.

Plus points

• Oats are an excellent source of soluble fibre, which can help to reduce high blood cholesterol levels. They also have a low Glycaemic Index.

• Up to 95 per cent of the calorie content of dates comes from natural sugars, but because of their fibre content – and because they are mixed with oats in this recipe – the body can keep the release of glucose into the bloodstream at a steady pace, resulting in a gentle and sustained rise in blood sugar levels for long-term energy, rather a sudden rise for a quick energy fix and then a fast dip.

• Sunflower seeds provide vitamin B_1, niacin and zinc, and are a rich source of vitamin E.

Each serving provides   **(one bar)** kcal 208, protein 3 g, fat 13 g (of which saturated fat 4 g), carbohydrate 22 g (of which sugars 11 g), fibre 2 g. Excellent source of vitamin E. Useful source of copper, vitamin B_1, zinc.

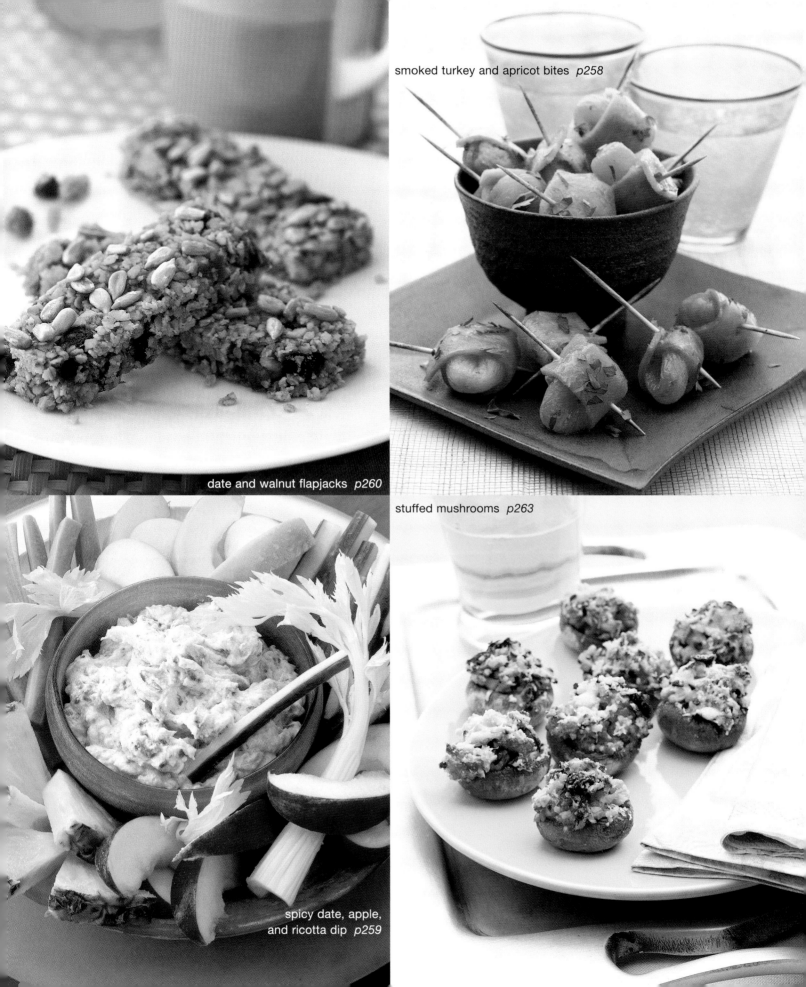

date and walnut flapjacks *p260*

smoked turkey and apricot bites *p258*

stuffed mushrooms *p263*

spicy date, apple,
and ricotta dip *p259*

Rosemary marinated olives

The flavour of olives is greatly enhanced by marinating them in fruity olive oil with fresh herbs and citrus juices. When served with colourful chunks of red and yellow pepper and little cherry tomatoes, they look and taste fabulous. For the best flavour, allow about 2 days marinating. These are great with warm pitta bread fingers.

Preparation time **10 minutes, plus 2 days marinating**   *Makes 800 g (1¾ lb), to serve 8*

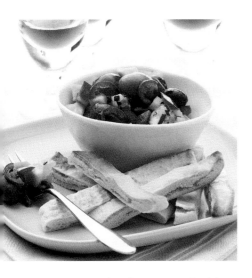

200 g (7 oz) olives, preferably a mixture of black and green

2 tbsp extra virgin olive oil

1 tbsp lemon juice

1 thin-skinned orange, scrubbed but not peeled, cut into small chunks

2 sprigs of fresh rosemary

1 fresh green chilli, seeded and thinly sliced

1 red pepper, seeded and cut into small chunks

1 yellow pepper, seeded and cut into small chunks

125 g (4½ oz) cherry tomatoes, halved or quartered

1 Place the olives in a large bowl and add the olive oil, lemon juice, chunks of orange, rosemary sprigs and chilli. Stir together, then cover (or transfer to a jar and seal). Place in the refrigerator.

2 For the next 2 days, every 12 hours or so, take the olive mixture from the fridge, uncover and stir. Cover again and return to the fridge to continue marinating.

3 When ready to eat, tip the olives into a serving bowl, add the peppers and tomatoes, and stir well together.

Some more ideas

Add the marinated olives to salads, such as young spinach leaves with chickpeas, or tuna and cucumber.

Make **garlicky marinated olives with feta**. Instead of orange, rosemary and chilli, add 2 roughly chopped garlic cloves, 30 g (1 oz) chopped sun-dried tomatoes and a small handful of roughly torn fresh basil leaves to the olive oil and lemon juice. Before serving the olives, toss them with 100 g (3½ oz) cubed feta cheese, the peppers, 125 g (4½ oz) halved baby plum tomatoes and some fresh basil leaves.

Plus points

• Olives are highly valued for their oil content, which is mostly the healthier monounsaturated type. Green olives provide more vitamin A than black olives.

• Extra virgin olive oil is the premium of all the olive oils. It has a low level of acidity and a wonderful aroma and flavour. As it is produced with minimal heat and refining processes, it retains more of its essential fatty acids and phytochemicals.

• The name rosemary comes from the Latin and means 'sea dew' – this strong, pungent herb was often found growing on the coast. In Roman times it was used mainly as a medicinal herb, to soothe the digestive system.

Each serving provides   **(100 g/3½ oz)** kcal 73, protein 1 g, fat 6 g (of which saturated fat 1 g), carbohydrate 5 g (of which sugars 4 g), fibre 2 g. Excellent source of vitamin C. Good source of vitamin A, vitamin E.

Stuffed mushrooms

Filled with a delicious combination of finely chopped courgette, spinach and hazelnuts, then topped with grated Parmesan cheese and baked, these mushrooms make a very tasty, hard-to-resist party bite. They look their best if the mushrooms used are all about the same size.

Preparation time **25–30 minutes**   Cooking time **15 minutes**   *Makes 16 mushrooms*

16 large closed-cap chestnut mushrooms or small field mushrooms, all about 4 cm (1½ in) diameter, about 250 g (8½ oz) in total

30 g (1 oz) butter

2 shallots, finely chopped

1 garlic clove, crushed

1 small courgette, finely chopped

15 g (½ oz) baby spinach leaves, finely shredded, plus extra leaves to garnish (optional)

30 g (1 oz) fresh wholemeal breadcrumbs

30 g (1 oz) hazelnuts, finely chopped

2 tbsp finely chopped parsley

45 g (1½ oz) Parmesan cheese, freshly grated

salt and pepper

1 Preheat the oven to 180°C (350°F, gas mark 4). Remove the stalks from the mushrooms and chop finely. Melt the butter in a frying pan, add the chopped mushroom stalks, shallots, garlic and courgette, and cook for 5 minutes, stirring occasionally.

2 Remove the pan from the heat and stir in the shredded spinach, breadcrumbs, hazelnuts, parsley, and season to taste.

3 Put the mushroom caps, hollow side up, in a single layer in a lightly greased shallow ovenproof dish or on a lightly greased baking tray. Heap some of the shallot and courgette mixture into each mushroom cap and sprinkle the Parmesan cheese over the top. (The mushrooms can be prepared 2–3 hours ahead and kept, covered with cling film, in the fridge.)

4 Bake for about 15 minutes or until the mushrooms are tender and the cheese has melted. Serve warm, on a bed of spinach leaves, if liked.

Some more ideas

For mushrooms stuffed with spring greens and walnuts, use spring greens in place of spinach, 1 red onion in place of shallots, chopped walnuts in place of hazelnuts, and fresh basil or coriander in place of parsley.

Make mushrooms with red pepper and pine nut filling. Sauté the mushroom stalks in 1 tbsp extra virgin olive oil with 4 finely chopped spring onions, ½ small seeded and finely chopped red pepper and 1 crushed garlic clove for 5 minutes. Stir in 30 g (1 oz) chopped pine nuts, 15 g (½ oz) chopped watercress, 30 g (1 oz) fresh breadcrumbs, 2 tbsp finely chopped parsley, and salt and pepper to taste. Fill the mushroom caps with this mixture and sprinkle with 45 g (1½ oz) finely grated mozzarella cheese. Bake as in the main recipe.

Plus points

● Mushrooms provide useful amounts of some of the B vitamins and are a good source of the trace mineral copper. This mineral has several functions – it is found in many enzymes, and is needed for bone growth as well as for the formation of connective tissue.

● Hazelnuts were known in China 5000 years ago and were also eaten by the Romans. They are a particularly good source of vitamin E and most of the B vitamins (with the exception of vitamin B_{12}).

photo, page 261

Each serving provides (one mushroom) kcal 46, protein 2 g, fat 4 g (of which saturated fat 2 g), carbohydrate 1 g (of which sugars 0.5 g), fibre 0.5 g. Useful source of selenium, vitamin E.

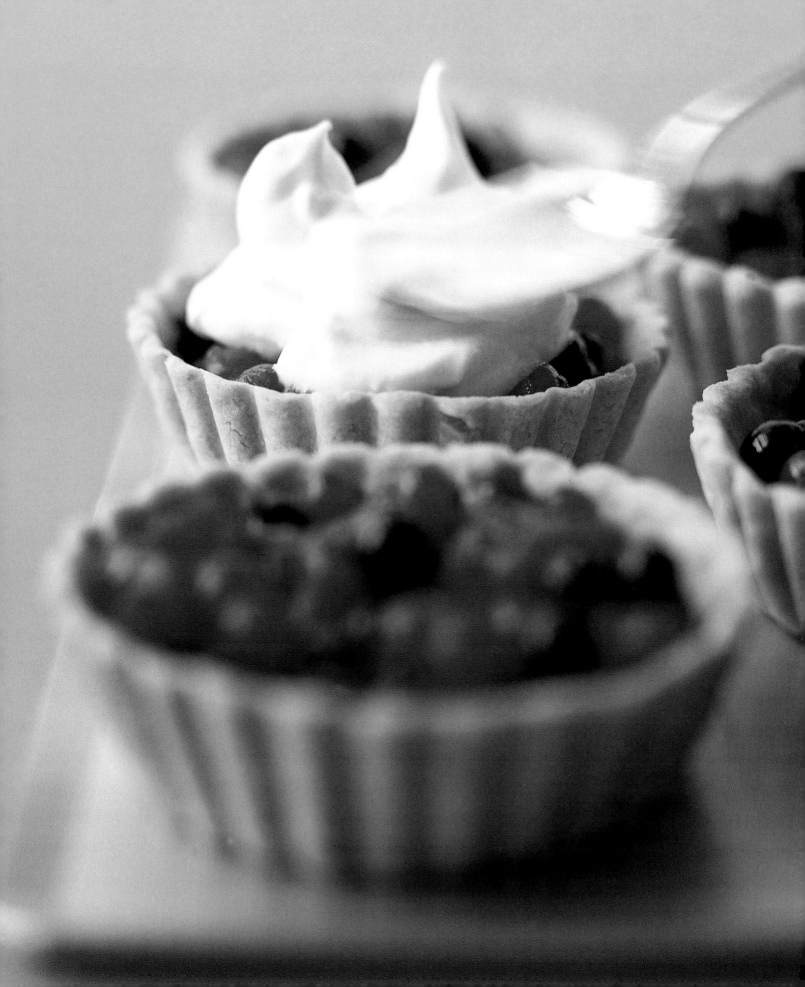

Desserts and drinks

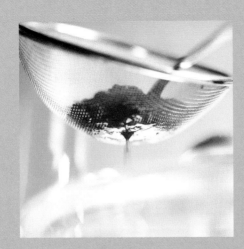

Mango smoothie

Smoothies are speedy and satisfying fruit drinks – as thick as a milk shake – that can either be made with milk and yogurt or just with pure fruit juices and fruit pulp. Almost any fresh fruit can be used, on its own or in combination. To serve more than 2, simply make a second batch of smoothies.

Preparation time **5 minutes**   *Serves 2*

1 ripe mango

150 g (5½ oz) plain low-fat yogurt, chilled

300 ml (10 fl oz) skimmed milk, chilled

1 tsp clear honey

seeds from 6 cardamom pods

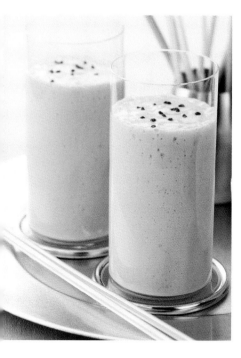

1 Peel the skin off the mango and cut the flesh away from the stone. Chop the flesh roughly and place it in a blender or food processor. Process until smooth.

2 Pour in the yogurt and milk, and continue to process until well mixed and frothy. Sweeten with honey.

3 Pour into 2 tall glasses and sprinkle the cardamom seeds over the top. Serve immediately.

Some more ideas

For a **tropical banana smoothie**, replace the mango and plain yogurt with 1 large sliced banana and 150 g (5½ oz) low-fat, tropical fruit-flavoured yogurt.

To make a **kiwi and raspberry smoothie**, use 2 peeled and chopped kiwi fruits, 225 g (8 oz) raspberries and 300 ml (10 fl oz) apple or white grape juice. Sweeten to taste with a little honey, if necessary.

Try a **pear and blackberry smoothie**, made with 2 peeled, cored and chopped ripe dessert pears, 125 g (4½ oz) blackberries, the pulpy flesh of 2 passion fruit and 300 ml (10 fl oz) cranberry juice.

Another delicious smoothie is **pineapple and strawberry**. Use 1 peeled, cored and chopped small pineapple with 225 g (8 oz) strawberries, 300 ml (10 fl oz) apple juice and 1 tbsp elderflower cordial.

Plus points

- Smoothies are made very quickly, using raw fruit, so they retain the maximum nutritional value of their ingredients.

- When made with milk and yogurt, a smoothie will also contain protein, calcium and many B vitamins – getting close to being a meal in a glass.

- Mango is an excellent source of the antioxidant beta-carotene, which the body can convert into vitamin A. This vitamin is essential for healthy skin and good vision, especially in dim light. Mangoes also provide substantial amounts of vitamin C as well as vitamins B_6 and E.

Each serving provides kcal 203, protein 10 g, fat 2.5 g (of which saturated fat 2 g), carbohydrate 37 g (of which sugars 37 g), fibre 4 g. Excellent source of vitamin A, vitamin C, vitamin E. Good source of calcium, vitamin B_2, vitamin B_6, vitamin B_{12}. Useful source of copper, folate, niacin, potassium, vitamin B_1, zinc.

Citrus wake-up

What an invigorating drink this is, made with fresh citrus, very lightly sweetened and flavoured with a little lime zest and mint. Squeezing your own juice makes all the difference in both nutrition and flavour, as vitamin C begins to dissipate as soon as a fruit or vegetable is cut. This mixed citrus drink makes a lively breakfast or brunch drink.

Preparation time **15–20 minutes**   *Serves 4*

4 juicy oranges, about 500 g (1 lb 2 oz) in total

1 pink grapefruit

1 lemon

1 lime

grated zest of 1 lime

1 tbsp caster sugar

2 tbsp finely shredded fresh mint leaves

To decorate (optional)

slices of lime

slices of lemon

1 Cut the oranges, grapefruit, lemon and lime in half crossways. Juice them using either an electric juicer or a simple citrus squeezer, preferably one that strains out the seeds but leaves in a generous quantity of pulp. If you have no squeezer at all, poke a fork into the flesh several times, then squeeze the juice from the fruit by hand, prodding with the fork now and again.

2 Combine the citrus juices in a jug with the lime zest, 4 tbsp water, the sugar and shreds of mint. Stir, then pour into glasses over a few ice cubes and, if you like, slices of lime and lemon.

Some more ideas

Any juicy oranges can be used – shamouti Jaffa oranges are particularly delicious with their balance of sweet and tart. Or use tangerines, satsumas, clementines, mandarins or ortaniques.

As a refreshing non-alcoholic alternative to wine or beer, dilute the mixture with sparkling mineral water – perfect for a sultry summer evening.

For a Mexican-inspired **citrus and mixed fruit 'zinger'**, omit the grapefruit and lime and use 2 lemons. Juice the citrus fruit and add the diced flesh of a ripe pineapple, 3 kiwi fruit

and ½ cucumber. Serve either chunky, as is, for a sort of fruit gazpacho, or whiz it all up with a hand-held electric blender until it is frothy. Adjust the sweetening to taste (you may prefer no sugar at all) and decorate with fresh mint.

Plus points

• Citrus fruit are one of the best sources of vitamin C. They also contain compounds called coumarins which are believed to help to thin the blood, thus preventing stroke and heart attacks. In addition, studies have shown a correlation between a regular intake of vitamin C and the maintenance of intellectual function in elderly people.

• Drinking sugary drinks with food slows down the rise in blood glucose, so aim to drink sweet drinks with meals rather than between meals.

photo, page 269

Each serving provides kcal 60, protein 1 g, fat 0 g, carbohydrate 14 g (of which sugars 14 g), fibre 2 g. Excellent source of vitamin C. Useful source of folate, vitamin B$_1$.

Frozen pineapple and berry slush

A cross between a breakfast sorbet and thick drink, this refreshing, virtually fat-free start to the day takes just seconds to whiz up. The secret of preparing it quickly is to keep a selection of chopped fruit in the freezer, then you can simply dip in to select a combination that suits your mood.

Preparation time 5–15 minutes, plus at least 1½ hours freezing of fruit   *Serves 4*

8 ice cubes

250 g (9 oz) hulled strawberries, frozen

250 g (9 oz) fresh pineapple chunks, frozen

120 ml (4 fl oz) pineapple juice

2 tbsp dried skimmed milk powder

1 tbsp vanilla sugar or caster sugar, or to taste

sprigs of fresh pineapple mint to decorate (optional)

1 Put the ice cubes in a food processor or heavy-duty blender and process until they are finely crushed. Alternatively, crush the ice cubes in a freezerproof bag, bashing them with a rolling pin, and then put them in the processor or blender.

2 Add the strawberries, pineapple chunks, pineapple juice and skimmed milk powder and process again until blended but still with small pieces of fruit and ice visible.

3 Taste and sweeten with sugar if necessary. (The amount of sugar needed will depend on the sweetness of the fruit.) Process briefly using the pulse button.

4 Spoon into tall glasses, decorate each with a sprig of pineapple mint, if you like, and serve with long spoons.

Some more ideas

This is even quicker to make if you buy 500 g bags of frozen mixed fruit.

Make a **summer fruit slush** with a 500 g bag of frozen mixed summer fruit, including blackberries, blueberries, redcurrants, cherries, raspberries and strawberries. Add 4 tbsp unsweetened orange juice and 2 tbsp skimmed milk powder and process. Sweeten with a little caster sugar to taste, if necessary.

For a **tropical slush** use 400 g (14 oz) frozen chopped mango flesh and 1 fresh banana, about 100 g (3½ oz). Add 4 tbsp coconut milk and 4 tbsp unsweetened orange juice.

Plus points

• Fresh (and frozen) pineapple contains a substance called bromelain, a digestive enzyme that can break down proteins. There is some evidence to suggest that bromelain may help to break up blood clots and may therefore be helpful in protecting against heart disease. Bromelain also has an anti-inflammatory action and has been used in the treatment of arthritis.

• A wide variety of fruit is now available frozen. These are convenient to have on hand and may well be a better source of vitamins than some 'fresh' fruits that have been poorly stored or badly handled or languished too long on the shelf. They are particularly useful for blended drinks, where the texture of the fruit is not important.

• Dried skimmed milk powder, which gives this slush body, provides calcium, essential for healthy bones and teeth, as well as protein, zinc, and vitamins B_2 and B_{12}.

Each serving provides kcal 95, protein 3 g, fat 0.3 g, carbohydrate 22 g (of which sugars 22 g), fibre 2 g. Excellent source of vitamin C. Useful source of calcium, folate, vitamin B_1, vitamin B_2.

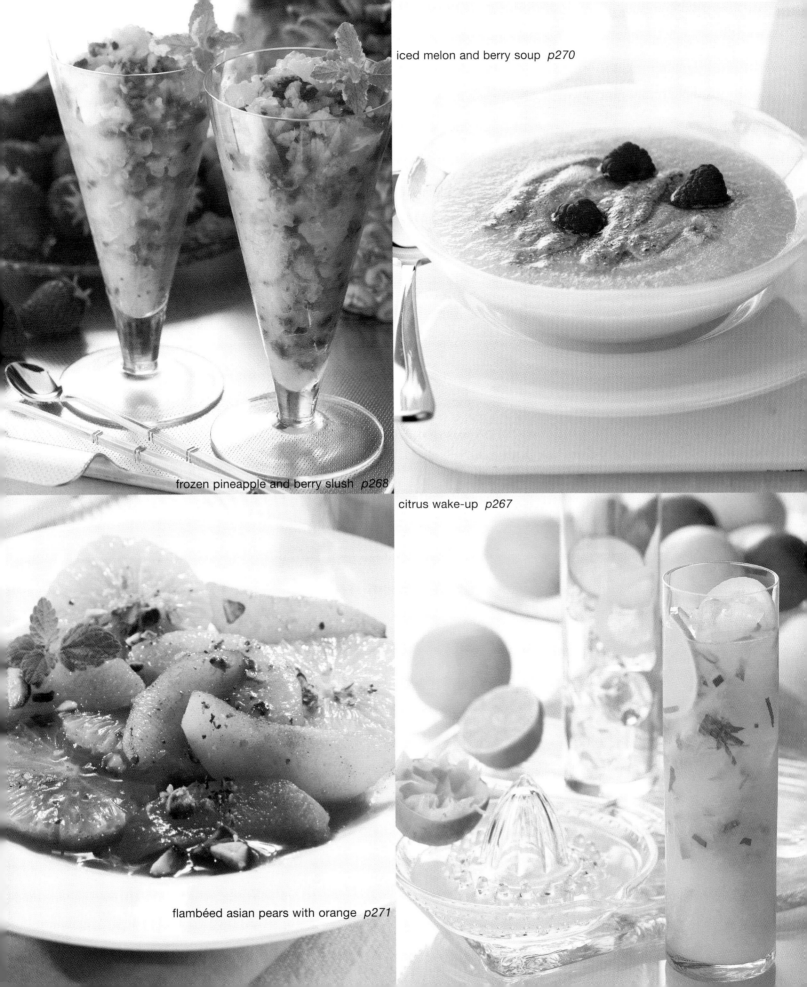

iced melon and berry soup *p270*

frozen pineapple and berry slush *p268*

citrus wake-up *p267*

flambéed asian pears with orange *p271*

Iced melon and berry soup

Almost any variety of green-fleshed melon, such as Galia or Honeydew, can be used for this very pretty soup, but it is essential that the melon be perfectly ripe and sweet. Serve the soup as a refreshing first course when the weather is hot, dressing up each bowlful with a swirl of berry purée and some whole berries.

Preparation time **20 minutes, plus 30 minutes chilling** *Serves 4*

1 large ripe green-fleshed melon, about 1.25 kg (2¾ lb)

juice of 1 lime

3.5 cm (1½ in) piece fresh root ginger, peeled and grated

150 g (5½ oz) blueberries

120 ml (4 fl oz) freshly squeezed orange juice

2 tbsp Greek-style yogurt

150 g (5½ oz) raspberries or strawberries

1 Halve the melon, discard the seeds and scoop the flesh out of the peel into a blender or food processor. Add the lime juice and ginger. Purée until smooth, stopping occasionally to push the pieces of melon to the bottom of the goblet or bowl. Pour the purée into a bowl, cover and chill for 30 minutes or until cold.

2 Put the blueberries into the blender or food processor. Add the orange juice and yogurt and purée until smooth. Transfer to a second bowl, cover and chill for about 30 minutes or until cold.

3 Divide the melon soup among 4 chilled shallow glass bowls or dishes. Spoon a quarter of the blueberry purée onto the centre of each in a decorative pattern. Scatter the raspberries or strawberries on top. Serve at once.

Some more ideas

Try orange-fleshed melon, such as Ogen, Charentais or Cantaloupe, and top the soup with sliced kiwi fruit instead of the red berries.

Use 2 kg (4½ lb) watermelon instead of the green melon. Chop the flesh, discarding the seeds, then purée with the lime juice and 1 seeded and chopped fresh green chilli instead of the ginger. Coarsely crush the blueberries with the raspberries and/or strawberries, adding 1–2 tbsp orange juice. Omit the yogurt.

Plus points

- All melons provide vitamins B and C, and are very low in calories. Their high water content makes them a delicious and refreshing thirst-quencher.

- Ginger is thought to be an anti-inflammatory agent that can help to ease some of the symptoms of arthritis.

- Blueberries are rich in vitamin C and a useful source of soluble fibre. They also contain several phytochemicals: flavonoids which strengthen blood capillaries and improve circulation, athocyanosides which help to fight infection and inflammation, and ellagic acid which can help to prevent cell damage that can lead to cancer. Like cranberries, blueberries also contain a natural antibiotic that can help to prevent urinary tract infections.

photo, page 269

Each serving provides   kcal 110, protein 3 g, fat 1 g (of which saturated fat 0.5 g), carbohydrate 24 g (of which sugars 24 g), fibre 4 g. Excellent source of vitamin C. Good source of potassium. Useful source of calcium, folate, vitamin B$_1$, vitamin B$_2$.

Flambéed Asian pears with orange

A delicious yet simple dessert, this is ready in just 25 minutes. Flaming the brandy burns off the alcohol, leaving a wonderful flavour which perfectly complements the oranges and pears. Even after cooking, Asian pears retain their crunchy texture, making a pleasant change from the more common dessert pears.

Preparation time **15 minutes**   Cooking time **10 minutes**   *Serves 6*

2 Asian pears

juice of ½ lemon

3 oranges

30 g (1 oz) butter

3 tbsp soft brown sugar

3 tbsp brandy

3 tbsp coarsely chopped pistachios

sprigs of fresh lemon balm to decorate

1 Peel, quarter and core the Asian pears. Cut them into slices and sprinkle with the lemon juice to prevent them from turning brown.

2 Peel the oranges, removing all the white pith. Cut them across into neat slices.

3 Melt the butter in a frying pan. Add the sugar and stir until dissolved. Add the pear slices and cook gently for about 3 minutes on each side or until they are just tender but still quite firm. Add the orange slices for the last minute of cooking, turning them to coat well with the juices in the pan.

4 Using a draining spoon, remove the pears and oranges to a shallow serving dish and keep warm. Boil the juices remaining in the pan to reduce a little, then pour over the fruit. Pour the brandy into the frying pan, heat it and set alight. Pour over the fruit.

5 Serve on warmed plates, sprinkled with the pistachios and decorated with lemon balm.

Some more ideas

Use sliced dessert pears instead of Asian pears. They will need only about 2 minutes cooking on each side to make them tender.

Use Poire William liqueur or Cointreau instead of brandy.

Replace the pears with apples, cut in rings. Cox's are particularly good prepared this way. Flambé with Calvados and sprinkle with chopped toasted hazelnuts.

Plus points

• Oranges are justly famous for their vitamin C content (54 mg per 100 g/3½ oz). This is one of the 'water-soluble' vitamins, which cannot be stored by the body, so it is essential that fruit and vegetables containing vitamin C are eaten every day. As scientists have increasingly recognised, this vitamin helps to prevent a number of degenerative diseases such as heart disease and cancer, through its powerful antioxidant activity.

photo, page 269

Each serving provides   kcal 150, protein 2 g, fat 7 g (of which saturated fat 3 g), carbohydrate 17 g (of which sugars 17 g), fibre 2 g. Good source of vitamin C. Useful source of folate, vitamin E.

Saffron and vanilla grilled fruit

This warm medley of luscious fruit is elegantly spiced with a marinade of saffron and vanilla. It is delicious on its own for a virtually no-fat dessert, or can be topped with a fruity sorbet, vanilla frozen yogurt or ice cream.

Preparation time **15 minutes, plus 1 hour optional marinating**   Cooking time **5 minutes**   *Serves 6*

small pinch of saffron threads

1 tsp pure vanilla extract

1 tbsp honey

2 tbsp Marsala wine or sweet sherry

juice of 1 orange

2 bananas

100 g (3½ oz) black grapes

1 papaya

2 kiwi fruit

1 Ugli fruit

To serve (optional)

6 scoops frozen yogurt, reduced-fat ice cream or sorbet

1 Heat a small dry pan over a high heat, add the saffron threads and toast for 30 seconds or until fragrant. Place the toasted saffron in a mortar and crush it with a pestle until fine. Add 4 tbsp hot water to the saffron and stir.

2 Transfer the saffron liquid to a mixing bowl and stir in the vanilla extract, honey, Marsala or sherry and orange juice.

3 Add the fruit to the saffron and vanilla marinade as you prepare it. Peel the bananas and cut them into bite-sized chunks. Pick the grapes from their stalks and add them whole to the marinade. Peel the papaya, remove the seeds and cut into bite-sized chunks. Peel the kiwi fruit and quarter it lengthways. Peel the Ugli fruit, removing all the white pith, and cut out the segments from between the membranes. Stir the fruit in the marinade. If time permits, cover the bowl tightly with cling film and leave the fruit to marinate for 1 hour before cooking.

4 Preheat the grill. Pour the fruit and marinade into a shallow ovenproof dish. Spread out the fruit in an even layer. Grill for 5 minutes or until all the fruit is heated through. Serve the fruit warm, topping each serving with a scoop of frozen yogurt, reduced-fat ice cream or sorbet, if you like.

Some more ideas

Make a tropical version of this dish by replacing the grapes with 2 thick slices of fresh pineapple, cut into chunks, and 3–4 fresh ripe apricots, halved and stoned. To make the marinade, omit the toasted saffron and hot water mixture and simply stir 1 tsp ground cinnamon with the vanilla extract and honey; use rum instead of Marsala or sherry, and the juice of 2 limes instead of orange juice.

Stone fruit, such as peaches, apricots and cherries, can be added to this warm fruit salad.

Plus points

● Long cooking will destroy a lot of the vitamin C in fruit, but most will survive the short cooking time in this recipe. Fibre and minerals are not affected by heat. The bananas, kiwi fruit and citrus fruit here provide potassium, which keeps body fluids in balance and blood pressure down.

● Papaya is a useful source of vitamin A (from the beta-carotene it contains), which is needed for good vision. This tropical fruit plays a vital role in preventing blindness in many parts of the world where those foods that provide most vitamin A in the UK (full-fat milk, cheese, butter and egg yolks) are not part of the average diet.

Each serving provides   (fruit alone) kcal 130, protein 2 g, fat 0.5 g, carbohydrate 30 g (of which sugars 26 g), fibre 2 g. Excellent source of vitamin C. Useful source of folate, potassium.

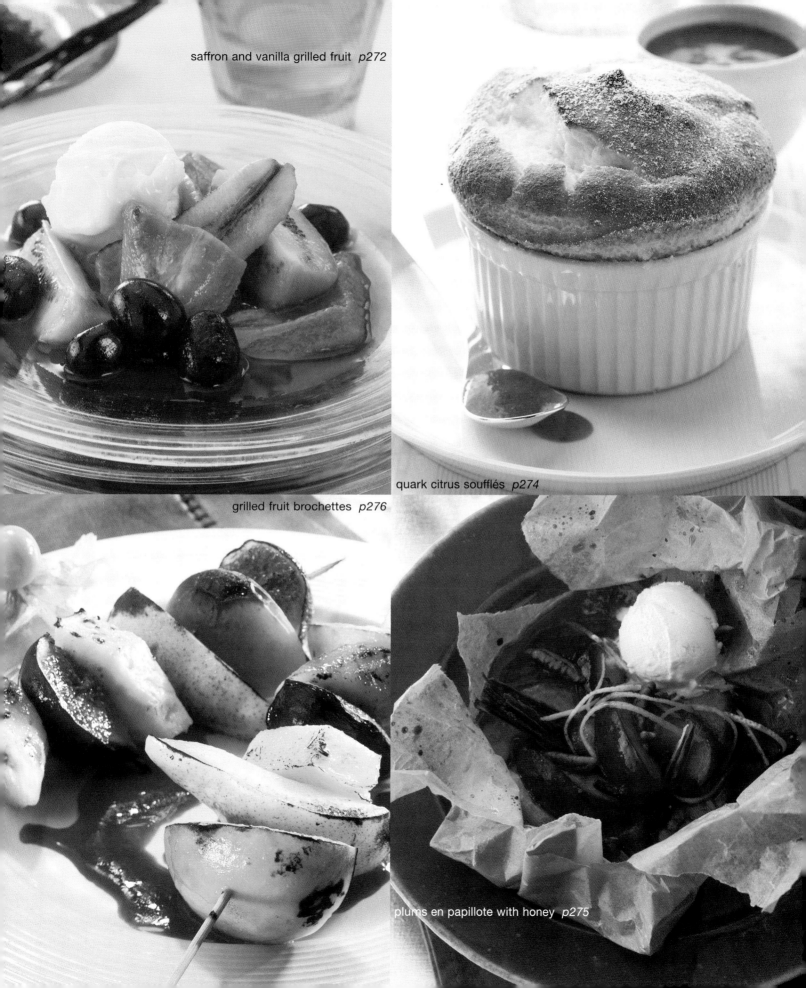

saffron and vanilla grilled fruit *p272*

quark citrus soufflés *p274*

grilled fruit brochettes *p276*

plums en papillote with honey *p275*

Quark citrus soufflés

These deliciously light, individual citrus soufflés will be a tempting and refreshing end to any meal. Quark cheese is low in fat and provides valuable nutrients such as calcium without adding too many calories. The accompanying strawberry coulis looks pretty and complements the soufflés perfectly, as well as contributing vitamin C.

Preparation time **30 minutes**   Cooking time **15–20 minutes**   *Serves 6*

15 g (½ oz) unsalted butter, melted

115 g (4 oz) caster sugar

4 eggs, separated

30 g (1 oz) cornflour

250 g (8½ oz) quark cheese

finely grated zest of 1 lime

finely grated zest of 1 small orange

sifted icing sugar to dust

Strawberry coulis

300 g (10½ oz) ripe strawberries, halved

2 tsp icing sugar, or to taste, sifted

dash of liqueur, such as kirsch (optional)

1 Preheat the oven to 190ºC (375ºF, gas mark 5). Brush 6 individual 200 ml (7 fl oz) soufflé dishes with the melted butter, then coat with caster sugar, using 30 g (1 oz) sugar in total. Set the dishes aside.

2 Put the egg yolks, 30 g (1 oz) of the caster sugar and the cornflour in a bowl and whisk together until creamy. Add the quark and the lime and orange zests, and whisk until thoroughly mixed.

3 In a clean mixing bowl, whisk the egg whites until stiff. Gradually whisk in the remaining 55 g (2 oz) caster sugar. Carefully fold the whisked egg whites into the quark mixture.

4 Spoon the mixture into the prepared soufflé dishes and set them on a baking sheet. Bake for 15–20 minutes or until well risen and golden brown.

5 Meanwhile, make the strawberry coulis. Purée the strawberries in a blender or food processor until smooth. Sweeten with the icing sugar, then stir in the liqueur, if using.

6 Serve the hot soufflés straight from the oven, dusted with a little icing sugar and with the coulis alongside.

Some more ideas

Use lemon and orange zests instead of lime and orange, or pink grapefruit and orange.

Coat the buttered dishes with 15 g (½ oz) finely crushed macaroons or ground hazelnuts instead of caster sugar.

For a **mixed berry soufflé**, grease a 1.7 litre (3 pint) soufflé dish with melted unsalted butter and dust with caster sugar. Make the soufflé mixture as in the main recipe, flavouring with the zest of 1 lemon and 1 lime. Put 350 g (12½ oz) mixed berries, such as raspberries, strawberries and blackberries, into the prepared soufflé dish. Spoon the soufflé mixture over the fruit, covering it completely, and bake for 30 minutes or until well risen and golden brown.

Plus points

• Quark is a soft curd cheese that can be made from skimmed or full-fat milk or from buttermilk. The fat content can therefore vary from low to virtually fat-free.

• Eggs are a good source of zinc, a mineral that is vital for growth, reproduction and efficient working of the immune system.

photo, page 273

Each serving provides (one soufflé) kcal 221, protein 12 g, fat 7 g (of which saturated fat 2 g), carbohydrate 31 g (of which sugars 27 g), fibre 0.5 g. Good source of vitamin B$_{12}$, vitamin C. Useful source of calcium, copper, folate, niacin, vitamin A, vitamin B$_2$, zinc.

Plums en papillote with honey

En papillote is a method of cooking food in the oven in parcels of paper, thus sealing in all the delicious juices. It is important to use baking parchment for the parcels as its coating is more moistureproof than greaseproof paper. When the parcels are opened for serving, a wonderful spicy perfume is released.

Preparation time **10 minutes**   Cooking time **20 minutes**   *Serves 8*

8 large dessert plums, stoned and thickly sliced

30 g (1 oz) unsalted butter

2 cinnamon sticks, each cut into 4 pieces

8 whole cloves

4 tbsp acacia honey, or another clear variety

1 large orange

To serve

4 scoops vanilla frozen yogurt or ice cream

3 tbsp coarsely chopped pecans

1 Preheat the oven to 200°C (400°F, gas mark 6).

2 Take 8 large squares of baking parchment and in the centre of each put one-eighth of the plum slices and butter, a piece of cinnamon stick and 1 clove. Drizzle ½ tbsp of honey over each portion of plums.

3 Use a citrus zester to take fine shreds of zest from the orange, or thinly pare off the zest with a vegetable peeler and then cut it into fine shreds. Squeeze the juice from the orange. Add one-eighth of the orange zest and juice to each portion of plums, sprinkling the zest and juice over the fruit evenly.

4 For each parcel, bring two opposite sides of the paper together over the fruit filling and fold two or three times. Fold over the other ends twice, then tuck them underneath, to make a neatly sealed parcel.

5 Place the parcels on a baking tray and bake for 20 minutes. The paper parcels will puff a little and brown slightly, and the fruit mixture inside will be bubbling hot.

6 Place the parcels on individual serving plates, carefully open up each one and top with a scoop of frozen yogurt or ice-cream. Sprinkle with the pecans and serve immediately.

Some more ideas

For **pineapple and banana en papillote**, replace the plums and spices with 1 small ripe pineapple, peeled, cored and chopped, and 4 bananas, thickly sliced. Add 2 star anise to each parcel, then drizzle with the honey and orange zest and juice.

Maple syrup makes a toffee-flavoured alternative to honey.

Plus points

* Plums contain a useful amount of vitamin E, an important antioxidant that helps to protect against degenerative diseases associated with ageing.

* Pecans, like other nuts, are rich in fat (70 g per 100 g/3½ oz), but little of this is saturated. They also provide generous amounts of vitamin E.

* Yogurt, along with other dairy products, is a valuable source of calcium. This mineral is essential for the structure of bones and teeth, which contain 99 per cent of all calcium in the body. But calcium is also important in a number of other vital processes, including blood clotting and the proper functioning of muscles and nerves.

photo, page 273

Each serving provides (one papillote) kcal 135, protein 1.5 g, fat 7 g (of which saturated fat 2.5 g), carbohydrates 17.5 g (of which sugars 17 g), fibre 1.5 g. Good source of vitamin C, vitamin E. Useful source of calcium, copper, potassium, vitamin A.

Grilled fruit brochettes

Cooking fruit on skewers, just long enough to heat the fruit through and slightly caramelise its sugars, is an easy and fun way of enjoying fresh fruit. If you are having a barbecue, cook the fruit brochettes over the charcoal fire – but take care not to char the fruit or leave it too long in the smoke.

Preparation time **20 minutes**   Cooking time **6–7 minutes**   *Serves 8*

½ medium-sized ripe pineapple

2 just ripe, firm bananas

2 ripe but firm pears

4 ripe but firm fresh figs

2 ripe but firm peaches

juice of 1 lemon

4 tsp sugar

cape gooseberries to decorate

Raspberry-orange coulis

225 g (8 oz) raspberries

grated zest and juice of ½ orange

1½ tbsp sugar, or to taste

1 Soak 8 bamboo skewers in cold water for 20 minutes.

2 Meanwhile, make the coulis. Purée the raspberries with the orange zest and juice and the sugar in a blender or food processor. If you like, sieve the purée to remove the raspberry pips. Set aside.

3 Preheat the grill. Prepare the pineapple, bananas, pears, figs and peaches, peeling as necessary and cutting into attractive bite-sized pieces. Thread the fruit onto the soaked skewers, alternating them to make a colourful arrangement.

4 Sprinkle the kebabs with half of the lemon juice and sugar. Grill them for 3–4 minutes or until lightly tinged with brown, then turn over, sprinkle with the remaining lemon juice and sugar and grill for a further 3 minutes or until the second side is lightly browned and caramelised a little.

5 While the kebabs are being grilled, pull back the papery skins on the cape gooseberries to form a star-like flower round the fruit.

6 Place a fruit kebab on each plate, drizzle round the coulis, decorate with cape gooseberries and serve hot.

Some more ideas

Use nectarines instead of peaches.

Use apples when peaches are not in season.

Serve the fruit kebabs raw, with the fresh fruit skewers resting in a pool of the coulis.

Plus points

● This delicious recipe provides useful amounts of important antioxidant vitamins – plenty of vitamin C from the raspberries and the orange and lemon juices, and vitamin A converted from the beta-carotene in the peaches. As the fruit is heated for only a very short time, most of the vitamin C is retained.

● There is plenty of dietary fibre – both soluble and insoluble – in this array of fruit, and this is essential to keep the digestive tract healthy. Insoluble fibre provides bulk and prevents constipation. The soluble fibre found in fruit can be fermented by bacteria in the gut, producing substances that help to protect against bowel cancer.

photo, page 273

Each serving provides (one brochette) kcal 87, protein 1 g, fat 0.3 g (of which saturated fat 0.1 g), carbohydrate 21 g (of which sugars 20 g), fibre 2.6 g. Excellent source of copper. Good source of vitamin B$_1$, vitamin C. Useful source of folate, niacin, potassium, vitamin B$_6$, vitamin E.

Peach and blackberry filo pizzas

These simple, attractive tarts have a crisp filo pastry base and a luscious fresh fruit topping. Filo pastry is made with very little fat, and most of it you add yourself when you brush the sheets sparingly with butter.

Preparation time **15 minutes**   Cooking time **15 minutes**   *Serves 4*

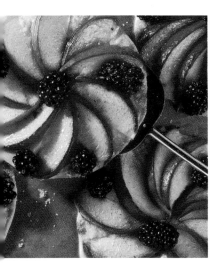

10 sheets filo pastry, about 30 x 20 cm (12 x 8 in) each, thawed if frozen

30 g (1 oz) unsalted butter, melted

2 tsp ground almonds or hazelnuts

4 peaches, about 115 g (4 oz) each

150 g (5½ oz) blackberries

2 tbsp vanilla caster sugar

To serve (optional)

0% fat Greek-style yogurt

1 Preheat the oven to 200°C (400°F, gas mark 6).

2 Place a sheet of filo on the work surface and brush very lightly all over with melted butter. Top with another sheet and brush with butter. Layer on 3 more filo sheets, brushing with butter each time, and finally brush the top surface. Using a saucer measuring about 13 cm (5½ in) as a guide, cut out 2 discs from the layered filo. Transfer to a baking tray. Repeat with the remaining filo pastry and butter to make 4 layered discs in total.

3 Sprinkle each disc with ½ tsp of ground almonds or hazelnuts, then set aside.

4 Cut the peaches in half, twist apart and remove the stones. Slice the peaches thinly. Place the peach slices on the filo pastry discs, arranging them so they leave a little of the pastry edge uncovered all round. Divide the blackberries among the pizzas. Sprinkle 1½ tsp sugar over each pizza.

5 Bake for 15 minutes or until the pastry is golden brown and the peaches are very tender and lightly caramelised. Transfer to individual plates and serve at once, with Greek-style yogurt, if liked. These filo pizzas are best served within 15 minutes of coming out of the oven as the pastry will quickly lose its crispness.

Some more ideas

Use raspberries instead of blackberries, and nectarines instead of peaches.

When berries are out of season, use well-drained preserved stem ginger, finely chopped – 2–3 tsp for each filo pizza.

To make **pear pizzas**, replace the peaches and blackberries with 2 dessert pears, peeled, cored and sliced. Toss the slices with 1 tsp ground coriander before arranging on the filo discs and baking.

Plus points

● Even though the filo pastry is brushed with butter, the quantity used here is small compared with that normally used in similar filo preparations, and the total fat content is lower than tarts made with shortcrust.

● Peaches are a good source of carbohydrate, with virtually no fat. Fresh peaches are also low in calories, with an average peach containing only 30 kcal.

● Blackberries provide lots of vitamins C and E, as well as being rich in bioflavonoids that work with vitamin C as antioxidants to boost immunity.

Each serving provides   **(one pizza)** kcal 200, protein 3 g, fat 9 g (of which saturated fat 3 g), carbohydrate 27 g (of which sugars 18 g), fibre 3 g. Good source of vitamin C, vitamin E.

Pear and redcurrant filo lattice

This lovely tart uses sweet and tangy redcurrants with juicy pears for a winning combination. The bright red juice of the currants tints the pears and looks most attractive under the pastry lattice. Although redcurrants only have a short season, they freeze well, so put some in the freezer to make a tart later in the year.

Preparation time **25 minutes**   Cooking time **15–20 minutes**   *Serves 6*

3 sheets filo pastry, 30 x 50 cm (12 x 20 in) each, about 90 g (3¼ oz) in total

20 g (¾ oz) unsalted butter, melted

Filling

2 tbsp redcurrant jelly

1 tsp lemon juice

3 ripe but firm pears, about 170 g (6 oz) each

125 g (4½ oz) redcurrants

45 g (1½ oz) ground almonds

1 Preheat the oven to 200°C (400°F, gas mark 6) and put a baking sheet in to heat. For the filling, place the redcurrant jelly and lemon juice in a small saucepan and heat gently until melted. Remove from the heat.

2 Peel the pears and slice thinly. Add to the jelly glaze and toss gently to coat. Stir in the redcurrants.

3 Lay out 2 sheets of filo on top of each other. (Keep the third sheet covered to prevent it from drying out.) Cut into quarters. Separate the 8 pieces and brush lightly with butter. Use to line a 23 cm (9 in) loose-bottomed, non-stick flan tin, overlapping them slightly, scrunching and tucking in the edges.

4 Sprinkle the ground almonds over the bottom of the tart case. Top with the pear and redcurrant mixture, spreading out the fruit evenly.

5 Cut the remaining filo sheet crossways in half and brush lightly with butter. Place one half on top of the other, then cut into 10 strips about 2 cm (¾ in) wide, trimming off excess pastry. Twist the doubled strips gently and arrange them in a lattice pattern over the filling, tucking in the ends neatly.

6 Place the tin on the hot baking sheet and bake for 15–20 minutes or until the pastry is crisp and golden brown. Serve warm.

Some more ideas

Make a **pear and raspberry filo lattice** by using raspberries instead of redcurrants, and seedless raspberry jam for the glaze rather than redcurrant jelly.

For a **mango and cape gooseberry filo tart**, sprinkle the bottom of the tart case with 30 g (1 oz) desiccated coconut. Peel and dice 2 ripe mangoes, about 350 g (12½ oz) each, and mix with 100 g (3½ oz) halved cape gooseberries. Toss gently with 2 tbsp each of lime juice and light muscovado sugar, then spoon into the pastry case and spread out evenly. Top with the pastry lattice; bake as in the main recipe.

Plus points

● Unlike most fruits, pears contain only a little vitamin C. However, in this recipe they are combined with redcurrants, which are a useful source of vitamin C. Pears do offer good amounts of potassium as well as soluble fibre.

● Redcurrants contain more beta-carotene than white currants but less than blackcurrants.

Each serving provides   kcal 164, protein 4 g, fat 7 g (of which saturated fat 2 g), carbohydrate 22 g (of which sugars 13 g), fibre 2 g. Useful source of copper, vitamin C, vitamin E.

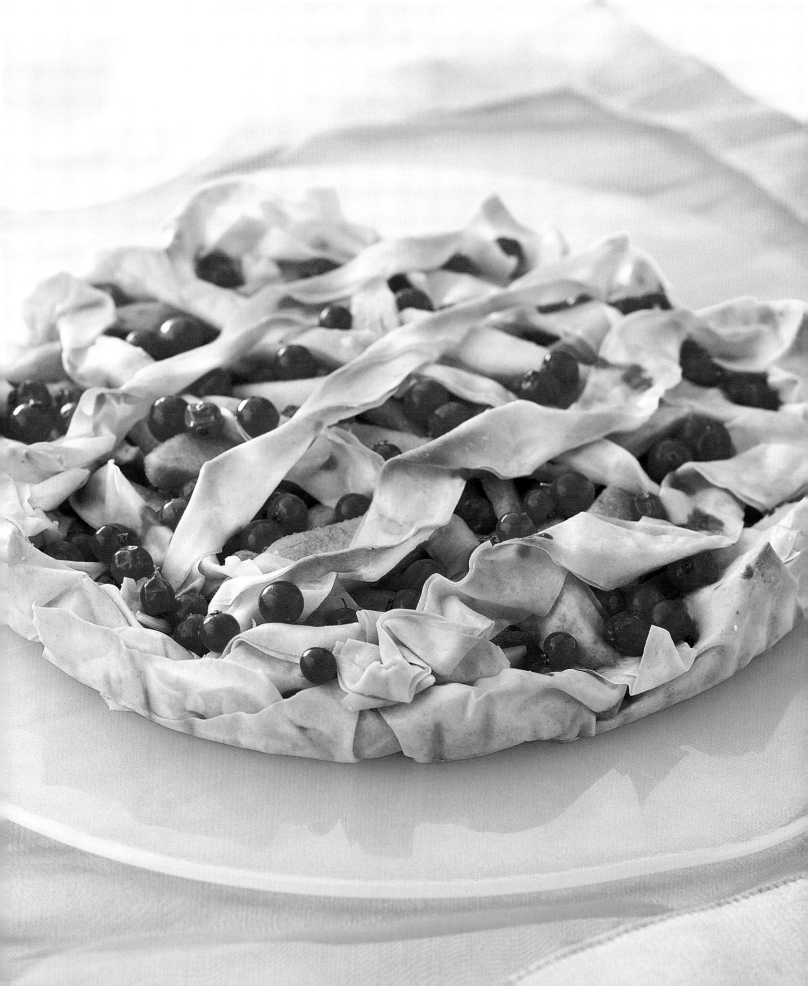

Vanilla angel cake

Almost fat-free, this very light cake really is the food of angels. It is made using egg whites only, no yolks, and during baking develops a delicious golden crust that hides the tender, pure white interior. Here, it is served with creamy fromage frais and summer berries, but it is just as lovely with juicy peaches, mango or apricots.

Preparation time **15 minutes**   Cooking time **35 minutes**   *Serves 10*

115 g (4 oz) plain flour

85 g (3 oz) icing sugar

8 large egg whites, at room temperature

150 g (5½ oz) caster sugar

¼ tsp salt

1 tsp cream of tartar

1 tsp pure vanilla extract

To serve

225 g (8 oz) strawberries, cut into quarters

225 g (8 oz) raspberries

225 g (8 oz) blueberries

300 g (10½ oz) fromage frais

1 Preheat the oven to 180°C (350°F, gas mark 4). Sift the flour and icing sugar onto a large plate and set aside.

2 Put the egg whites in a large bowl and whisk until quite frothy. Add the sugar, salt, cream of tartar and vanilla extract, and continue whisking until the mixture forms stiff peaks.

3 Sift the flour mixture over the egg whites and fold in very gently with a large metal spoon until well blended.

4 Spoon the mixture into an ungreased 25 cm (10 in) non-stick tube tin, making sure there are no air pockets. Bake for 35 minutes or until well risen, golden brown and springy to the touch.

5 Invert the cake, still in the tin, onto a wire rack and leave to cool completely, upside down. When it is cold, slide a long knife around the side of the tin to loosen the cake, then invert it onto a serving plate. (The cake can be kept, wrapped in cling film or stored in an airtight container, for 1–2 days.)

6 Just before serving, mix together the strawberries, raspberries and blueberries. Spoon the fruit into the hollow in the centre of the cake. Serve with the fromage frais in a bowl.

Some more ideas

To make a **lemon and lime angel cake**, add the finely grated zest of 1 lemon and 1 lime to the beaten egg white with the sifted flour and icing sugar. While the cake is cooling, peel 2 small Cantaloupe melons and remove the seeds. Cut the melon into small chunks and place in a bowl. Squeeze the juice from the lemon and lime, sprinkle it over the melon and toss to coat well. Serve the cake with the melon pieces piled up in the centre.

For a **chocolate angel cake**, sift 2 tbsp cocoa powder with the flour and icing sugar. Decorate the cake with a mixture of 1 tbsp each cocoa powder and icing sugar, sifted together.

To make a **coffee angel cake**, sift 1 tbsp instant coffee powder (not granules) with the flour and icing sugar. Decorate with icing sugar.

Plus point

• Fromage frais is a useful source of calcium, which is an essential component of bones and teeth – the adult skeleton contains 1.2 kg (nearly 3 lb) calcium, and 99 per cent of this is present in the bones. Calcium also plays an important role in the regulation of blood clotting, muscle contraction and nerve function.

photo, page 283

Each serving provides kcal 190, protein 6 g, fat 2 g (of which saturated fat 1 g), carbohydrate 39 g (of which sugars 30 g), fibre 2 g. Excellent source of vitamin C. Useful source of vitamin B_2, vitamin B_{12}.

Baked almond-stuffed peaches

Baking fruit brings out its flavour wonderfully, and a stuffing is a simple way of making baked fruit special. Here peaches are filled with a mixture of dried apricots, almonds and amaretti biscuits. Many other fruits – nectarines, apples, pears or quinces – can be prepared in the same way, to ring the seasonal changes.

Preparation time **20 minutes**   Cooking time **about 40 minutes**   *Serves 8*

5 large ripe but firm peaches

10 ready-to-eat dried apricots, finely diced

6 amaretti biscuits, crumbled

2 tsp pure almond extract

1 tbsp brandy

1 egg white

55 g (2 oz) whole blanched almonds

1 Preheat the oven to 180°C (350°F, gas mark 4).

2 Cut the peaches in half and remove the stones. Arrange 8 of the halves, cut side up, in a shallow baking dish. Set aside. Finely dice the remaining 2 peach halves.

3 Combine the diced peach with the dried apricots, crumbled amaretti, almond extract, brandy and egg white. Stir to mix thoroughly.

4 Heat a small heavy ungreased frying pan and lightly toast the almonds, turning and tossing every so often, until they are lightly browned in spots. Remove and chop, in a food processor or by hand, to make a mixture of small chunks of nuts and ground nuts.

5 Add the chopped almonds to the fruit and amaretti mixture and mix well. Use the mixture to fill the hollows in the peach halves, heaping up the filling and pressing it gently together. Cover the baking dish with a tent of cooking foil.

6 Bake for 25–30 minutes, then remove the foil. Increase the oven temperature to 200°C (400°F, gas mark 6) and bake for a further 5–10 minutes or until the nutty topping is lightly browned. The peaches are best when warm, but they can be chilled before serving.

Some more ideas

Nectarines can be used instead of peaches, with pistachios instead of almonds.

Macaroons can be used instead of amaretti, but fewer according to size.

For **baked stuffed apples or pears**, substitute sultanas for the diced dried apricots and add a few shakes of ground cinnamon to the filling. Allow 10 minutes longer baking time before removing the foil.

Use quinces instead of peaches, allowing 15 minutes extra baking time.

Plus points

• Peaches contain plenty of vitamin C (31 mg per 100 g/3½ oz) and this can help the body to absorb iron present in other foods – in this case from dried apricots. Iron deficiency anaemia is probably the most common deficiency disease in the UK, so every little bit helps. Dried apricots also provide vitamin A and plenty of potassium for regulating blood pressure.

• Almonds not only have a delicious and distinctive flavour, but also contain protein and plenty of vitamin E.

photo, page 283

Each serving provides   kcal 100, protein 3 g, fat 4.5 g (of which saturated fat 0.5 g), carbohydrate 12 g (of which sugars 10.5 g), fibre 2.5 g. Good source of vitamin C, vitamin E. Useful source of copper, niacin, potassium, vitamin B$_2$.

Black Forest mousse cake

This very light cake is almost fat-free, being based on egg whites whisked to firm peaks and folded together with flour, sugar and cocoa powder. Cocoa delivers a rich chocolate flavour without the fat of chocolate.

Preparation time **15 minutes, plus cooling**   Cooking time **20–25 minutes**   *Serves 6*

45 g (1½ oz) plain flour

5 tbsp cocoa powder

100 g (3½ oz) caster sugar

small pinch of salt

5 large egg whites

1 tsp pure vanilla extract

340 g (12 oz) sweet dark cherries, stoned and halved

1 tbsp icing sugar

To serve (optional)

3 tbsp fromage frais

1 tbsp cherry conserve

1–2 tbsp kirsch or rum (optional)

1 Preheat the oven to 180°C (350°F, gas mark 4). Line the bottom of a 23 cm (9 in) round deep cake tin with greaseproof paper.

2 Sift the flour, cocoa powder, half of the sugar and the salt into a bowl.

3 In another large bowl, which is perfectly clean and grease-free, whisk the egg whites until they are foamy. Continue whisking until they will hold a soft peak. Add the remaining sugar, 1 tbsp at a time, and the vanilla extract, while you continue to whisk the egg whites. Whisk until they are glossy and smooth, and will hold a firm peak.

4 Sprinkle the flour and cocoa mixture over the egg whites and fold in gently but thoroughly, taking care not to deflate the egg whites too much. Spoon the mixture into the tin. Smooth the surface gently. Sprinkle the cherries evenly over the top of the cake.

5 Bake for 20–25 minutes or until the cake has risen and is just firm to the touch yet still moist on top (a skewer inserted into the centre should come out clean). Remove from the oven and leave to cool.

6 Sprinkle the cake with the icing sugar before serving. If you want to serve with the fromage frais accompaniment, simply combine the fromage frais with the cherry conserve and optional kirsch or rum to taste.

Some more ideas

Canned stoned cherries in juice, drained, can be used if fresh cherries are not in season.

Instead of cherries, use a combination of soft red fruits such as raspberries or small strawberries, or mixed fruit of the forest.

For a **vanilla cake**, omit the cocoa powder and replace with the same amount of cornflour. To give an almond flavour instead of vanilla, use pure almond extract.

Plus points

- Egg white still provides protein (9 g per 100 g/3½ oz), but has none of the fat or cholesterol found in egg yolk.

- Cocoa powder contains less fat than plain or milk chocolate, and five times as much iron. This iron is not as well absorbed as the iron in meat, but the vitamin C in the cherries will help the body to absorb it.

- Each serving is quite sugar-rich, so this cake is best saved for special occasions.

Each serving provides   kcal 180, protein 6 g, fat 3 g (of which saturated fat 2 g), carbohydrate 34 g (of which sugars 27 g), fibre 2 g. Good source of copper. Useful source of iron.

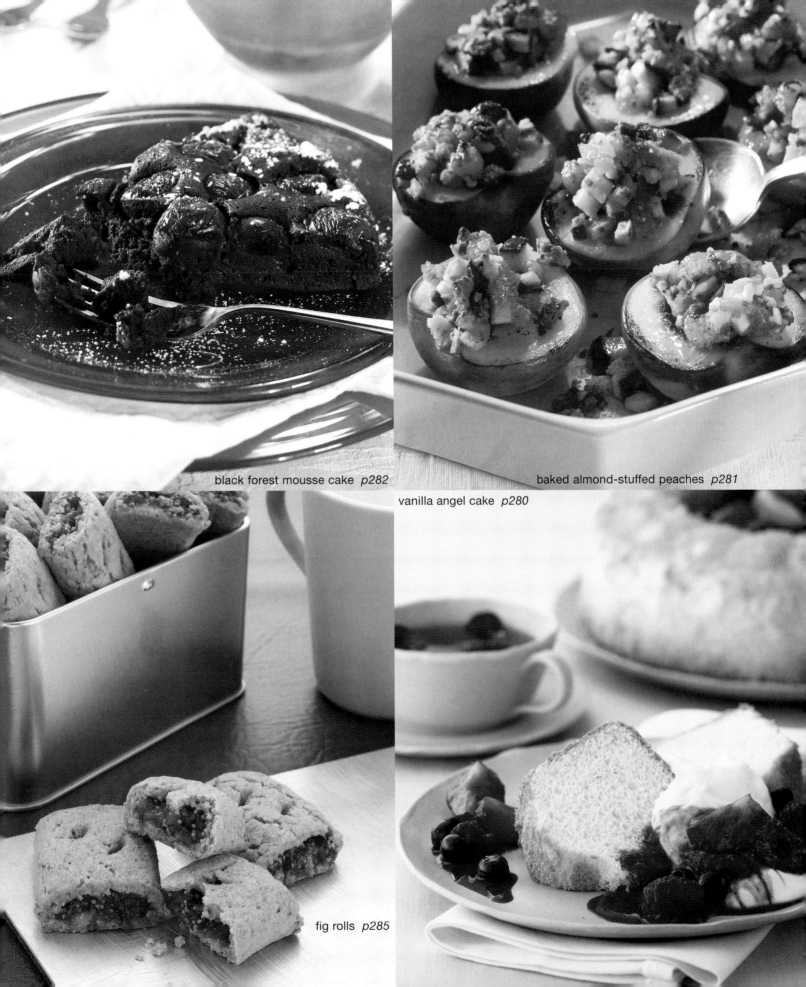

black forest mousse cake *p282*

baked almond-stuffed peaches *p281*

vanilla angel cake *p280*

fig rolls *p285*

Cranberry and almond biscotti

Biscotti means twice baked, a reference to the technique that gives these Italian biscuits their characteristically hard texture. Traditionally they are served after dinner, with a glass of Vin Santo for dipping, but they are also delicious with fresh fruit salad or a cup of coffee or tea at any time of day.

Preparation time **30 minutes**   Cooking time **30–40 minutes**   *Makes 20 biscotti*

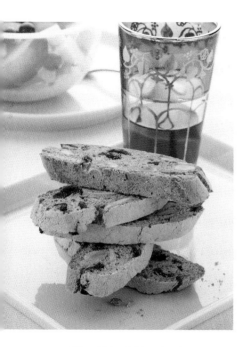

50 g (1¾ oz) blanched almonds

1 large egg

85 g (3 oz) caster sugar

140 g (5 oz) plain flour

½ tsp baking powder

1 tsp ground cinnamon

55 g (2 oz) dried cranberries

1 Preheat the oven to 180°C (350°F, gas mark 4). Spread the almonds in a baking tin and toast them in the oven for about 10 minutes or until lightly browned. Set aside to cool.

2 Put the egg and sugar in a bowl and whisk with an electric mixer until very thick and pale; the mixture should be thick enough to leave a trail on the surface when you lift out the beaters. (If using a hand whisk or rotary beater, set the bowl over a pan of almost boiling water, making sure the water is not touching the base of the bowl.)

3 Sift the flour, baking powder and cinnamon onto a sheet of greaseproof paper, then sift the mixture again onto the whisked egg mixture. Using a large metal spoon, gently fold the sifted mixture into the egg mixture, then stir in the toasted almonds and cranberries to make a stiff dough.

4 Spoon the dough onto a greased baking tray and, with floured hands, form it into a neat brick shape about 25 x 6 x 2 cm (10 x 2½ x ¾ in). Bake for 20–25 minutes or until golden brown. Cool on the baking tray for 5 minutes, then transfer to a board.

5 Using a serrated bread knife, cut the brick across, slightly on the diagonal, into 20 slices. Arrange the slices flat on the baking tray and return to the oven. Bake for

10–15 minutes or until golden brown. Cool on the baking tray for about 5 minutes, then transfer to a wire rack and cool completely. The biscotti can be kept in an airtight tin for up to 2 weeks.

Some more ideas

Substitute dried cherries or sultanas for the cranberries.

To make **chocolate biscotti**, replace the cranberries with 55 g (2 oz) coarsely chopped good dark chocolate (at least 70 per cent cocoa solids). Add 1 tsp pure vanilla extract when you whisk the egg and sugar.

Plus points

• Almonds provide a good source of protein and also contain several vitamins and minerals, including vitamin E, several of the B-group vitamins, magnesium, copper, zinc, iron and phosphorus. They are a particularly useful source of calcium for people on dairy-free diets, and have been shown to be useful in diabetes as part of a healthy diet.

• Both fresh and dried cranberries are a good source of vitamin C.

Each serving provides   (one biscotti) kcal 70, protein 1 g, fat 2 g (of which saturated fat 0 g), carbohydrate 12 g (of which sugars 6 g), fibre 0.5 g.

Fig rolls

Here's a classic – a crisp, shortbread paste wrapped around a rich fig filling. The natural sweetness and full flavour of dried figs need little embellishment other than lemon juice to add a zesty tang.

Preparation time **35 minutes, plus 30 minutes chilling**   Cooking time **12–15 minutes**   *Makes 20 rolls*

115 g (4 oz) plain white flour

115 g (4 oz) plain wholemeal flour

150 g (5½ oz) unsalted butter, cut into small pieces

65 g (2¼ oz) light muscovado sugar

1 tsp pure vanilla extract

2 egg yolks

250 g (8½ oz) ready-to-eat dried figs, finely chopped

2 tbsp lemon juice

1 Sift the two flours into a mixing bowl, tipping in any bran left in the sieve. Rub in the butter with your fingertips until the mixture resembles breadcrumbs.

2 Add the sugar, vanilla extract and egg yolks, and mix to a firm dough, adding 1–2 tsp water if necessary to bind. (Alternatively, blend the flours and butter in a food processor, then add the sugar, vanilla and egg yolks, and blend briefly to make a dough.) Wrap in cling film and chill for 30 minutes.

3 Put the figs in a small, heavy-based saucepan with 6 tbsp water. Bring to the boil, then reduce the heat, cover and simmer gently for 3–5 minutes or until the figs have plumped up slightly and absorbed the water. Transfer to a bowl and mash lightly with a fork. Add the lemon juice and stir, then leave to cool.

4 Preheat the oven to 190°C (375°F, gas mark 5). Roll out the dough on a lightly floured surface to a 50 x 15 cm (20 x 6 in) rectangle. Cut the dough rectangle in half lengthways to make 2 strips.

5 Spoon half the fig purée evenly along each strip, near one of the long sides. Bring the opposite long side up and over the filling, to form a 'log' shape, and press the edges of the dough together to seal.

6 Flatten each of the logs slightly. Using a sharp knife, cut each log across into 10 biscuits and transfer to a greased baking sheet. Prick each biscuit with a fork or score with a sharp knife. Bake for 12–15 minutes or until slightly darkened in colour.

7 Transfer the biscuits to a wire rack to cool. They can be kept in an airtight container for 2–3 days (the shortbread might go soft if mixed with other biscuits).

Another idea

To make **cherry and apple rolls**, gently simmer 100 g (3½ oz) dried cherries in a saucepan with 5 tbsp water and 1 cored and finely chopped dessert apple until the water is absorbed. Use instead of the fig filling.

Plus point

• Dried fruits are a useful source of iron in the diet, particularly for those eating little or no red meat. In addition to iron, dried figs also offer good amounts of calcium. Just 3 dried figs (55 g/2 oz) will provide around 20 per cent of the RNI (reference daily intake) of calcium and 17 per cent of the RNI of iron for a woman aged 19–50.

photo, page 283

Each serving provides   **(one fig roll)** kcal 130, protein 2 g, fat 7 g (of which saturated fat 4 g), carbohydrate 17 g (of which sugars 10 g), fibre 1.5 g. Useful source of vitamin A, vitamin B$_6$.

Little custard pots

These creamy baked custards, delicately flavoured with vanilla and accompanied by a fresh cherry compote, are easy to make and sure to be popular with all ages. Take care not to overcook the custards – they should be just set when you take them out of the oven. This dessert can be prepared well ahead of serving.

Preparation time **15 minutes**   Cooking time **25–30 minutes**   *Serves 6*

600 ml (1 pint) semi-skimmed milk

½ vanilla pod, split

2 eggs

2 egg yolks

40 g (1¼ oz) caster sugar

½ tsp cornflour

Cherry compote

1 tbsp demerara sugar

450 g (1 lb) fresh cherries, stoned

2 tsp arrowroot

1 Place the milk and vanilla pod in a saucepan and heat until almost boiling. Remove from the heat, cover and set aside to infuse for 15 minutes.

2 Preheat the oven to 160ºC (325ºF, gas mark 3). Put the whole eggs, egg yolks, caster sugar and cornflour into a bowl and lightly whisk together.

3 Bring the milk back to boiling point, then remove the vanilla pod and pour the hot milk over the egg mixture, whisking all the time. Strain the mixture into a jug, then divide among 6 lightly buttered 120 ml (4 fl oz) ramekin dishes.

4 Set the ramekins in a roasting tin and pour enough hot water into the tin to come halfway up the sides of the ramekins. Bake for 30–35 minutes or until lightly set – the custards should still be slightly wobbly, as they will continue cooking for a few minutes after being removed from the oven. Lift them out of the tin of hot water and place on a wire rack to cool. Once cold, chill until ready to serve.

5 For the cherry compote, put the demerara sugar and 6 tbsp water in a saucepan and heat gently until the sugar has dissolved. Bring to the boil, then reduce the heat and add the cherries. Cover and simmer gently for 4–5 minutes, stirring occasionally, until tender. Lift out the cherries with a draining spoon and put them into a serving bowl.

6 Mix the arrowroot with 1 tbsp cold water. Stir into the cherry juices in the saucepan and simmer for 1 minute, stirring, until thickened and clear. Allow to cool for a few minutes, then pour over the cherries. (The compote can be served warm or at room temperature.)

7 Spoon a little of the cherry compote over the top of each custard pot, and serve the rest of the compote in a bowl.

Some more ideas

If you want to turn out the custards for serving, line the bottom of each ramekin with a circle of baking parchment, and add an extra egg yolk to the mixture. After baking, chill for at least 4 hours or, preferably, overnight. To turn out, lightly press the edge of each custard with your fingertips to pull it away from the dish, then run a knife around the edge. Put an inverted serving plate on top of the ramekin, then turn them both over, holding them firmly together, and lift off the ramekin.

Each serving provides kcal 178, protein 7 g, fat 6 g (of which saturated fat 2 g), carbohydrate 26 g (of which sugars 23 g), fibre 1 g. Good source of vitamin B_{12}. Useful source of calcium, vitamin A, vitamin B_2, vitamin C, zinc.

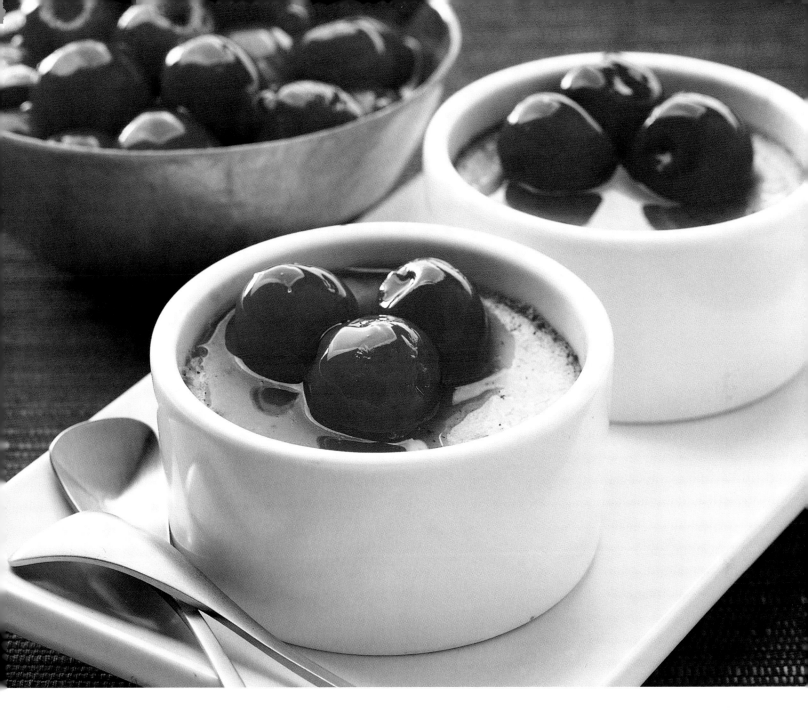

For **chocolate custard pots with poached pears**, flavour the milk with a thin strip of pared orange zest instead of the vanilla pod. In step 2, replace the caster sugar with light soft brown sugar, and add 1 tbsp sifted cocoa powder. Continue as in the main recipe. For the pears, heat 300 ml (10 fl oz) water with 85 g (3 oz) caster sugar and a split vanilla pod until the sugar dissolves, then bring to the boil and simmer for 2–3 minutes. Add 4 firm dessert pears, peeled, cored and thickly sliced. Cover and simmer for 12–15 minutes or until just tender, turning the pear slices in the syrup occasionally. Lift out the pears with a draining spoon and transfer to a serving dish. Simmer the syrup for 5 minutes to reduce slightly, then cool for 5 minutes. Remove the vanilla pod and pour over the pears.

Plus points

- Adding extra egg yolks in this recipe boosts the content of vitamins A and D and most of the B vitamins, as these nutrients are concentrated in the yolk of the egg rather than the white.

- Cherries are rich in potassium and provide useful amounts of vitamin C.

Five-star cookies

These nutty, moist cookies will cheer up mid-morning coffee or an afterschool snack. They are satisfying and packed full of healthy ingredients to restore flagging energy levels, without being too sweet. Barley flakes, which are slightly crisper than oatflakes, are available from most healthfood shops.

Preparation time **20 minutes**   Cooking time **10–15 minutes**   *Makes 16 cookies*

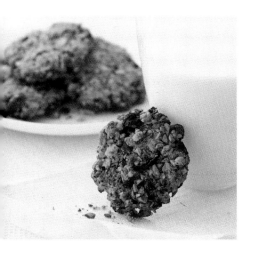

50 g (1¾ oz) hazelnuts, finely chopped

50 g (1¾ oz) sunflower seeds, finely chopped

50 g (1¾ oz) ready-to-eat dried apricots, finely chopped

50 g (1¾ oz) stoned dried dates, finely chopped

1 tbsp light muscovado sugar

50 g (1¾ oz) barley flakes

50 g (1¾ oz) self-raising wholemeal flour

½ tsp baking powder

2 tbsp sunflower oil

4 tbsp apple juice

1 Preheat the oven to 190°C (375°F, gas mark 5). Mix the chopped hazelnuts, sunflower seeds, apricots and dates together in a bowl. Add the sugar, barley flakes, flour and baking powder, and stir until all the ingredients are thoroughly combined.

2 Mix together the sunflower oil and apple juice, and pour over the dry mixture. Stir until the dry ingredients are moistened and clump together.

3 Scoop up a large teaspoon of the mixture and, with dampened fingers, lightly press it together into a ball about the size of a large walnut. Then press it into a small, thick cookie about 5–6 cm (2–2½ in) in diameter. Neaten the edge with your fingers. Place on a large greased baking sheet. Repeat with the remaining mixture.

4 Bake the cookies for 10–15 minutes or until slightly risen and browned on top. Transfer to a wire rack and leave to cool. They can be kept in an airtight container for up to 4 days.

Some more ideas

Use unsalted cashew nuts instead of hazelnuts.

Use ready-to-eat dried peaches and figs instead of the apricots and dates.

Substitute oatflakes or wheatflakes for the barley.

Plus points

• Sunflower seeds are a good source of the antioxidant vitamin E, which helps to protect cell membranes from damage by free radicals. Sunflower seeds are rich in polyunsaturated fats and also provide good amounts of vitamin B_1 and the minerals copper, iron, magnesium, phosphorus, selenium and zinc.

• Barley is thought to be the world's oldest cultivated grain. It is rich in starch and contains a type of dietary fibre called fructoligosaccarides (FOS), which is believed to stimulate the growth of friendly bacteria in the gut while inhibiting the growth of harmful bacteria.

Each serving provides **(one cookie)** kcal 90, protein 2 g, fat 5 g (of which saturated fat 1 g), carbohydrate 9 g (of which sugars 4 g), fibre 1 g. Useful source of copper.

Orange and pecan biscuits

These are 'slice-and-bake' biscuits – the roll of dough can be prepared in advance and kept in the fridge. Then, whenever biscuits are wanted, you simply slice the roll into rounds, top with pecan nuts and bake.

Preparation time **15 minutes, plus 2 hours chilling**　Cooking time **8–10 minutes**　*Makes 24 biscuits*

55 g (2 oz) plain wholemeal flour, plus extra for kneading

55 g (2 oz) self-raising white flour

85 g (3 oz) light muscovado sugar

55 g (2 oz) ground rice

30 g (1 oz) pecan nuts, chopped

grated zest of 1 orange

4 tbsp sunflower oil

1 large egg

24 pecan nut halves to decorate

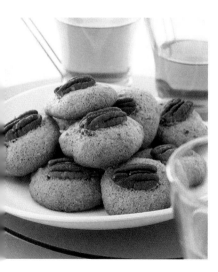

1　Put the wholemeal and self-raising flours, sugar, ground rice, chopped pecan nuts and orange zest in a bowl, and stir until well combined.

2　In a small bowl, beat the oil and egg together with a fork. Add this mixture to the dry ingredients and mix with a fork until they come together to make a dough.

3　Knead the dough very lightly on a floured surface until smooth, then roll into a sausage shape about 30 cm (12 in) long. Wrap in cling film and chill for 2 hours. (The dough can be kept in the fridge for 2–3 days before slicing and baking.)

4　Preheat the oven to 180°C (350°F, gas mark 4). Unwrap the roll of dough and lightly reshape to a neat sausage, if necessary.

5　Cut the roll across into 24 slices using a sharp knife. Arrange the slices, spaced apart, on 2 large non-stick baking sheets. Top each slice with a pecan nut half, pressing it in slightly.

6　Bake for about 10 minutes or until firm to the touch and lightly golden. Transfer the biscuits to a wire rack to cool completely. They can be stored in an airtight tin for up to 5 days.

Another idea
To make **almond polenta biscuits**, mix 55 g (2 oz) instant polenta with 85 g (3 oz) icing sugar and 115 g (4 oz) self-raising flour. Rub in 55 g (2 oz) butter until the mixture resembles breadcrumbs. Beat 1 large egg with ½ tsp pure almond extract, add to the crumb mixture and mix to form a soft dough. Roll, wrap and chill as in the main recipe. Before baking, scatter 30 g (1 oz) flaked almonds over the slices.

Plus points
● Like other nuts, pecans are rich in fat – up to 70 g per 100 g (3½ oz) – but little of this is saturated fat, the majority being present as polyunsaturated fat. Pecans also provide generous amounts of vitamin E.

● Sunflower oil is one of the most widely used vegetable oils because of its mild flavour, and it works well in biscuits and other baked goods in place of saturated fats such as butter. It is a particularly good source of vitamin E, a powerful antioxidant. Polyunsaturated fats, such as are found in sunflower oil, are more susceptible to rancidity than saturated fats, but the vitamin E content helps to stop the oil going rancid.

Each serving provides　(one biscuit) kcal 106, protein 2 g, fat 7 g (of which saturated fat 1 g), carbohydrate 9 g (of which sugars 4 g), fibre 1 g. Good source of vitamin E. Useful source of copper.

Mocha ricotta tiramisu

This delectable version of the popular Italian dessert includes the traditional sponge biscuits soaked in coffee and liqueur for the base, but rather than a rich topping there is a light and creamy mixture of sweetened ricotta cheese and Greek-style yogurt. A sprinkling of grated dark chocolate is the finishing touch.

Preparation time **20 minutes, plus at least 30 minutes chilling**   *Serves 4*

8 savoiardi or boudoir biscuits (sponge fingers), about 65 g (2¼ oz) in total

1 tsp Continental roast coffee granules

120 ml (4 fl oz) boiling water

2 tbsp coffee liqueur or brandy

1 tsp caster sugar

200 g (7 oz) ricotta cheese

200 g (7 oz) 0% fat Greek-style yogurt

25 g (1 oz) icing sugar, sifted

1 tsp pure vanilla extract

25 g (1 oz) good dark chocolate (at least 70% cocoa solids), grated, to decorate

1 Break each of the sponge fingers into 3 pieces, then divide evenly among four 240 ml (8 fl oz) glass tumblers or dessert glasses.

2 Place the coffee in a measuring jug and add the boiling water. Add the liqueur or brandy and caster sugar, and stir to dissolve. Pour evenly over the sponge fingers. Leave to soak while you make the topping.

3 Beat the ricotta with the yogurt, icing sugar and vanilla extract until smooth and creamy. Pile on top of the soaked sponge fingers.

4 Sprinkle the top of each dessert with grated chocolate. Cover and chill for at least 30 minutes (but no more than 3–4 hours) before serving.

reserving 12 for decoration. Sprinkle each dessert with 1 tbsp dark rum, brandy or orange liqueur. Make a thick custard using 1½ tbsp custard powder, 2 tbsp caster sugar and 300 ml (10 fl oz) semi-skimmed milk, following the instructions on the label. Flavour with 1 tsp pure vanilla extract. Allow to cool, then blend with 100 g (3½ oz) Greek-style yogurt. Spoon on top of the biscuit and raspberry mixture. Crush 8 more biscuits and scatter the crumbs over the top of the desserts, then decorate them with the reserved raspberries. Chill for 30 minutes before serving.

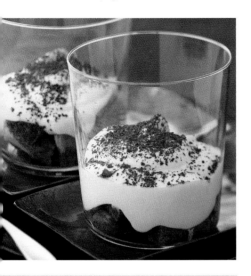

Some more ideas

Replace the Greek-style yogurt with fromage frais or vanilla-flavoured low-fat yogurt.

Instead of grated chocolate, decorate the tops of the desserts by dusting each with ½ tsp of cocoa powder.

To make an **amaretti and raspberry dessert**, 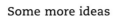 divide 28 amaretti (or ratafia) biscuits, about 75 g (2½ oz) in total, among 4 glass tumblers or dishes. Add 250 g (8½ oz) raspberries,

Plus points

● Ricotta is very much lower in fat and calories than the creamy mascarpone that is traditionally used for this pudding. Adding Greek-style yogurt to the ricotta provides creaminess without loading the fat content.

● Dark chocolate is a good source of copper, a mineral that helps the body to absorb iron. Grating it finely, as in this recipe, helps to go further.

Each serving provides   kcal 228, protein 9 g, fat 8 g (of which saturated fat 5 g), carbohydrate 24 g (of which sugars 20 g), fibre 0.5 g. Good source of calcium, vitamin A. Useful source of vitamin B₂, vitamin B₁₂, zinc.

Rich fruit ring cake

Most rich fruit cakes are high in fat and added sugar, but this one is an exception. It's relatively low in fat, and depends mainly on dried fruits soaked in apple juice for natural sweetness. Decorated with nuts, and glacé and crystallised fruits, it makes a healthy cake that would be festive enough for Christmas.

Preparation time **about 30 minutes, plus soaking and 2–3 weeks maturing**   Cooking time **1¼–1½ hours**   *Serves 18*

85 g (3 oz) dried cranberries

85 g (3 oz) sultanas

85 g (3 oz) dried pears, chopped

85 g (3 oz) stoned prunes, chopped

85 g (3 oz) dried figs, chopped

85 g (3 oz) stoned dried dates, chopped

250 ml (8½ fl oz) apple juice

50 g (1¾ oz) pecan nuts, chopped

50 g (1¾ oz) candied ginger, chopped

finely grated zest and juice of 1 lemon

5 tbsp sunflower oil

1 egg

75 g (2½ oz) molasses sugar

115 g (4 oz) self-raising white flour

115 g (4 oz) self-raising wholemeal flour

1 tsp baking powder

2 tsp ground mixed spice

3–4 tbsp semi-skimmed milk, as needed

Decoration

2 tbsp apricot jam

55 g (2 oz) glacé cherries

30 g (1 oz) hazelnuts

40 g (1¼ oz) pecan nut halves

40 g (1¼ oz) walnut halves

55 g (2 oz) candied ginger, sliced

icing sugar to dust

1 Place all the dried fruit in a medium-sized saucepan. Add the apple juice, place over a moderate heat and bring slowly to the boil. Cover and simmer gently for 3–4 minutes or until the fruit begins to absorb the liquid.

2 Remove the pan from the heat and leave, covered, until completely cold. Stir in the pecan nuts, ginger, and lemon zest and juice.

3 Preheat the oven to 150°C (300°F, gas mark 2). Brush a 23 cm (9 in) ring tin with a little oil. In a bowl, beat together the sunflower oil, egg and sugar until smooth.

4 Sift the white and wholemeal flours, baking powder and mixed spice into a large bowl, tipping in any bran in the sieve. Add the soaked fruit and the egg mixture, and stir well to combine thoroughly. Stir in enough milk to make a fairly soft mixture.

5 Spoon the mixture into the prepared tin and smooth the top. Bake for 1¼–1½ hours or until risen, firm and golden brown, and just beginning to shrink away from the sides of the tin.

6 Leave the cake to cool in the tin for at least 1 hour before running a knife around the edge and turning it out. Wrap in greaseproof paper and foil, and store for 2–3 weeks before serving, to allow the flavours to mature.

7 To decorate the cake, gently heat the jam with 1 tsp water, then press through a sieve. Brush the top of the cake with the jam. Arrange the cherries, nuts and candied ginger on top, pressing them gently into the jam. Finally, dust with sifted icing sugar.

Plus points

● Dried figs are a good source of fibre and also contain compounds known to have mild laxative effects. Drying the fruit concentrates their nutrients, making them a useful source of calcium and iron.

● Pecans are a good source of protein and unsaturated fats, and they provide useful amounts of vitamin E, folate and fibre.

Each serving provides   kcal 250, protein 4 g, fat 10 g (of which saturated fat 1 g), carbohydrate 38 g (of which sugars 29 g), fibre 3 g. Useful source of copper, vitamin B$_6$.

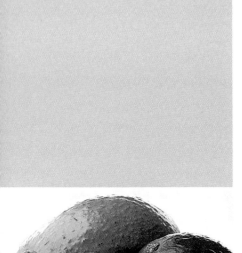

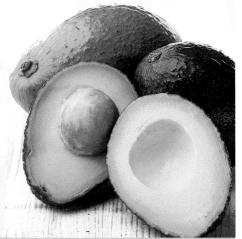

Buying and stocking food

Supermarkets can be treacherous places. Cake displays here. Piles of quiches and pies there. Rich desserts, high-fat salty ready-meals, sugary cereals everywhere! Grocery-store owners are in the business of getting you to buy on impulse. And they're good at it.

But you are better. And after you read this, you'll be better still. Your goal, of course, is to buy healthy, tasty foods, in the right quantities, at good prices, without succumbing to the temptations around you. Here is your guide.

General shopping principles

Shop from a list. First plan your meals for the week, then outline a list – this will save time and help to avoid impulse buying. Although it is fun to explore new stores, try to find a shop you are comfortable with. This way you can get to know the store well, and you can organise your shopping list according to the layout of the store.

Focus on the aisles you want. Go only to those areas that stock what you're looking for. Begin your shopping with the fruits and vegetables and then work your way around – usually, it's the meats, the seafood, the dairy, the juices and the breads.

Don't be tempted by the end displays. Every business uses psychology to get you to buy, and supermarkets are no exception! The end displays on the aisles are usually highly processed, not-so-nutritious foods that are packaged brilliantly. Despite their allure, if they aren't on your list and aren't everyday staples of your home, walk on by.

Start with a full stomach. Never shop when you are hungry. The temptation is too great to rip open a bag of something you'll later regret, and to fill your trolley with foods you don't need but that look awfully tempting in the moment.

Ponder the P foods. That is: prepared, presliced, precooked. Basically, these tend to be processed. You pay a lot for that extra service, and often prepared foods are oversalted, oversugared, and over-additived for cheapness and flavour. That said, convenience is important. You are safest in the fresh produce section. Prewashed and sorted mixed greens might very well be worth the extra pennies if it's the difference between a healthy vegetable side dish and no side dish at all.

Create a shopping system. For example, once a month, buy the staples: the canned goods, frozen vegetables, oils, dried herbs that you use regularly for cooking. In the in-between weeks, only buy perishables that you'll need that week – meats, seafood, fruits, vegetables, milk. This approach keeps you out of the central aisles of the supermarket (where processed foods tend to be) three weeks out of four, and saves you lots of time and temptation.

Shop for value. More and more people are buying in bulk at cash-and-carry outlets. But buying in bulk doesn't always mean buying more frugally. With a coupon or supermarket offer, you may find that a supermarket price is cheaper than the cash-and-carry price. Likewise, the supermarket's own-brand may be the cheapest route, even in small quantities. How do you measure? Get acquainted with the price of food per kilo. Many shelf labels now give this cost. It's the only way to comparison-shop effectively.

Don't be too good. Ever buy lots of produce, and ten days later, end up throwing out half of it because it's no longer good for eating? Don't feel alone – it happens all the time. Again, use your weekly planner as a guide. If you are throwing out more produce than you are eating, consider purchasing frozen and canned fruits and vegetables. Nutritionally, there's very little difference between fresh, frozen and canned.

Just check the label for added sugars and sodium, and avoid them.

Near is better than far. When it comes to fresh produce, locally grown food is typically tastier and healthier than produce shipped in from thousands of miles away. So while many vegetables and fruits are now available year-round thanks to more open trade agreements, aim to buy foods in season.

Shopping for fruit and vegetables

Perhaps no other place will give you more variety and abundance of nutrition than the supermarket fresh produce area. The dizzying array of selections can confuse anyone. Here is what you need to be a savvy consumer.

Take your time. Many shoppers go to the same old bins, buy the same old things, and head off to the next section of the store. If time permits, and your food plans are somewhat flexible for the week, slow down and give the entire section a once-over. What looks fresh? What looks interesting? What's on sale? The produce section is the one area of a grocery store where you should be willing to shift from the shopping list and buy based on what's available.

Fear no fruit. Break out of your rut! Add a new fruit or vegetable to your trolley once every other week. The key to a well-balanced food programme is variety. Ask the fresh foods manager for

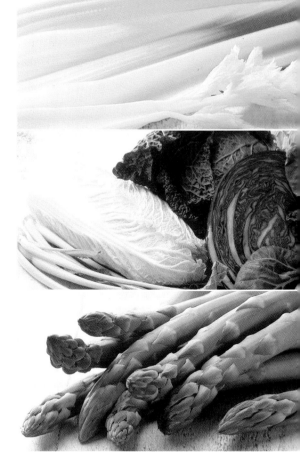

tips on how to use an unusual fruit or vegetable – that's what they're there for.

Look for quality. Avoid any fruit or vegetable that is bruised or looks old. There is often a separate shelf in the market labelled 'Reduced for Quick Sale'. Although it may be appealing to purchase really inexpensive produce, the nutritional value of these foods is less than that of their fresher equivalents.

Look for nutrition. Most vegetables will not come with nutritional labelling, but this information is often available. Many shops now offer nutritional information in the form of posters and pamphlets displayed in the produce department. So if you want to find out if broccoli has more fibre than green beans do, the answer is probably available right there.

Vegetables

Asparagus Choose tender, straight green stalks. Avoid spreading or woody stems. Store in plastic bags in the refrigerator vegetable compartment for one to three days. Best season: April to June.

Broccoli Look for dark green heads with tightly closed buds. Stalks should be tender yet firm, and the leaves should be fresh and unwilted. Avoid yellow buds or rubbery stems. Store in plastic bags in the refrigerator vegetable compartment for two to four days.

Brussels sprouts Buy firm, bright sprouts with tightly packed leaves. Avoid yellowing vegetables. Store in the fridge for up to three days.

Cabbage Choose heads that are solid and heavy for their size. Avoid heads with splits or yellowed leaves. Store in the refrigerator vegetable compartment for three to seven days.

Carrots Choose well-shaped, firm, bright orange carrots. Avoid those with blemishes or splits. Store in the refrigerator vegetable compartment for one to four weeks.

Cauliflower Select firm, compact heads with white florets and bright green leaves. Avoid heads with brown spots or yellow leaves. Store in the refrigerator vegetable compartment for two to four days.

Celery Choose celery that has crisp stalks. Leaves should be light or medium green. Avoid limp or yellowing leaves. Can be stored in the refrigerator vegetable compartment for one week.

Courgettes The youngest courgettes taste the best. Look for courgettes that are about 12–18 cm (5–7 in) long. They should be firm, heavy for their size with bright vivid colour and free of brown spots or cuts. Keep in a loose bag in the refrigerator. Use in two to three days.

Green beans Search for smooth, crisp pods. Avoid limp, wrinkled or fat, overmature pods. Can be stored in plastic bags in the refrigerator vegetable compartment for one to three days.

Greens Greens for cooking include spinach, kale, collards and Chinese cabbage (napa and bok choy are the best known). They should be crisp and fresh looking, with good colour and no brown spots or yellowing leaves. Keep greens in a plastic bag in the refrigerator. They keep for two to four days, but try to use as soon after purchase as possible.

Mushrooms Should be firm and white and relatively clean. Avoid dark, bruised ones. Can be stored unwashed, loosely covered, on a refrigerator shelf for four days. Avoid placing mushrooms in the vegetable comparment, as they have a tendency to become soft.

Onions Select onions that do not appear to be ready to sprout. They should be heavy for their size. Store in a cool, dry place but not in the refrigerator.

Parsnips Choose young, straight, firm roots without blemish. Avoid large roots; they tend to be woody. Can be stored unwashed in a perforated bag in the refrigerator for one week.

Peas, mange-tout and sugarsnap peas Fresh pea pods should be bright green and firm. Store in the fridge for up to five days. Shell peas just before use.

Peppers (red, orange or green) Peppers should be firm and well shaped, with shiny flesh. Avoid limp, soft or wrinkled peppers. Can be stored in the refrigerator vegetable compartment for four to five days.

Potatoes and sweet potatoes Look for firm, well-shaped potatoes. Avoid any that are blemished, sprouted, or cracked. They should be stored in a cool, dry place away from the sunlight. Most potatoes will keep for two weeks at room temperature.

Pumpkin and other squashes Should be firm and heavy for their size. Store whole pumpkins and other hard-skinned squash in a cool, dry, airy place, ideally hanging in a net bag; in the right conditions it will keep for several months. Store cut pieces and squashes with edible skin in the fridge for up to five days.

Shallots Choose firm, well-shaped bulbs that are heavy for their size. The papery skins should be dry and shiny. Store in a cool, dry place. They will keep for several months.

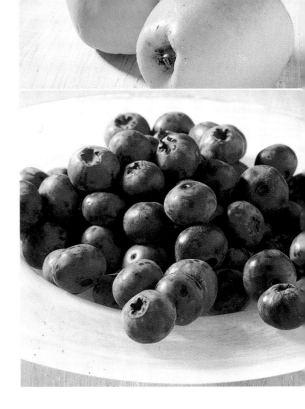

Spring onions Should have firm white bulbs with crisp green tops. Avoid those with withered or yellow tops. Can be stored in plastic bags in the refrigerator for two to three days.

Sweetcorn Choose cobs with firm, plump kernels. Avoid any that look dried and withered. Store in the fridge for up to five days.

Tomatoes Should be firm and fully coloured, and feel heavy for their size. Flavour is best in tomatoes that are stored at room temperature; avoid buying from refrigerated sections of shop. Best season: late spring through early autumn.

Turnips Choose small, firm, slightly rounded turnips. Avoid large ones, as they tend to be strong-flavoured and woody. Can be stored unwashed in the refrigerator for one week.

Fruit

Apples Fruit should be firm and of good colour for the variety. Keep cold and humid. Buy apples with a fresh fragrance; they should not smell musty. All varieties of apple except for Red Delicious can be used for cooking as well as eating raw. Available all year.

Avocados Colour ranges from purple to black to green according to variety. Irregular brown marks on surface are superficial and don't affect the quality. Hold at room temperature until fruit yields gently to pressure, then refrigerate. Available all year.

Bananas Fruit should be plump. Colour varies from green to dark yellow with brownish flecks, according to degree of ripeness. Avoid greyish yellow fruit, which indicates chilling injury. Ripen at room temperature. When at the stage of preferred ripeness, eat or refrigerate. Skin colour turns brown on refrigeration, but flesh keeps well for several days. Available all year.

Berries Choose plump, firm, full-coloured berries. All varieties, with the exception of strawberries, should be free of their hull. Avoid any baskets showing signs of bruised or leaking fruit. Cover and refrigerate. Use within a few days. Available mainly June to August.

Cantaloupes They should be free of any stem and should 'give' when pressed gently. Keep at room temperature for a few days, then refrigerate and use as soon as possible. Available May to September.

Cherries Sweet cherries are bright and glossy, ranging from deep red to black in colour. They should be attached to fresh green stems. Avoid cherries that are hard, sticky, or light in colour. Refrigerate and use within a few days. Available mainly May to August.

Clementines Clementines are a type of mandarin orange grown primarily in Spain. They are small, with a thin skin and a sweet orange flesh. Store in refrigerator like oranges. Mostly available in the winter months. Late-season clementines are often sweeter than the first of the season (this is generally true for oranges as well).

Cranberries Select plump, firm, lustrous red to reddish black berries. Refrigerate and use within two weeks. Can be frozen in original package. Available mainly September to December.

Dates Fruit should be soft and a lustrous brown. Refrigerate after opening packet, and keep well wrapped to avoid drying and hardening. Available all year.

Grapefruit Should be firm, not puffy or loose-skinned. Look for fruits that are heavy for their size, indicating juiciness. Green tinge does not affect eating quality. Refrigerate or keep at room temperature. Available all year.

Grapes Choose plump, well-coloured grapes that are firmly attached to green, pliable stems. Green grapes are sweetest when yellow-green in colour. Red varieties are best when rich, red colour predominates. Grapes won't increase in sweetness, so there's no need to hold them for further ripening. Refrigerate and use within one week. Available mainly June through February.

Honeydew melons Look for a creamy or yellowish white rind with a velvety feel. Avoid stark-white or greenish tinged rinds. Keep at room temperature for a few days, then refrigerate. Peak: June to October.

Kiwi fruit Choose firm fruit that yields only slightly when pressed. Avoid fruit that is damaged or soft. Keep at room temperature until ripe, then refrigerate. Available year-round.

Lemons/Limes Look for a fine-textured skin, indicating juiciness. Should be heavy for their size. Keep at room temperature or refrigerate. Available all year.

Mangoes Skin colour generally green with yellowish to red areas. Red and yellow colour increases with ripening. Avoid any with greyish skin discoloration, pitting, or black spots. Keep at room temperature until soft. When fully soft, refrigerate. Peak: May to August.

Oranges Should be firm and heavy with a fine-textured skin. A green skin colour does not affect eating quality. Store at room temperature or refrigerate. Available all year.

Papayas Select medium-sized, well-coloured fruit – that is, at least half yellow. Ripen at room temperature until skin colour is primarily golden, then refrigerate. Peak: October to December.

Peaches and nectarines Background colour of peaches should be yellowish or cream-coloured; nectarines are yellow-orange when ripe. Fruit should be firm with a slight softening along the 'seam' line. Avoid green or greenish tinged fruits and any that are hard, dull or bruised. Peak: June to September.

Pears Colour varies according to variety. Generally require additional ripening at home. Hold at room temperature until stem end yields to gentle pressure, then refrigerate. Year-round availability due to different varieties.

Pineapple Select large fruit with fresh green leaves. Shell colour is not an indicator of maturity. Pineapples don't 'ripen' after harvest, so may be eaten immediately. Keep at room temperature or refrigerate. Available year-round. Peak: March to June.

Plums Appearance and flavour differ widely by variety. Hold at room temperature until they yield gently to pressure. Peak: June to September.

Pomegranates Rind should be pink or bright red with a crimson seeded flesh. Avoid any that appear dry. Keep cold and humid. Available mainly September to November.

Strawberries Choose berries that are fresh, clean, bright and red. The green caps should be intact, and the fruit should be free of bruises. Strawberries are best eaten immediately, but if they must be stored, refrigerate them with

their caps intact. Available year-round with peak supply April through June.

Tangerines Choose fruit heavy for its size. A puffy appearance and feel is normal. Refrigerate and use as soon as possible. Peak: November to January.

Watermelons Difficult to determine ripeness of uncut melons. Choose firm, smooth melons with a waxy bloom or dullness on the rind. Underside should be yellowish or creamy white. Avoid stark white or greenish coloured underside. With cut melons, select red, juicy flesh with black seeds. Keep at room temperature or refrigerate. Peak: May to August.

Shopping for frozen foods

Since you may not have the opportunity to grocery shop each week, stocking up on frozen foods can be a good idea. There are many healthy foods to choose from in today's freezer case.

Vegetables Although many people believe that fresh vegetables are the only way to go, frozen vegetables can be equally tasty and sometimes have more nutrients than fresh, as they are frozen very soon after picking. Often vegetables at the supermarket or greengrocer's can be on the shelf for a few days, and then you may store them at home a few more days before you cook them. Vitamins and minerals will be lost during this delay to the table. Frozen vegetables have been flash-frozen, thus preserving the nutrients.

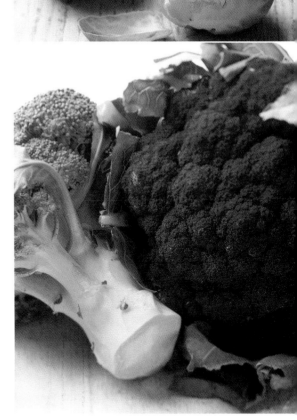

- Always choose vegetables that are plain, not dressed with cream, butter or cheese sauces.
- If possible, buy vegetables in bags versus boxes. It is much easier to seal up whatever you do not use.
- Try to use up frozen vegetables within four months. Rotate the vegetables every time you purchase more. Place older vegetables up front and new ones in the back.

Fruits When berries or other fruits are out of season, consider purchasing them frozen. Buy these fruits with no sugar added. Berries are a great source of vitamin C and fibre that you should be able to enjoy all year long.

Ready-meals It would be great to have a home-cooked meal every night, but for many of us, this may never be a reality. Today's frozen ready-meals can give you convenience and often taste, saving you time and washing up. Check the nutritional labelling for calories, fats, saturated fat and sodium. Many can be laden with extra fat and salt, so they may not be such a good choice. Be sure to check the portion size too – will it be enough or would you be better off boiling some pasta? Supplement frozen entrées with a fresh salad or other vegetables.

Desserts Ice cream and frozen yogurt are always a treat. Today there are myriad options, and fortunately for people with diabetes, there are low and no-sugar brands as well as fat-free brands. Make sure to read the labels and compare fat and calories.

Shopping for the larder

The shelves today are bursting with so many everyday foods as well as more unusual ethnic foods that were formerly only available in speciality shops. Reading the label will be your key to whether or not a product would be a healthy choice. Let's go aisle by aisle and explore what's on the shelves.

Canned fruits and vegetables For many people, purchasing canned fruits and vegetables is a time-saver. Try to use canned fruits and vegetables within a year of purchase. Canned fruits are packed many ways. Look for fruit that is unsweetened and packed only in its own juice or water. Fruits in syrup – heavy or light – will probably add unnecessary sugar to your meals.

For vegetables, just be sure the label states 'No Salt Added'. Often salt is added during the processing. If you can't get salt-free canned vegetables, drain and rinse them well.

Canned beans These are a wonderful addition to your food plan. They are more convenient than dried beans, which must be soaked and cooked. Read the label and look for no added fats or sodium (salt). Use them to extend meat dishes, as in Chilli con carne or Spanish rabbit and chickpea stew (page 92).

Tomatoes To many cooks, canned tomatoes are indispensable. They add flavour to cooked rice, pasta and numerous other dishes. Another bonus:

research indicates that eating cooked tomato products gives you a cancer-fighting phytochemical called lycopene. Look for no-salt-added tomatoes. Any of the common forms will do: whole tomatoes, diced tomatoes, crushed tomatoes, tomato paste, tomato purée and tomato pasta sauce.

Condiments Bottled condiments add lots of flavour yet contain little, if any, fat. Here are some to keep on hand:

- Chili sauce
- Tomato ketchup
- Reduced-fat mayonnaise
- Dijon mustard
- Salsa
- Low-sodium soy sauce
- Worcestershire sauce

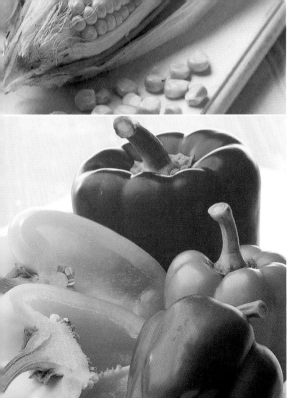

Oils and vinegars

All oils are 100 per cent fat and thus contain about 13 g (½ oz) of fat per tablespoon. But certain fats are healthier for you than others. Seek out monounsaturated fats such as olive and rapeseed oils. The less saturated fat you can eat, the better; this means cutting down on butter and other animal fats.

Keep oils stored in a cool, dry place or in the refrigerator for best freshness. Remove oil from the refrigerator 15 minutes prior to preparing your recipe to allow it to decloud.

Vinegars can add great flavour to your foods. Many vinegars are wine vinegars, but some – like apple cider vinegar – are made from fruits other than grapes. Once opened, vinegars should

be used within a year. Keep vinegars in a cool, dry place.

Here are more specifics on both oils and vinegars:

Spray oils Whether you purchase the aerosol cans of vegetable sprays or place your own oil in a pump spray, the advantage of using the sprays is that you will use far less oil than if pouring from a bottle. Spray oils can be used for sautéing, stir-frying, roasting and grilling.

Rapeseed oil Use rapeseed oil for cooking, including sautéing and baking. Rapeseed oil has a lighter taste than olive oil does, so it can be an alternative choice to get your monounsaturated fats.

Olive oil Renowned for its taste, olive oil is probably the best loved of the oils. You can select olive oil according to its grade; most cooks prefer an extra-virgin oil, from the first pressing of the olives. This is the best tasting of the olive oils and has the lowest acidity and richest flavour.

Flavoured oils Oils can be flavoured with lemon, garlic, herbs and spices. Just a dab on foods can give them great flavour.

Balsamic vinegar Balsamic vinegar is made from dark grapes that produce a dark, sweet, mellow and highly aromatic vinegar. Balsamic vinegar is aged in wooden casks for years. Add it to salad dressings or use as part of a marinade for poultry.

Wine vinegar Wine vinegar can be made from red or white wine. Its flavour can vary from mild to strong. Sherry vinegar is especially tasty and can be used as a substitute for balsamic vinegar.

Rice vinegar Rice vinegar is East Asian and is clear and mild. It has a nice sweet-and-sour taste. Splash rice vinegar on salads.

Herb vinegars Often herbs, spices or fruits are added to vinegar. Products like these are great because you do not need oil to accompany them, since the vinegar is so tasty to begin with.

Prepared soups

Buying ready-made soup is certainly convenient when you don't have the time to make a home-made pot. There are so many to choose from, so here is what you should look for. In any and all cases, consider tossing in extra vegetables (frozen work fine) to add fibre and extra nutrition.

Dehydrated soups These are great, because they store well in a desk drawer and also pack well for travelling. Just add water, stir – and in less than 7 minutes you have soup. Be aware that some brands are very high in sodium, so check the label. Many are now available in low-calorie varieties.

Ready-to-eat soups Look for more vegetable, bean, and non-cream-based soups. For a main meal, look for a heartier soup without too much salt added.

Canned soup Look for canned low-fat, lower-sodium versions wherever possible.

Ready-made stocks Fresh stock from the chiller cabinet tend to be higher in nutrients than dried stock cubes. Be aware of salt content, especially in stock and bouillon cubes; although convenient, they are packed with sodium. If you do use them, omit adding salt to the recipe.

Pasta, rice and other grains

Everyone loves a bowl of pasta or nutty rice, and there are so many varieties to choose from. But all are carbohydrates, so you need to be selective and particularly careful about portion sizes. In general, use grains as a side dish, accompanying a large helping of a vegetable dish. Here's a smart way to approach it: mentally split your dinner plate into quarters. One quarter should be a protein like lean meat or fish; of your meal just over a quarter should be a healthy, fibre-rich starchy food like pasta; the remaining section should be non-starchy vegetables such as green beans and carrots.

Here's what you need to know to make smart choices:

Pasta Wholewheat pasta has about three times the fibre of regular pasta made with white flour. Coloured pastas such as carrot, beet or spinach are certainly pretty and add variety, but they don't count as a vegetable serving. Get into the habit of adding at least one vegetable to the pasta dish to enrich it with valuable antioxidants. Keep your pastas in a cool, dry pantry; use them within a year. Cook until 'al dente' (still slightly firm) rather than soft and almost mushy.

As for fresh pasta: It cooks in as little as 1–3 minutes, a time-saver indeed. The disadvantage is that you have to use it up within 24 hours of purchase. Fresh pasta may also contain more eggs, which ups the calories. If you can find fresh wholewheat pasta, so much the better!

Rice Try Basmati rice instead of standard long-grain or other rice. Basmati has a lower Glycaemic Index and a wonderful aroma. Brown rice has more nutrients than white, and more fibre. Wild rice is actually a long-grain marsh rice and has more protein, zinc and riboflavin than brown rice. If you buy rice mixes, use half the seasoning packet or omit it entirely, because it is usually heavy in salt. To get rid of excess external starch, rinse rice several times. Of all the grains, rice freezes the best.

Other grains From couscous and barley to quinoa and wheatberries, grains are making a comeback in kitchens and restaurants everywhere. Consider them for healthy, fibre-rich side dishes. While each has its own personality and cooking needs, there are some commonalities. Most come in a dry form that needs cooking in a liquid to plump and soften it. Use water or low-sodium, low-fat chicken broth. Do not stir during cooking: that will loosen the starch and the grain will be gummy. Cooking time will vary from grain to grain; millet will usually be tender in 20 minutes, tougher grains may take an hour or more. Most grains can be found in health-food stores and major supermarkets. Buy in bulk to save money. Store in glass containers either in the refrigerator or in a cool, dry place.

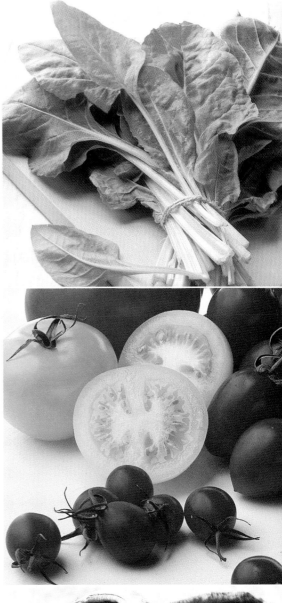

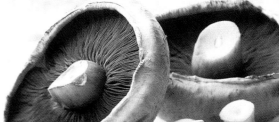

How to plan meals

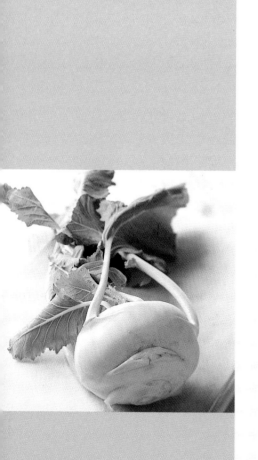

Did you know that by late afternoon, most of us probably still won't know what we are going to have for dinner? It sounds surprising – but that's because we make the false assumption that everyone else is better organised than we are.

The truth is, for the majority of people, life is busy, life is unpredictable, and many of us leave such mundane issues of 'what's for dinner?' to the last moment.

There are lots of benefits to planning your week's meals: less time wasted shopping, one less daily chore to worry about, and money saved by buying just what you need. Then there are the health reasons. For those with diabetes, getting the right mix of nutrients is crucial. And not just some days – it matters every day.

But don't think that meal planning means spending your Saturday mornings picking seven dinner recipes, a full week of lunch menus, and a daily breakfast. Your meal plans need not be so restrictive. Merely by keeping lots of fresh, healthy foods to hand and planning the main ingredient for your main meals – fish on Monday, chicken breasts on Tuesday, a bean soup on Wednesday, fresh or frozen vegetables to accompany them – you will have gone a long way towards getting your nutrition in balance.

The key is variety and choice. Choose foods that you enjoy, foods that are quick and easy enough for you to prepare so that it's not an effort making dinner, and foods that offer a range of nutrients.

Restrictive and prescriptive food lists can be limiting, though if you prefer this approach, speak to your state-registered dietitian and work together to create a plan that suits you. But the beauty of a general healthy-eating approach for diabetes is that it rarely tells you what specific food you have to eat. Rather, it encourages you to think about the types of food you are choosing. So 'vegetable' on a menu plan gives you the flexibility to decide whether that means broccoli, green beans or artichoke. This type of freedom is often preferable, since we all have unique food preferences.

Writing down what you eat is another helpful measure. This helps you to discipline yourself to eat more consistently and shop more effectively; your notes become a food diary that helps you to see how your diet is affecting your weight, your mood, your health, and of course, your blood glucose levels (see Daily food and health tracker, page 305, and Food and mood diary, page 306). By looking at your food diary, you will see at a glance which foods should become a more regular part of your diet, and which you should cut down on. It will help you with planning, as you will come to know if you actually need a snack at 4pm or if it's better to have one at 10am, or both. If you take insulin, by planning, you will know how much insulin you will need and whether you should delay eating – or eat sooner.

People newly diagnosed with diabetes are strongly encouraged to consult a registered dietitian to discuss their nutritional needs and preferences. Not only will a dietitian advise you on what types of food are appropriate in diabetes, but you may also be given a rough time schedule for when to eat, in order to better control your blood glucose levels. By using a meal-planning system, you can work through challenges like having an irregular work schedule, meeting the food needs of people you live with, food budgets, business lunches and so on. You can write on a planning sheet (see page 308) each week to plan your meals. Or perhaps you'll want to use your computer. Whichever method you choose, writing down your plan, rather than simply planning your week's meals in your head, is a much more organised approach. You're more likely to meet your diabetes-management goals using a written plan and referring to it often.

Eating healthily is not a life sentence; it's a way of ensuring that you make the right choices today that will shape a better future for you tomorrow.

Eating regular meals

Rule number one is: eat regular meals, based on starchy foods such as breads, pasta, potatoes, rice and cereals. This helps you to control your blood glucose levels, particularly if the foods have a low Glycaemic Index (see page 8). Whenever possible, choose high-fibre varieties of these foods, such as granary bread and whole-grain cereals. Fibre maintains the health of your digestive system and prevents problems such as constipation.

Start the day with breakfast, and take a mid-morning snack if you need one. Stop to have lunch, rather than eating a quick sandwich at your desk while you work. A mid-afternoon snack may help to keep you going till dinner time. And if your main meal of the day is a ready-meal, balance it with extra vegetables or salad. End a meal with fruit-based desserts.

With diabetes the emphasis should be on enjoying a variety of tasty foods, based on your current condition and treatment. When planning your meals, think about balance. Remember that you always have a choice in the decisions you make. Choosing wellness will have positive effects for you, both physically and mentally. Although your diet is best tailored to your particular needs with the help of a qualified dietitian, the following sample menu plan outlines the types of foods that should be eaten by anyone who wants to follow a healthy and varied diet. Recommended amounts vary from person to person.

Breakfast
- Small glass of unsweetened fruit juice, or a portion of fresh, dried or canned fruit in unsweetened juice
- Fibre-rich breakfast cereal, such as muesli, bran flakes, wheat biscuits or porridge
- Semi-skimmed or skimmed milk
- Artificial sweetener or a little sugar or honey
- Wholemeal, granary, or other whole-grain bread
- Unsaturated margarine or low-fat spread
- Reduced-sugar jam or pure fruit spread

Mid-morning snack
- Oat or wheat-based biscuits, preferably reduced-fat
- Fresh fruit

Lunch
- A portion of wholemeal, granary, or other whole-grain bread, pitta bread or chapattis; or pasta, rice or potatoes (preferably whole and with the skin)
- A portion of a low-fat main dish, such as chicken or turkey, lean ham, drained tuna in brine, beans (such as baked beans or mixed bean salad), boiled egg, reduced-fat cheese (such as half-fat Cheddar, Brie or low-fat soft cheese) or a little full-fat Cheddar cheese (grated goes further)
- Mixed salad with fat-free dressing or reduced calorie mayonnaise; or large portion of vegetables
- Fresh or dried fruit

Mid-afternoon snack

- Plain biscuits, a few nuts and raisins, or low-fat yogurt or fresh fruit

Dinner

- Rice, pasta, potatoes as lunch
- Mixed salad or large portion of vegetables
- Lean meat, fish, egg, cheese or pulse vegetables, cooked in the minimum amount of fat
- Fruit-based dessert, such as the recipe for Baked almond-stuffed peaches on page 281
- Reduced-fat custard made with skimmed milk, or fresh fruit, or low-fat yogurt, or a scoop of ice cream with canned fruit in unsweetened juice

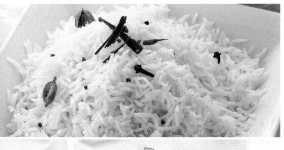

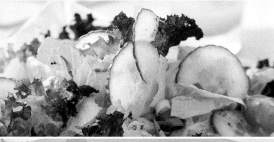

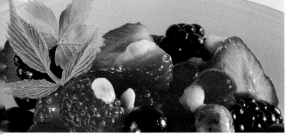

What's on a label?

When choosing packaged foods and drinks, the nutrition panel on the label can provide useful information about the calories, fat and sugar they contain. Amounts are given per 100 g of food and sometimes also per average serving. Some labels give even more information, such as the amount of saturated fats and sodium. The following are examples of what you might see on the label:

Energy is represented as kJ (kilojoules) and kcals (kilocalories). Kilocalories are equivalent to 1000 calories. Because 1 calorie is minuscule, values are usually expressed as kcals, and in everyday language the term 'calories' is used to refer to kilocalories.

Carbohydrate includes both sugar and starches. The figure given for sugars includes both added sugar and natural sugar content. See also page 7.

Fat There are three main types of fat listed on a label – saturates, polyunsaturates and monounsaturates. The information will show the amount of total fat and sometimes also the different types. Try to avoid foods that are high in unhealthy saturated fats. See also page 9.

Guideline Daily Amounts (GDA)

A guide to the daily amount of calories, fat and salt recommended for good health for adults: calories 2500 a day for men, 2000 for women; fat 95 g for men, 70 g for women; salt 7 g a day for men, 5 g for women. Comparing these against the values in a serving of the product can help you to decide if the product would make a good choice in your overall daily diet.

Health claims on labels – what do they mean?

When looking for lower-fat and lower-sugar packaged food options, it pays to know the meaning of various claims:

- **Low fat** – the food contains less than 3 g fat per 100 g/100 ml of foods.
- **Reduced fat** – the food must contain 25 per cent less fat than a similar product. This does not mean the product is 'low-fat'.
- **Less than 5% fat (or 95% fat free)** – the food contains less than 5 g fat per 100 g. For example, if the claim appeared on a ready-meal in which the serving size was 400 g, then the portion would contain 20 g fat. Use these claims as a guide and always check the nutrition panel for the total amount of fat in a serving. You can then compare this with the Guideline Daily Amount (GDA).
- **X% less fat than the standard product** – shows the fat reduction made to a product compared with a standard named product, for instance, 20 per cent less fat than a comparable product. This type of claim can help you to choose lower-fat options; however, always check to see how much fat the product contributes to

your GDA – it may still be high in fat.

- **No added sugar** – no sugars from any source have been added. May still contain a lot of natural sugar, such as fruit sugar in fruit juice.
- **Low sugar** – contains no more than 5 g of sugar per 100 g/100 ml.
- **Reduced sugar** – must contain 25 per cent less sugar than the regular product.

Putting it all together

It's one thing to aim for consistently healthy eating. But putting it into practice takes more than discipline – it takes clever thinking and specific actions. With that in mind, here is a collection of hints and tips to help you on your road to eating to beat diabetes.

- **Have regular meals**, preferably of a similar size each day. Keep to the amounts as recommended by your dietitian or diabetes health care professionals. Missing meals will affect your blood glucose and under-eating can make you suddenly feel hungry and reach for the less healthy foods.
- **Eat at least five portions** of fruit and vegetables each day. The health benefits are important, and if you are watching your weight these foods can help to fill you up at a low calorie cost.
- **Plan meals ahead** when possible, have the right foods to hand, and less healthy foods out of sight.
- **Limit the fat you eat**, particularly saturated (animal) fats, as this type of

fat is linked to heart disease. Choose monounsaturated fats, such as olive oil and rapeseed oil. Eating less fat and fatty foods will also help you to lose weight. Use less butter, margarine, cheese and fatty meats. Choose low-fat dairy foods, such as skimmed milk and low-fat yogurt. Use low-fat cooking methods: bake, grill, roast without fat, microwave, steam, poach, char-grill, stir-fry and griddle.

- **Limit sugar and sugary foods**. This does not mean that your diet has to be sugar-free. Sugar can be used as an ingredient in foods and in baking as part of a healthy diet. But keep to sugar-free, low-sugar or diet fizzy drinks and squashes, as sugary drinks cause blood glucose levels to rise quickly.
- **Eat more fish**, and try to choose oily fish (such as herring, salmon, and mackerel) once a week.
- **Opt for foods with a low Glycaemic Index** (see page 8). For bulk and fibre, choose starchy foods such as potatoes in their skins, pasta and Basmati rice, and whole-grain bread and cereals.
- **Try to get to a healthy weight** and stay there.
- **If you have a food craving**, it can help to know that it will pass. The longer you can resist the craving, the weaker it will become. Think how you might deal with a similar situation differently next time. For instance, have to hand some vegetable or fruit nibbles such as carrots, melon and strawberries. Sugar-free jelly, a glass of tomato juice, a chilled sugar-free drink or a mug of low-calorie soup can also be helpful.

The medical term for low blood sugar is 'hypoglycaemia', often referred to as a 'hypo'. Generally speaking, a hypo is most likely to occur in people treated with insulin. It can be caused by missing a meal or snack, engaging in strenuous physical activity without having eaten enough beforehand, injecting more insulin than is needed, or drinking alcohol on an empty stomach. Sometimes, however, there may be no obvious reason for a hypo. Symptoms of a hypo vary, but the common ones are light-headedness, feeling faint, sweating, shaking, hunger and confusion.

A hypo should be treated by taking a dextrose tablet, sugared water or a sugar lump to quickly raise your blood sugar, followed within half an hour by something more substantial (such as a glass of milk and a slice of toast) to maintain a good blood sugar level.

- **Enhance the natural flavours** in your cooking with herbs, spices, garlic, chilli, lemon or lime juice, flavoured vinegars, tomato purée, a splash of wine, hot pepper sauce, capers, a few olives or mustard. These will help you to reduce added salt.
- **Drink alcohol in moderation only** – the guidelines for diabetes are three units of alcohol a day for men, two units a day for women. For example, a small glass of wine or half a pint of normal-strength beer is 1 unit. Never drink on an empty stomach, as alcohol can make hypoglycaemia (low blood glucose levels) more likely to occur.

Shaping up

Physical activity will help you to stay fit, and if you are wanting to control or reduce your weight, it will help towards that goal. In addition, during exercise our body's natural pharmacy releases endorphin and serotonin into the bloodstream. These natural painkillers enhance mood and promote a general feel-good factor. If you exercise when you have been feeling tired or lethargic, you will notice the benefits physically, in terms of your energy levels, and psychologically, in terms of your mood.

You don't need to jog ten times round the park, and you don't need to exercise for 30 minutes at a time: it's fine to have three 10-minute bursts of activity. Even walking up a few flights of stairs instead of taking the lift, or running up and down the stairs at home a few times a day, can make a big difference to your general fitness levels. However you do it, be sure to incorporate simple physical activities into your daily life, with a goal of reaching 30 minutes' exercise five times a week.

A week of great eating

Good, healthy food: you should know it when you see it. Usually, it's colourful. Usually, the portions are modest. Usually, there are lots of vegetables. If the meat takes up more space on your plate than the vegetables, you might want to

think again – as you might if the dish mainly consists of noodles, rice or potatoes.

When it comes to eating healthily, you cannot beat visual training. If you can see a good plate of food, then you are more likely to eat a good plate of food. And if you see a not-so-good plate of food, with the right knowledge, you are more likely to eat the healthy parts of it, and politely pass on the remainder.

There's a second intuition you need to develop to be truly on top of your diet: what a healthy day of food looks like. To eat well with diabetes, you need to eat sensibly throughout the day in order to keep blood glucose stable and your nutrient mix optimal.

Look at the checklist on the opposite page and also at the Food and mood diary on page 306. Use this as a guide to take some positive steps. You may want to photocopy the pages first so you can use them again and log your progress. Doing this will give you invaluable insight into your eating habits. If they serve you well, make lots more copies and create a notebook. They will also help you to prepare a weekly food planner (see page 308).

How this book helps

Using the recipes in this book, you will be able to keep to a healthy diet without spending hours in the kitchen. The dishes use convenient and healthier alternatives to

standard ingredients, making them low in fat and sugar while being high in fibre. Meals are cooked in only a small amount of oil, and the oils chosen are unsaturated. Each recipe has been carefully considered for its nutritional quality. All are much lower in fat (particularly saturated fat) than standard recipes, and ingredients high in soluble fibre have been used wherever appropriate.

When preparing meals, try to use only small amounts of salt; a high salt intake has been linked to high blood pressure. And choose good non-stick cookware so that you can cook in the minimum of oil, without difficult washing-up.

The recipes in these pages include a wide variety of fruits and vegetables prepared in tasty ways, and some meat and fish dishes already contain vegetables, but go the next step by 'fortifying' your everyday meals with extra helpings. Some ideas include:
- Add fruit to breakfast cereal and yogurt.
- Add slices of tomato and cucumber to sandwiches.
- Use salsa (home-made or bought) as a salad dressing.
- Add orange slices or tangerines to green salads, or chopped apples to coleslaw.
- When preparing pasta, add vegetables to the cooking water.
- Top a baked potato with stir-fried vegetables.
- Add vegetables to omelettes.
- Drink low-sodium vegetable juices.

Daily food and health tracker

monday ●

tuesday ●

wednesday ●

thursday ●

friday ●

saturday ●

sunday ●

monitoring your day

Fruit and vegetables

1 2 3 4 5 6 7 8 9 10

Glasses of water

1 2 3 4 5 6 7 8 9 10

Times ate out of boredom, stress, habit

1 2 3 4 5 6 7 8 9 10

Rate your energy today:

1 2 3 4 5

Rate your attitude today:

1 2 3 4 5

Rate your health today:

1 2 3 4 5

Rate the quality of your eating today:

1 2 3 4 5

How was breakfast?

☐ Skipped it

☐ Balanced

☐ Not so balanced

☐ Correct portions

☐ Too much

How was lunch?

☐ Skipped it

☐ Balanced

☐ Not so balanced

☐ Correct portions

☐ Too much

How was dinner?

☐ Skipped it

☐ Balanced

☐ Not so balanced

☐ Correct portions

☐ Too much

Achievement checklist

☐ Ate a fibre-rich cereal

☐ Chose whole-grain bread

☐ Had fruit instead of dessert

☐ Skipped dressing on salad

☐ Took the skin off poultry

☐ Said no to an extra helping

☐ Used a low-calorie mixer with my drink

☐ Went for a walk

☐ Joined the gym or a regular physical activity class

☐ Had consistently good blood glucose readings

☐ Kept my appointment at the clinic

Now add some of your own:

_____

_____

_____

daily comments

_____

_____

_____

_____

_____

_____

_____

_____

_____

_____

_____

_____

_____

_____

_____

_____

_____

_____

_____

_____

_____

_____

_____

_____

FOOD AND

The chart below is designed to help you to keep track of what you eat at different times of the day and how these foods are linked to your mood. For example, you might tick 'working day' and note that at 8am you ate 1 slice of white toast with a scraping of butter and jam, plus a banana and drink of orange juice. You record, perhaps, that you were sleepy but forced yourself to eat. Later that morning at 10am you might eat 2 chocolate biscuits, noting that you 'needed' them after a staff meeting and commenting that you tend to reach for chocolate when you feel under

Date_____   Working day ☐   Non-working day ☐

Time	Food eaten and quantity	Fruit and vegetables	Drink

MOOD DIARY

pressure. (In this case, it would be better to combat the urge by eating a few nuts and raisins before the meeting, as these are digested more slowly). The fruit and vegetable column will help you to check that you're eating at least five portions of these a day. Photocopy the page so that you can keep your own Food and mood diary. Compare what you eat and how you feel at different times and in different situations on working and non-working days. The diary will show you how emotions play a role in what you eat and will help you to make healthier choices.

Emotions, e.g. tired, hungry, feeling low	Comments and conclusions

Weekly planner

meals

shopping

trip 1

*when*_____

list

_____

_____

_____

_____

_____

_____

_____

_____

trip 2

*when*_____

list

_____

_____

_____

_____

_____

_____

_____

_____

	monday	tuesday	wednesday
breakfast			
lunch			
dinner			
snacks			
social activities involving food			

thursday	friday	saturday	sunday
breakfast	breakfast	breakfast	breakfast
lunch	lunch	lunch	lunch
dinner	dinner	dinner	dinner
snacks	snacks	snacks	snacks
social activities involving food	social activities involving food	social activities involving food	social activities involving food

Glossary

Acesulfame potassium, or Ace-K A sugar substitute, 200 times sweeter than sugar, that contains no calories.

Allergen A substance foreign to the body that causes an allergic reaction.

Allicin The chemical responsible for garlic's odour and health effects.

Amino acids Organic (carbon-containing) acids that the body links to make proteins. Nine amino acids are termed essential, because they must be provided in the diet; the body produces the remaining 11 as they are needed.

Anaemia A condition in which there is a shortage of red cells in the blood or a deficiency of haemoglobin (the oxygen-carrying pigment) in these cells.

Anthocyanins Antioxidant flavonoids found in many plant pigments.

Anticarcinogens Compounds that are thought to counteract certain cancer-causing substances.

Antioxidant A substance that protects cells from the damaging effects of free radicals. Some antioxidants are made by the body; others, such as vitamins C and E, are obtained through diet or supplements.

Asparagine An amino acid found in certain plants, especially legumes.

Aspartame An artificial sweetener that is 200 times sweeter than sugar.

Bacteria Single-celled microorganisms that are found in air, food, water, soil and other living creatures, including humans. 'Friendly' bacteria support your body's own gut bacteria in preventing infections and synthesising certain vitamins; others cause disease.

Basal metabolic rate The energy required to maintain vital processes in the human body.

Beta-carotene One of a group of nutrients known as carotenoids. An immune-system booster and powerful antioxidant, beta-carotene neutralises the free radicals that can damage cells and promote disease.

Beta-glucans The soluble dietary fibre component of barley and oat bran.

B-group vitamins Although not chemically related to one another, many of the B vitamins occur in the same foods, and most perform closely linked tasks within the body. B vitamins are known either by numbers or names, or both: B_1, thiamine; B_2, riboflavin; B_3, niacin; B_5, pantothenic acid; B_6, pyridoxine; B_{12}, cobalamin; biotin; and folate.

Biotin One of the B vitamins.

Calcium The most plentiful mineral in the body; a major component of bones, teeth and soft tissues. Calcium is needed for nerve and muscle function, blood clotting and metabolism.

Calorie The basic unit of measurement for the energy value of food and the energy needs of the body. Because 1 calorie is minuscule, values are usually expressed as units of 1,000 calories, properly written as kilocalories (kcal).

Capsanthin A carotenoid. Capsanthin contributes to the red colour in paprika.

Carbohydrates *Simple carbohydrates* are foods that are easily digested into glucose, such as table sugar and bleached flour. *Complex carbohydrates*, which make up the bulk of whole grains and vegetables, are starches composed of complex sugars, fibre and other nutrients. They take longer to digest and have more beneficial ingredients in them.

Carcinogen A substance that can cause cancer.

Carotenes Yellow and red pigments that colour yellow-orange fruits and vegetables and most dark green vegetables. They are among the antioxidants that protect against the effects of ageing and disease. The human body converts one such pigment – beta-carotene – into vitamin A.

Carotenoids A group of red and yellow pigments similar to carotenes.

Chromium A trace mineral that ensures proper glucose metabolism.

Cobalamin (see B-group vitamins; Vitamin B_{12}).

Complex carbohydrates (see Carbohydrates).

Copper A trace mineral necessary for the production of red blood cells, connective tissue and nerve fibres. Component of several enzymes.

Cruciferous vegetables Members of the mustard family of plants, which includes broccoli, cabbage, cauliflower, cress, mustard, radish and turnips.

Diabetes (diabetes mellitus) A disorder of carbohydrate metabolism, characterised by inadequate production or utilisation of insulin and resulting in excessive amounts of glucose in the blood and urine. There are two main forms: *Type 1 diabetes* occurs when the body's immune system destroys the insulin-producing cells in the pancreas, which can cause a total halt in insulin production. In *type 2 diabetes*, the pancreas produces insulin, but the body's cells begin to 'resist' insulin's message to let blood glucose in the cells – a condition called insulin resistance.

Diuretic A substance that causes the body to excrete excess urine.

E. coli (Escherichia coli) Bacteria that occur naturally in the intestines of humans and other animals; one of the common causes of diarrhoea and urinary tract infections.

Electrolytes Substances that separate into ions that conduct electricity when fused or dissolved in fluids. In the human body, sodium, potassium and chloride are electrolytes essential for nerve and muscle function and for maintaining the fluid balance as well as the acid-alkali balance of cells and tissues.

Essential fatty acids The building blocks that the body uses to make fats.

Fats A class of organic chemicals, also called fatty acids or lipids. When digested, they create nearly double the energy of the same amount of carbohydrates or protein.

Fibre Indigestible material in food that stimulates peristalsis in the intestine.

Flavonoids Plant pigments that are potent antioxidants.

Folate One of the B vitamins, also known as folic acid.

Free radicals Waste products of oxygen metabolism that can damage cell components.

Fructose A naturally occurring, simple (monosaccharide) fruit sugar.

Glucose A simple sugar (monosaccharide) that the body converts directly into energy; blood levels of glucose are regulated by several hormones, including insulin.

Glucosinolates A group of phytochemicals found in cruciferous vegetables.

Gluten The tough nitrogenous substance remaining when wheat or other grain is washed to remove the starch.

Glycaemic Index A scale of numbers for foods with carbohydrates that have the lowest to highest effects on blood sugar. There are currently two indexes. One uses a scale of 1–100, with 100 representing a glucose tablet, which has the most rapid effect on blood sugar. The other common index uses a scale with 100 representing white bread (so some foods will be above 100).

Glycogen A form of glucose stored in the liver and muscles, which is converted back into glucose when needed.

Gram (g) A metric unit of weight; 1 g is equal to 1000 milligrams. There are 28.4 g to an ounce.

High-density lipoproteins (HDLs) The smallest and 'heaviest' lipoproteins, they retrieve cholesterol from the tissues and transport it to the liver, which uses it to make bile; called 'good cholesterol', because high blood levels of HDLs do not increase the risk of a heart attack.

Hormones Chemicals that are secreted by the endocrine glands or tissue; they control the functions of all the body's organs and processes, including growth, development and reproduction.

Hydrogenation The process for transforming an oil (unsaturated liquid fat) into a hard fat by incorporating hydrogen. Hydrogenated fat is similar to saturated fat and linked to an increased risk of heart disease.

Hypertension Elevation of the blood pressure.

Hypoglycaemia An abnormally low level of glucose in the blood.

Indoles Nitrogen compounds found in vegetables and believed to protect against certain cancers by accelerating the elimination of oestrogen.

Insulin A hormone that regulates carbohydrate metabolism.

Insulin resistance (see Diabetes).

Iodine A mineral that is essential for the formation of thyroid hormones.

Iron A mineral that is essential for the manufacture of haemoglobin and the transport of oxygen.

Lactose The natural sugar in milk.

Lipid A fatty compound made of hydrogen, carbon and oxygen. Lipids are insoluble in water. The chemical family includes fats, fatty acids, carotenoid pigments, cholesterol, oils and waxes.

Lipoprotein A combination of a lipid and a protein that can transport cholesterol in the bloodstream. The main types of lipoprotein are high density (HDL), low density (LDL), and very low density (VLDL).

Low-density lipoproteins (LDLs) These abundant, so-called 'bad' lipoproteins carry most of the circulating cholesterol; high levels are associated with atherosclerosis and heart disease.

Lutein A phytochemical found in spinach and other dark green leaves.

Lycopene The main pigment in certain fruits, such as tomato and paprika.

Lysine A basic amino acid essential in human nutrition.

Macronutrients Nutrients the body requires in large amounts for energy – specifically, carbohydrates, proteins and fats.

Magnesium A trace mineral that is needed for healthy bones, the transmission of nerve signals, protein and DNA synthesis, and the conversion of glycogen stores into energy.

Metabolism The body's physical and chemical processes, including conversion of food into energy, that are needed to maintain life.

Microgram (mcg) A unit of weight equivalent to 1/1000 milligram.

Micronutrients Essential nutrients that the body needs in only trace or very small amounts.

Milligram (mg) 1/1000 gram.

Monosaccharide (see Fructose; Glucose).

Monounsaturated fats Fats that are liquid at room temperature and semisolid or solid under refrigeration. They are believed to help to protect against heart disease.

Niacin (see B-group vitamins; Vitamin B_3).

Oestrogen A female sex hormone produced in both sexes, but in much greater quantities in females.

Omega-3 fatty acid (see also Essential fatty acids). A polyunsaturated fatty acid, essential for normal retinal function, that influences various metabolic pathways, resulting in lowered cholesterol and triglyceride levels, inhibited platelet clotting, and reduced inflammatory and immune reactions.

Oxalic acid A potentially toxic chemical found in certain plants that inhibits the absorption of calcium, iron, zinc and other minerals. Can promote the development of oxalate kidney stones.

Oxidation A chemical process in which food is burned with oxygen to release energy.

Pancreas A large gland, situated near the stomach, that secretes a digestive fluid into the intestine and also secretes the hormone insulin.

Pantothenic Acid (see B-group vitamins).

Pectin Soluble dietary fibre that regulates intestinal function and can help to lower blood cholesterol levels.

Peristalsis Wavelike muscle contractions that help to propel food and fluids through the digestive tract.

Phosphorus A mineral needed for healthy bones and teeth, nerves, muscles and for many bodily functions.

Phthalides A group of secondary phytochemical compounds. A component of celery, 3-n-butyl phthalide, gives this plant its characteristic smell and taste.

Phytochemicals Chemicals derived from plants; some have powerful effects, including both the prevention and the promotion of certain cancers, heart disease and degenerative conditions linked to ageing.

Polyphenols Organic compounds, including tannins, that combine with iron and can hinder its absorption; found in a number of foods, tea and red wines.

Polyunsaturated fat A fat containing a high percentage of fatty acids that lack hydrogen atoms and have extra carbon bonds. It is liquid at room temperature.

Potassium A trace mineral that is needed to regulate fluid balance and many other functions (see Electrolytes).

Protein Part of a large class of chemicals called amino acids. The body uses proteins to build and repair muscles and tissues. Proteins are in plant foods – vegetables, grains, beans, nuts, soy products – and are the main ingredient in animal foods like beef, poultry, seafood and dairy products.

Pyridoxine (see B-group vitamins; Vitamin B_6).

Recommended daily amount (RDA)
The value used on food labels that refers to the recommended daily amounts of vitamins, minerals and major nutrients needed for good health.

Reference nutrient intake (RNI) The amount of a nutrient that should be taken daily in order to meet the requirements of the majority of a specified population group – for example, children aged 7–10 years, women aged 19–50 years.

Resveratrol A phytochemical derived from grape skin.

Riboflavin (see B-group vitamins; Vitamin B_2).

Saccharin A sugar substitute. Saccharin is not metabolised by the body and provides little or no calories.

Saturated fat A lipid with a high hydrogen content; the predominant fat in animal products and other fats that remain solid at room temperature. A high intake of saturated fat is linked to an increased risk of heart disease, certain cancers and other diseases.

Selenium An essential trace mineral with antioxidant properties.

Serotonin A neurotransmitter that helps to promote sleep and regulates many body processes, including pain perception and the secretion of pituitary hormones.

Simple carbohydrates (see Carbohydrates).

Sodium A trace mineral essential for maintenance of fluid balance; it combines with chloride to form table salt.

Soluble fibre A dietary fibre that becomes sticky when wet and dissolves in water.

Starch A complex carbohydrate that is the principal storage molecule of plants and the major source of carbohydrate and energy in our diet.

Sucralose The only sugar substitute made from sugar. It has no calories and is 600 times sweeter than sugar.

Sucrose A sugar composed of glucose and fructose. The sugar obtained from cane and beets; it is also present in honey, fruits and vegetables.

Sugar substitutes (see Acesulfame potassium, Aspartame, Saccharin, Sucralose).

Sulforaphane An antioxidant phytochemical compound.

Tannin An astringent substance derived from plants that can contract blood vessels and body tissues.

Thiamine (see B-group vitamins; Vitamin B_1).

Triglycerides The most common form of dietary and body fat; high blood levels have been linked to heart disease.

Tryptophan An essential amino acid found in many animal foods; a precursor of serotonin. Its use as a dietary supplement has been linked with serious illness, most likely due to contamination during the manufacturing process.

Very low density lipoproteins (VLDLs)
Fat-carrying proteins that transport mostly triglycerides in the blood.

Vitamin A A fat-soluble nutrient occurring in foods such as green and yellow vegetables and egg yolk, essential to growth and the prevention of night blindness.

Vitamin B_1 (thiamine) A water-soluble compound of the vitamin-B complex essential for the normal functioning of the nervous system. Found in natural sources such as green peas, liver and the seed coats of cereal grains.

Vitamin B_2 (riboflavin) A vitamin-B complex factor, essential for growth, found in milk, fresh meat, eggs, leafy vegetables and enriched flour.

Vitamin B_3 (niacin) Also called nicotinic acid, it controls blood sugar, keeps skin healthy, and maintains the proper functioning of the nervous and digestive systems.

Vitamin B_6 (pyridoxine) Found in foods such as whole-grain cereals, meats and fish. Among other functions, this vitamin forms red blood cells, helps cells to make protein, and manufactures brain chemicals (neurotransmitters) such as serotonin.

Vitamin B_{12} (cobalamin) Obtained from liver, milk, eggs, fish, oysters and clams. Important for red blood cell production, maintains the protective sheath around nerves, helps to convert food to energy and plays a critical role in the production of DNA and RNA, the genetic material in cells.

Vitamin C (ascorbic acid) A water-soluble vitamin occurring in citrus fruits and green vegetables.

Vitamin D A fat-soluble vitamin found in milk and fish-liver oils.

Vitamin E An important antioxidant found in vegetable oils, whole-grain cereals, butter and eggs.

Water-soluble vitamins Vitamins that dissolve in water, specifically vitamin C and the B-group vitamins.

Zeaxanthin A carotenoid found in collards, kale, mustard greens and spinach.

Zinc A trace mineral that is essential for many processes, including metabolism, the healing of wounds and normal growth.

Index

Titles in *italics* are for recipes in 'Some more ideas'.

Diabetes Cookbook was adapted from Eat to Beat Diabetes, published byThe Reader's Digest Association, Inc., USA

This edition was published by
The Reader's Digest Association Limited, London

First edition copyright © 2004
The Reader's Digest Association Limited,
11 Westferry Circus, Canary Wharf,
London E14 4HE

Reprinted 2004

We are committed to both the quality of our products and the service we provide to our customers. We value your comments, so please feel free to contact us on **08705 113366** or via our web site at: **www.readersdigest.co.uk**

If you have any comments or suggestions about the content of our books, email us at: gbeditorial@readersdigest.co.uk

Copyright © 2004 Reader's Digest Association Far East Limited
Philippines Copyright © 2004 Reader's Digest Association Far East Limited

PHOTOGRAPHERS

Sue Atkinson, Martin Brigdale, Gus Filgate,
Amanda Heywood, Graham Kirk, William Lingwood,
Sean Myers, Simon Smith

The recipes in the *Diabetes Cookbook* were drawn
from the Reader's Digest Eat well, Live Well series

Concept Code	US4414H/G
Book Code	400-202-02
ISBN	0 276 42848 X